Health and Sugar Substitutes

Proceedings of the ERGOB Conference on Sugar Substitutes,
Geneva, October 30 to November 1, 1978

Health
and Sugar Substitutes

Editor

B. Guggenheim, Zurich

Chairman of the Department for Oral Microbiology
and General Immunology, Dental Institute, University of Zurich

40 figures and 35 tables, 1979

S. Karger · Basel · München · Paris · London · New York · Sydney

© Copyright 1979 by S. Karger AG, 4011 Basel (Switzerland), Arnold-Böcklin-Strasse 25
Printed in Switzerland by Walter Hauri & Co., Buch- und Offsetdruck, Zürich
ISBN 3-8055-2961-9

Contents

III. Practical Problems in Substituting Sugar in Various Foods

IV. New Sweeteners

V. Sugar Substitutes in Oral Health – Metabolic Criteria Indicative for Cariogenicity 191

VI. Factors in Safety, Benefit/Risk Assessment and Legal Aspects 259

Preface

The International Conference on Sugar Substitutes was organized to commemorate the tenth anniversary of the European Research Group for Oral Biology (ERGOB). During the Basel Congress of the European Organization of Caries Research (ORCA) in 1968, a number of young researchers felt frustrated with the customary ten minutes paper sessions, because they did not leave enough time for the free exchange of scientific information. Immediately after the congress, a small circle of enthusiastic youngsters searched for an alternative. It was evident that such an ambitious task was not to be achieved within the rather inflexible institution of a large established scientific organization. They therefore decided to create a new body. A constitution was written which included the following organizing principles:

To guarantee permanent revitalization and regeneration of the group, permanent membership was excluded. Because a certain continuity was thought to be desirable, an executive committee of four members including a secretary-treasurer with an unlimited term of office was proposed. The term of office of the other committee members was limited to two years. Two meetings were to be held annually. The size of the group was limited to a maximum of twelve participants to allow the free exchange of thoughts and the informal discussion of developments in basic research related to oral biology. Unlike the United States, where the National Institute of Dental Research organized similar meetings, no supranational institution existed in Europe which would have been able to support our activities. Therefore, two companies were invited to sponsor the meetings on a long-term basis. Each sponsoring company was to be granted the privilege of sending a qualified researcher to the meetings. We are very grateful for the generous help of Elida Cosmetics Ltd. and Akzo Consumenten Produkten bv, in providing grants for the regular activities of ERGOB.

During the past ten years in 19 meetings a great number of active scientists have profited from these friendly gatherings. On the occasion of the 20th meeting, the executive committee decided to organize an open conference to introduce this rather unique group to a wider scientific community. Besides being of pressing importance at the present time, the topic "Sugar Substitutes" was chosen as an example of our desire to communicate interdisciplinarily on matters of broad interest. Following our usual custom, experts working on related problems outside the field of oral biology were invited to attend.

Although there are no doubts whatsoever that even the partial replacement of sucrose by nutritive or non-nutritive sugar substitutes is a valid means of reducing dental caries, there is no unanimity with regard to the criteria to be applied for the assessment of the cariogenicity of sweeteners or foodstuffs. This has created a great deal of confusion, that has been nourished by a merciless battle for shares of the market. The struggle for truth about the safety of non-nutritive sweeteners has much more bearing to the public health than being merely a concern of preventive dentistry, however important it may be. People in the western hemisphere are more and more losing faith in the benefits of unlimited technological progress in general and have become specifically sensitized against possible side effects of "chemicals", be it drugs or food additives. This malaise has had consequences on the political level for example in the rather unfortunate all or nothing approach of the Delaney clause in the United States. In the field of sugar substitutes, cyclamate and saccharin have run into massive crossfire because of reports branding these compounds as bladder carcinogens in rodents.

It is one of the paradoxses of our time that most of the sugar substitutes are consumed to reduce caloric intake while a large segment of the world's population is threatened by starvation. Nevertheless, the great many diabetic patients having a legitimate and vital interest in the regular use of sugar substitutes were intimidated by such alarming reports.

There is little doubt today that no act of authority will settle this dilemma. Practical alternatives can only be proposed by tackling these important problems by competent, honest and ethical research. The necessity to protect our environment – and at long last ourselves – is one of the major contemporary demands of our society. However, the way out of this vicious circle cannot be found by apodictic actions but only by clear-headed, competent benefit/risk assessments.

Within the limited area of sugar substitutes, we hope that the Geneva Conference and the new material presented in this volume will introduce some more clarity into this highly controversial field. If it contributes to the resolution of only a few of the pertinent questions and consequently brings back some of the lost credibility to sugar substitute research, the anniversary conference of ERGOB and this volume will have served their purpose.

August 1, 1978   B. Guggenheim

I. The reasons for substituting or not substituting sugar

Moderator: K.G.M.M. Alberti, London
Co-Moderator: H. Keen, London

Health and Sugar Substitutes
Proc. ERGOB Conf., Geneva 1978, pp. 2-9 (Karger, Basel 1978)

SUCROSE IN HUMAN NUTRITION - IMPORTANCE OF DELINEATION OF SAFE INGESTANT
LEVELS - A current Survey

G.D. Campbell

The Durban Diabetes Study Project, P.O. Box 30048,
4058 Mayville, Rep. of South Africa

ARE THERE ANY INDICATIONS FOR SUCROSE INGESTION IN HUMANS?

Though 90 million tons of sucrose were made in the world last year, it
can hardly be regarded as an essential human nutrient. Local workers[1] have
suggested that largely due to availability there are only 3 real indications
for its use. (a) In marathon runners, (b) in convalescence from disease,
(c) in treating hypoglycaemia. These indications from only a minute part of
this vast crop.

"CONSUMPTION" OF SUCROSE

Recently, Czarnikow, the London Brokers[2] asked:- "Why is it so difficult
to estimate sucrose consumption?". In many countries, large amounts of
sucrose and high-sucrose molasses are made into alcohol, complicating any
assessments of consumption. In S. Africa, most of our potable alcohol comes
from the Grape Industry (even the 'white' spirits made from ethyl alcohol)
and our task here is easier. However, even the strictest studies from this
Project tend to give lower figures than the Sugar Industry's meticulous
records. Most people under-estimate sucrose intakes, possibly as many
believe that a high sucrose intake is "a bad thing". Inaccurate census
records also contribute to these difficulties. It is probable that the
Industry's figures, though higher, are more accurate, and thus the annual
"Sugar Yearbook"[3] can be unreservedly recommended to the preventive
nutritionist.

THE "SUCROSE RULES"

Paradoxically, diabetes and obesity are seen in Natal Indians with daily
energy intakes of as low as 6,400 - 8,400 kJ. However, in the same area,
these disorders are absent in Natal Sugar Cane Cutters with energy intakes

exceeding 24,600 kJ. I have shown a remarkably constant period of time
of exposure to city life before diabetes emerges in migrants. The "Rule of
20 Years" is based upon the fact that the period of exposure of city life
in migrant Zulus peaks at between 18 and 22 years. The "Rule of 20%" is
based upon there being sucrose energy intakes of more than 20% in people
with low energy intakes who suffer from obesity or diabetes. The "Rule of
32 kg (70 lb)" results from the observation that the threshold of sucrose
intakes between countries where diabetes is either common or uncommon is
32 kg (70 lb) annual per capita intake.

HOW TOXIC IS SUCROSE?

Using the S. African Sugar Industry's computerised direct cane analysis
system to assess sucrose intake from chewing cane, I have shown that of
a minimum daily energy intake of 24,600 kJ , that most cane cutters ingest
a minimum intake of 530 g of sucrose. Though we have studied many who have
been exposed to this massive intake for many years, degenerative disorders
are totally absent, though in one worker we did detect a pre-beta band[5]. The
argument given is that with the tremendous energy expenditure necessitated
in cutting and stacking several tons of cane, that they work this intake off.
As humans cannot metabolise sucrose directly, what they work off must be
glucose and fructose. Thus sucrose cannot be regarded as being toxic per se
as the body uses it only as invert sugar. I showed earlier[6] that glucose
tolerance peaks after 50 g of glucose or sucrose by mouth were twice as high
with glucose. In the term I first used, the "impact" of glucose is twice
that of sucrose. Degenerative disorders are seen chiefly in populations who
eat foods causing high, speedy and sustained rises in blood glucose levels.
This has been shown clearly with respect to insulin rises recently when Scots
with 3 times the rate of myocardial infarction were compared with Swedes[7].
I must add that the sugar cane cutter study may have been affected by the
fact that there is a high level of "glucose tolerance factor" in our canes.
Recent studies by ourselves[8] in healthy volunteers, have shown no significant
differences in blood glucose and insulin responses when a pure sucrose
solution was compared with an amount of equal polarity sugar cane juice
expressed under laboratory conditions. One other remarkable finding in the
Project's Sugar Cane Juice Study is, that there are factors in fresh juice
which have a massive potentiating effect upon prostaglandin action in vitro,

as compared with a similar pure sucrose solution. What relevance this has to the remarkable tolerance of the cane cutter to sustained sucrose loads is not clear. Incidentally, the feeding of 900 g (2 lb) of sucrose to these people in less than 10 minutes, gave us quite unusual blood glucose curves, with 2 peaks in a 2 1/2 hour profile - the socalled "Bactrian" curve.

AN ANTI-SUCROSE CAMPAIGN

In the consideration of lowering human sucrose intakes, it is important to know whether or how an anti-sucrose campaign can be run. In 1965, I became so totally convinced that sucrose intakes in Zulus and Indians in Durban had become disproportionate for their health, that I started a one-man campaign against the powerful and not always necessarily accurate advertising of the Sugar Industry. Firstly, I used to lecture in English, Urdu, Tamil and Zulu to the crowds in the large waiting room of the Diabetic Clinic, about the genetic and environmental connotations of diabetes, and suggested that all members of the families of diabetics should be on CHO-food restriction, and especially that of sucrose. Secondly, I drew up a propaganda sheet both in English and Zulu, in the simplest terms reiterating what I had said in my lectures in the waiting room, and every diabetic was handed several of these to be handed out at home and to neighbours. This included simple phrases such as "When one person in any house is taking saccharin, then all should do so". Every day when the Clinic rush was over, the Clinic Orderly, Mr. M. Abdulla, in his white coat, would stand upon local street corners and hand out copies of my document to all passers-by, and at the same would deliver homilies in the street to interested people about the possible prevention of diabetes by food restriction. In all 26,000 of these "tracts" were handed out. Thirdly, in my capacity as Radio Doctor of the Zulu Programme (Radio Bantu Port Natal) in 1970, and of the Natal Indian Radio Programme in 1972, I was able to repeat much of what I had set out before, to an eventual total of millions of people as the Zulu Talks were translated into 7 other African languages, and indeed were actually being delivered again in 1976 in the Radio Tswana Programme in Bophutaswana. There is little doubt, based upon local dietary surveys, that these talks had most meaningful effects, especially in the families and friends of diabetics, but less in the general population. This shows how effective simple one-man campaigns can be organised, especially where sucrose intakes are considered to be inordinately large.

GOVERNMENTAL ACTION AGAINST SUCROSE

At last, one country, Norway, has become concerned about its high level
of sucrose intake. In the New York Academy of Sciences monthly "London
Letter" by the Editor of the "New Scientist", Bernard Dixon spoke about
food advice upon a national scale: "....... Other Government moves in Norway
may be more obvious and less welcome. One is a decision not to subsidise
sugar, so that the retail price will reflect the true import price. The plan
is for consumption to stabilise at around 32 kg (70 lb) per head per year.
This is the figure which G. D. Campbell of the Durban Diabetes Study Project
in S. Africa, reports to be dividing countries where diabetes is common,
from those were diabetes is a rarity".
This lead will need to be followed as (see below) world stocks of sucrose
are about 8 million tons too high, and thus urgent efforts will be made to
stimulate human sucrose ingestion upon a global scale.

CERTAIN ECONOMIC AND AGRICULTURAL ASPECTS

In many countries consumption is largely governed by retail price. In
S. Africa, we have the extraordinary state of affairs where sucrose is
being sold for less than it costs to produce. Inept governmental planning
relied upon very high export prices to support the local market which was
hardly wise in the light of large fluctuations in world sucrose prices
since 1962. In an article upon "Sugar as an Addictive Agent", I ended by
saying that the case was 'not proven'. However, sucrose is a remarkable
sedative agent and eating it gives enormous pleasure to many people,
paricularly to very poor people, who will often sacrifice more nutritious
foods to obtain it, as it is generally much cheaper. Thus people are going
to eat sucrose whether we like it or not, often in the largest quantities
that they can get, and I feel that we must restrict such intake to reasonable
limits.

THE "HUMAN RIGHTS" QUESTION

Lengthy membership of the International and S. African Associations of
Sugar Cane Technologists has given me contact with forces not possibly
recognised by many nutritionists. Firstly, the global Sugar Industry employs
vast numbers of people possibly in the region of 8 million[10], secondly,

sucrose is an extremely expensive material for use on an industrial basis.
Profound industrial competition to sucrose as a sweetener has appeared in
the form of the high fructose corn syrups which are being made in vast
quantities by the brilliant immobilised enzyme process, and which may
supplant 70% of the industrial sucrose usage in the next decade. There is
a critical level of global sugar stocks as regards sustaining of export
prices - 24 million tons. As this stock exceeds 32 million tons, prices
have plummeted, and cannot rise until the stock level falls again to
24 million tons. Thus with these low prices, great hardship is in store for
a great many workers especially those not sustained by "welfare" states.
Vast plans are afoot in Brazil to produce more sugar cane for making power
ethanol and these may go far to helping that country to become independent
of oil. Today it costs S.A. Rands 245 - 275 (U.S. $ 270 - 303) to produce a
ton of crystal sucrose, which can be made into 600 l of power alcohol -
enough to fill the tanks of 12 large cars - hardly an economical feasibility.
Recent experiments in Durban to run cars on mixtures of ethyl and methyl
alcohol and furfuraldehyde have been exciting, but rewarding in every way
other than economic. In the small province in which I live, Natal, we are
the 7th largest sucrose exporter in the world. Even a slight cut-back can
be disastrous for many workers. In 1979 a cut-back of 23% of cane originally
to have been harvested, has been proposed. Thus we cannot think of dramatic
and widespread cuts in human sucrose intake, but must try as hard as we can
to define an optimum highest per capita national annual intake threshold,
which will not harm the consumer who wants and will get sucrose, and yet will
not put many workers out of work. Matters are not made easier by the reluctance
of farmers to turn from sucrose to less easy and remunerative crops.

CONCLUSIONS AND RECOMMENDATIONS

Thus huge amounts of sucrose are made every year in the world and there
is now a disproportionately massive stockpile. In many countries, intake is
far too high and there is little doubt that this has contributed towards the
emergence of a spectrum of diseases of advancement first referred to as
the "Saccharine Disease" by T. L. Cleave and myself[11]. Sucrose can be widely
applied to industrial usage as a raw material, but is prohibitively expensive. Production of sucrose by beet or cane is a factor of the sunshine that

falls upon the leaves of the plant. It might therefore be rational for countries in warmer climates to suggest to those in colder regions that they might convert their massive beet acreages to alternative crops, and leave the growing of sucrose to where sunlight is more abundant. However, if we consider Russia, which is the largest producer of sucrose in the world, not only is sugar beet a short-term and productive crop, but its season fits in well with rotation of other crops. Further, the USSR could hardly replace their huge import of grain crops from the USA upon beet acreages as temperatures there are not so suitable for the growing of such grains. Again in spite of this massive sucrose crop, Russia still imports more. The fact remains that the world has far too much sucrose on its hands and I'm sure that we are going to witness determined efforts to get humans to eat more of it. Further, any efforts by preventive nutritionists to decrease will be all the more forcefully resisted. The sucrose forces are thus powerful interests, who have an enormous surplus of their product. The face gigantic competition on an industrial basis from the high fructose corn sweeteners: they face consumer resistance in those countries where cyclamates and saccharin are still available, and they face a future squeeze from aspartame and the dihydrochalcone sweeteners: their commodity is too expensive for widespread use as a raw material. Thus we can expect a vigourous campaign to increase human consumption as we experienced in 1967. Measures to lower disproportionately high national sucrose intakes may include:

1. National avoidance of subsidisation of sucrose, as in Norway.
2. Restriction of TV and other advertising of sucrose, and sucrose-sweetened foodstuffs.
3. Concerted cut-back of sucrose production upon an international scale – this year's International Agreement has been a failure, unfortunately.
4. Crops alternative to sucrose should be planted.
5. Determined efforts should be made to funnel sucrose into the automotive fuel and animal feeds sectors – as well as other industrial applications.
6. Retail prices should rise to limit sales: this is happening now.
7. Attempts should be made by the Sugar authorities to rationalise supplies and avoid maldistribution. For instance, should every person on mainland China eat an extra 10 kg sucrose annually the surplus would disappear in a year.

8. There is obviously scope for harmless increase of sucrose in countries
   where intakes are very low.

9. The entirely safe sweeteners - saccharin and cyclamate - should once
   again be made freely available as they are in S. Africa. Bear in mind
   that the restriction of cyclamate resulted in a 13% increase in sucrose
   consumption in USA.

FINAL NOTE

It is not really possible to delineate accurately at present an "optimum
highest per capita annual national intake" other than to suggest that this
should not exceed 32 kg (70 lb), as this earlier figure suggested by myself
has the merit of epidemiological backing, and has been supported by one
distinguished authority. It can certainly be regarded as a reasonable mean
of 'desirable' figures of the "No-sucrose-at-any-cost" people (0.0 kg) and
the Sugar Authorities (45 kg). It is hoped that this congress will stimulate
attempts to decide upon some such figure, based upon further epidemiological
work on the relationship between long-term dietary studies and emergence of
the disorders of advancement. Not only the World Public, but its Governments
are in fairly urgent need of such advice, especially in the light of the
massive sucrose surplus.

REFERENCES

1. Jackson, W.P.U. and Vinik, A. in Diabetes, Clinical and Metabolic
    p. 179, Juta and Son, Cape Town, 1977.

2. Czarnikow Report, S.A. Sugar Journal 5: 62-220, 1978.

3. Sugar Year Book (I.S.O.) pp. 28, Haymarket, London SW1, 1978.

4. Campbell, G.D. Hearings of the Select Committee on Nutrition and
    Human Needs of the U.S. Senate (93rd Congress), Part. 2,
    Series 73/ND 2, pp. 214, 1973.

5. Truswell, A.S., Mann, J.I. and Campbell, G.D. Lancet I,
    p. 602, 1971.

6. Campbell, G.D. Diabetes, ICS/231, Excerpta Medica Series,
    p. 325, 1970.

7. Logan, R.L. et al Lancet I, p. 953, 1978.

8. Kloppers, P.J., Meiring, L. and Campbell, G.D. unpublished
    observations, 1978.

9. Campbell, G.D. Acceptable Addictions, Documenta Geigy (Basle)
    p. 7, 1971.

10. S.A. Sugar Association, Economic Section estimate, 1978.

11. Cleave, T.L. and Campbell, G.D. in Diabetes, Coronary Thrombosis
    and the Saccharine Disease, 1st Ed., John Wright and Sons,
    Bristol, 1966.

Health and Sugar Substitutes
Proc. ERGOB Conf., Geneva 1978, pp. 10-16 (Karger, Basel 1978)

PSYCHOLOGICAL CORRELATES OF SUGAR CONSUMPTION

Howard R. Moskowitz

MPi Sensory Testing, Inc., 770 Lexington Avenue
New York, N.Y. 10021, USA

INTRODUCTION - THE SWEET TASTE

Current research suggests that we are innately sensitive to, and prefer, sweetness. Studies of newborn infants[1] show that neonates 6 hours old exhibit reflex reactions (gustofacial reflex) indicating differences between sweet, sour and bitter solutions. Consumption studies of sweetened solutions[2] show differential ingestion of varying sweetened solutions. Finally, Nowlis[3] discovered neonatal reflexive tongue movements to sweeteners correlated with the concentration of these sweeteners which parallel previously published data on perceived sweetness[4].

Faced with this early acceptance of sweetness, and with the large industrial applications of sweeteners as flavoring agents and as non-tasted functionality agents, let us consider the three basic aspects of sweetness: Quality, Intensity and Hedonics. Each of these aspects is critical to understand consumption of sweetened foods.

QUALITY

A century ago Fick[5] postulated four primary tastes: Sweetness, Saltiness, Sourness, and Bitterness. Tied in with the notion of sweet quality is that sweeteners provide different spectra of taste perceptions. No sweetener provokes the pure sensation of sweetness, nor has any researcher except von Békésy ever reported a "pure sweetness" perception. For sugars as well as artificial sweeteners, sweetness co-occurs with other taste/smell/touch sensations.

Within the sugar family, sweetness quality varies. Glucose,

galactose, fructose, etc., differ qualitatively from sucrose.
The qualitative difference is hard to define. It may be the
presence of various levels of odor perception, textural differences, heats of solution (especially for xylitol), viscosity,
etc.[6] The qualitative differences in sugar substitutes show up
both in model aqueous solutions which lack a background taste and
in actual food products. Table I shows the degree of 'off-after-
taste, and sweetness present in cola beverages sweetened with
various levels of saccharin, cyclamate, aspartame and their
combinations.[7]

TABLE 1

SWEETNESS, OFF-TASTE AND HEDONICS OF COLA BEVERAGES SWEETENED WITH:

SAMPLE	CYCLAMATE (AMT)	SACCHARIN (AMT)	ASPARTAME (AMT)	SWEET-NESS	LIKING	AFTER-TASTE
1	0	0	3.8	6.3	-40.0	44.7
2	0	0	6.6	29.3	-44.7	44.3
3	0	0	16.0	75.0	+38.0	37.3
4	0	2.6	3.5	56.7	+13.3	52.3
5	0	2.6	7.0	92.0	+57.0	40.0
6	0	2.9	15.5	128.5	+14.8	65.7
7	0	5.2	3.5	72.0	+40.0	35.0
8	0	4.8	6.4	109.0	+44.7	50.0
9	0	11.2	3.7	103.6	+24.0	70.3
10	0	12.1	16.1	133.3	-40.5	66.7
11	6.2	0	3.0	18.0	-83.3	46.7
12	8.1	0	7.8	73.3	+33.3	43.3
13	7.6	5.5	3.6	100.0	+42.3	65.0
14	7.7	5.5	7.4	115.0	+50.0	44.7
15	6.9	5.0	13.3	140.0	-20.0	71.7
16	7.7	11.0	3.7	127.7	+22.3	70.7
17	6.6	9.5	6.3	149.0	-25.0	73.3
18	7.4	10.6	14.1	157.7	-50.0	86.5
19	13.4	0	3.2	43.0	-26.7	42.3
20	16.5	0	7.9	78.0	+55.6	46.7
21	14.7	0	14.1	126.7	+16.7	67.5
22	16.3	2.9	3.9	100.1	+44.3	36.7
23	16.3	5.9	7.8	158.5	-53.3	83.3
24	0	0	9.8	33.3	-113.3	44.7
25	0	3.3	0	33.3	-75.0	53.3
26	0	11.9	0	62.3	-22.0	58.3
27	8.3	0	0	1.5	-179.7	48.7
28	13.4	0	0	7.4	-122.3	46.7
29	7.9	11.4	0	100.0	+60.0	45.3
30	16.8	7.1	2.4	106.0	-49.0	36.7

AMT = mg sweetener/oz

INTENSITY

Since 1953, psychophysicists have used scales for sensory measurement possessing ratio properties. By magnitude estimation scaling, [8,9] judges assign numerical ratings to reflect sweetness. Magnitude estimation allows panelists to assign numbers so that ratios of numbers reflect ratios of sweetness. Psychophysicists use magnitude estimation to relate perceived sweetness to physical concentration. For carbohydrate sweeteners (e.g., sucrose, glucose, sorbitol, etc.) the relation between sweetness (s) and concentration (c) is a power function: $s = k(c)^n$.

The estimates of <u>n</u> for carbohydrate sweeteners are approximately 1.3 of the taste solution is evaluated by sipping the sweetener and swirling it in the mouth and approximately 0.5 if the taste solution is flowed over the tongue in a continuous stream.

This psychophysical relation for sweetness vs. concentration does not generalize to 'artificial sweeteners'.[10] Saccharin sweetness grows as a decelerating function of concentration (n = 0.65). The reason for this difference in growth rates is not clear. Possibly the <u>observed</u> or <u>phenotypical</u> sweetness of artificial sweeteners may be a <u>compromise</u> sensory percept, generated as a result of suppression by bitter. Artificial sweeteners generate perceptions of bitterness and sweetness. The observed bitterness and sweetness is the perceptual equilibrium. They result from an ongoing competition between the sweetness of artificial sweetener and the underlying bitterness which suppresses that sweetness.

SWEETNESS MIXTURES

An important research area is the measurement of the sweetness of mixtures of sweeteners, or mixtures of a sweetener with a non-sweet substance (e.g., sodium chloride, citric acid).

These studies show that:

- Sweeteners add to produce increased sweetness intensity. The sensory system may sum the two physical concentrations (after first converting the disparate concentrations into a commensurate unit) and then transforms the higher concentration into sweetness. [11,12]

- In heterogenous mixtures both tastes suppress each other. The mixture taste is lower than expected on the basis of additivity.[10]

- In commercial food products (e.g., cola beverages) similar equations hold.

SWEETNESS HEDONICS

Published scientific studies reveal that:

- In laboratory studies aqueous solutions of sugars are liked. Compared directly with food, however, simple aqueous solutions are disliked. Cognitive factors are critical for sweetness hedonics.[13]

- Sweetness acceptability varies with concentration and type of sweetener. For carbohydrate sweeteners, acceptance rises as the sweetness of a solution increases from 0 to that of 9% sucrose or equally sweet 18% glucose[10].

- At 9% w/v, acceptability peaks, and for increasing concentration, acceptability diminishes.

- The same general rules govern products which are equally sweetened beverages, puddings and cakes[13].

- Artificial sweeteners in aqueous solution show different and more variable relations between acceptability and sweetness[12].

- An artificial sweetener must be more sweet than a sugar to be equally liked.

- Age may influence sweetness liking. Table II compares adults, and children's liking ratings for several variations of a beverage. The children were 8-12 years old, and the adults were women. Panelists tested one of the beverages at home for 2-3 weeks and rated liking of sweetness and sweetness itself by magnitude estimation. The children prefer a sweeter product than do adults. Just as 9% w/v sucrose is optimally acceptable to adults, there may well be a region of optimal liking for children, albeit probably a higher concentration.

TABLE II
SWEETNESS AND LIKING RATINGS FOR BEVERAGES

PRODUCT	ADULTS		CHILDREN (8-12)	
	SWEETNESS	LIKING OF SWEETNESS	SWEETNESS	LIKING OF SWEETNESS
A	78.4	47.4	84.5	73.3
B	84.8	66.5	83.9	79.0
C	90.8	46.1	93.9	78.5
D	95.0	43.9	96.6	81.9
E	100.2	31.8	105.7	83.3

- Health and body state modify sweetness hedonics. Research suggests that obese individuals may not show a peak liking at 9% weight/volume sucrose. Rather, obese individuals may report a breakpoint in liking at a concentration approximately 18% w/v sucrose (or 36% w/v glucose). In other studies, the obese person may report disliking all sweet substances. In those cases, disliking of sweetness directly tracks the sweetness of the sugar stimulus.[14]

SOME UNANSWERED QUESTIONS

There are questions pertaining to behavior that need answers, for two reasons:

- Scientific, archival records for our understanding of sweetness perception.

- Applications of scientific knowlegde to better satisfy the consumer.

1. Sweetness Quality:

What is the relation between chemical structure and sweetness quality?

What are the precise qualitative aspects of the off-tastes which are inherent in artificial sweeteners

How can we mask these off-tastes without changing structure?

2. Sweetness Intensity:

Can a general sweetness index be developed to reflect the true perceived sweetness of alternative sweeteners, and what are the sweetness indices of different sweeteners at varying concentrations, for the sweeteners that are currently used?

3. Sweetness Hedonics

What is the relation between sweetness, concentration and acceptability for new sweeteners being developed?

Can we develop food products that trade off better flavor for sweetness (especially for children's foods)?

What are the long-term prospects for training consumers to accept foods with low or no sugar, or with low or no sweetness?

Is there a pervading 'sweet tooth' in man that is trainable to accept low sweetness?

REFERENCES

1. Steiner, J. Annals of the New York Academy of Sciences, 237: 229, 1974.

2. Desor, J.A., Maller, O., & Turner. Journal Comparative & Physiological Psychology, 84: 406, 1973.

3. Nowlis, G.H. In: Taste and Development (edited by Weiffenbach, J.) Government Printing Office, Washington, D.C. p. 190, 1977.

4. Moskowitz, H.R. American Journal of Psychology, 84: 387 1971.

5. Boring, E.G. Sensation and Perception in The History Of Experimental Psychology, N.Y., Appleton-Century Crofts, 1942.

6. Moskowitz, H.R. Journal of Food Science, 37: 624, 1972

7. Moskowitz, H.R., Wolfe, K. & Beck, C. Food Product Development in press, 1978

8. Stevens, S.S. Science, 118: 573, 1953.

9. Stevens, S.S. Psychophysics: An Introduction To Its Perceptual, Neural and Social Prospects, New York, John Wiley, 1975.

10. Moskowitz, H.R. In: Sugars in Nutrition (edited by Sipple, H. & McNutt, R.) p. 37, Academic Press, New York 1974.

11. Moskowitz, H.R.   Journal of Experimental Psychology, <u>99</u>: 88, 1973.

12. Moskowitz, H.R. & Dubose, C.   Canadian Journal of Food Science & Technology, <u>10</u>: 126, 1977.

13. Moskowitz, H.R., Kluter, R.A., Westerling, J. & Jacobs, H.L.   Science, <u>184</u>: 583, 1974.

14. Moskowitz, H.R.   In: Taste and Development (edited by Weiffelbach, J.) Government Printing Office, Washington, D.C. p. 282, 1977.

OBESITY AND DIABETES

A.E. Renold*, M, Berger and B. Jeanrenaud

University of Geneva Medical School, Department of Medicine
1211 Geneva 4, Switzerland.

That diabetes and obesity are mutually related is quite generally accepted, so much so that the relationship deserves regular re-examination since the near-unanimity of its acceptance must be considered suspect[1].

Indeed, some of the difficulties involved in dealing with this subject within the framework of knowledge available to us today are emphasized all too easily: After many years of resisting the obvious, diabetologists in general have accepted the evidence that diabetes mellitus is but a syndrome, and that its multifactorial nature must be recognised before real understanding of its pathogenesis can be achieved[2]. Similarly, although it is customary to speak of obesity as a single entity, much discussion being exercised in defining its quantitative beginning, most of us are intuitively aware that multifactorial genesis is again a most likely complication with which we will have to deal. There are many clinicians and medical biologists interested in obesity who do take into consideration such aspects as the distribution of excess adipose tissue (e.g. gynoid or android type)[3], the presence or absence of an abnormally large number of adipose tissue cells and/or the mean fat cell size[4], but there are still more who do not. It is my opinion, that understanding of pathogenetic events will advance only with increased recognition of the different types of diabetes and also of obesity. Indeed, the recent acceptance of the need to differentiate among types of diabetes, has already resulted in

* Address : Institut de Biochimie Clinique, Sentier de la Roseraie,
            CH 1211 Geneva 4.

significant improvements in their etiologic understanding, including the realisation that the role of genetics is different in
juvenile onset diabetes (JOD), and in maturity-onset diabetes
(MOD), especially when the latter type occurs in the young (MODY)[2].

With regard to the relationship of obesity to diabetes,
it has already been emphasised that the "android" distribution of
obesity more frequently results in carbohydrate intolerance and
diabetes[3,5]. Also, certain otherwise unrelated genetic backgrounds
seem to favour the correltation of obesity and diabetes more than
others: thus the relationship between the prevalence of diabetes
and obesity is poor in Bantu women[6], and especially in Pima
Indians[7]. In the latter example, however, there is a relationship between the weight at the time of diabetes onset and diabetes;
in other words, there is a relationship between the incidence of
obesity and diabetes, even though there is none between prevalence
of obesity and diabetes.

From epidemiological studies in many countries, nothing
has emerged that clearly relates the frequency of carbohydrate
intolerance to the type of food that resulted in overweight[8,9].
It would seem, therefore, that the type of food may rather be
involved in facilitating overeating and the onset of the obesity
syndrome, because of intrinsic appeal of some foods to the population concerned, but that the development of glucose intolerance
in a given obese population is not controlled by the type of food
which led to the obesity. Needless to say, all of these statements are tentative ones, since truly "hard" data is most difficult to obtain in this field.

When dealing with the relationships between diabetes and
obesity, it is also important to remember that the study of a
given population of grossly obese individuals has almost always
resulted in the observation that approximately 50% exhibit normal,
or near-normal glucose tolerance. It would therefore seem mandatory to deal, at some time, not only with the question of why
approximately half of a grossly obese population develops glucose
intolerance, but also with that of why the other half does not.

We are fully aware of the fact that this conference is primarily interested in information directly applicable to man. I must nevertheless point out that much of what is presently being considered in the pathogenesis of diabetes as related to obesity has been heralded by either observations on experiments of nature, that is on laboratory animal mutants characterized by over-eating and obesity, or by observations involving experimental manipulation.

The first conclusion which became evident when spontaneously obese animals were bred and observed, was the multiplicity of genetic anomalies, even of types of hereditary transmission, that may underly either a spontaneous diabetic or a spontaneous obesity syndrome[10,11,12].

Secondly, and perhaps most important, a general pattern or sequence appears to apply to the majority of animal syndromes associated with obesity, whether spontaneous and presumably genetic in origin, or experimentally or environmentally induced[13,14]. That sequence, as interpreted by the senior author, is listed below:

1. Functional anomaly of the hypothalamic centres relating to food intake, either of intrinsic hypothalamic origin, or resulting from signals initiated in higher CNS centres, or from the periphery.

2. Over-eating, even if of mild nature, with at least two immediate consequences: relative (and probably minor) hyperglycemia and greater stimulation of release of intestinal insulinogenic factors.

3. Increased insulin secretion as the result of either direct hypothalamic influence via the autonomic nervous system, or the result of over-eating.

4. Resistance to insulin action, possibly and partly the result of insulin-induced reduction of the density of insulin receptors (negative adaptation).

5. Hyperplasia and/or hypertrophy of insulin producing cells
    as a result of continued stimulation through over-eating
    and/or hypothalamic stimulation, further enhanced by the
    lesser effectiveness of the insulin produced because of
    the established resistance to insulin action.
6. There now follows a self-enhancing cycle, with increased
    insulin production leading to an increased proportion of
    absorbed food being deposited as fat, while appetite and
    food intake are preserved, thereby resulting in still
    further...
7. ... secretion of insulin, whether mediated by greater
    hyperglycemia or greater release of intestinal factors
    favouring insulin secretion.

It should be noted that the sequence just listed does
not necessarily represent the only sequence of metabolic events
considered, beginning by the metabolic event listed under 1.
Rather, the initiation of the cycle leading to obesity could
occur, and has been suggested to occur, at four points at least:

at metabolic event no 1,[15] hypothalamic defect being primary;

at metabolic event no 2, over-eating being primary; difficult
    to separate from 1;

at metabolic event no 3,[16,14] excess insulin secretion being
    primary;

at metabolic event no 4, the resistance to insulin action
    being primary, for example in skeletal muscle[17].

REFERENCES

1. Berger, M., Muller, W.A. and Renold, A.E. in Advances in
    Modern Nutrition, vol. 2: Diabetes, Obesity, and Vascular
    disease, edited by Katzen, H.M. and Mahler, R.J., pp. 211-228,
    Hemisphere Publishing Corporation, Washington, D.C., 1978.
2. Fajans, S. Heterogeneity of Diabetes mellitus in man.

Banting Lecture 1978.   Diabetes, 1978, in press.

3. Vague, J.   Am. J. Clin. Nutr. 4: 20-34, 1956.

4. Salans, L.B., Knittle, J.L. and Hirsch, J.   J. Clin. Invest.
    47: 153-165, 1968.

5. Vague, J., Vague, P., Boyer, J. and Cloix, M.C.   Excerpta
    Med. Int. Congr. Ser. 231: 517-525, 1971.

6. Jackson, W.P.V.   Postgrad. Med. J. 48: 391-398, 1972.

7. Bennett, P.H., Rushforth, N.B., Miller, M. and Lacompte, P.M.
    Recent Prog. Horm. Res. 32: 333-376, 1976.

8. West, K.M.   Acta Diabetol. Lat. 9 (Suppl. 1): 405-431, 1972.

9. Baird, J.D.   Acta Diabetol. Lat. 9 (Suppl. 1): 621-639, 1972.

10. Renold, A.E.   Adv. Metab. Disord. 3: 49-84, 1968.

11. Cameron, D.P., Stauffacher, W. and Renold, A.E.   in Handbook
    of Physiology, Sect. 7: Endocrinology, Vol. 1: Endocrine
    Pancreas, edited by Steiner, D.F., Freinkel, N. and Geiger,
    S.R., pp. 611-624, American Physiological Society,
    Washington, D.C.

12. Herberg, L. and Coleman, D.L.   Metabolism 26: 59-99, 1977.

13. Kahn, C.R., Neville, D.M. Jr, Gorden, P., Freychet, P. and
    Roth, J.   Biochem. and Biophys. Res. Communications 48: 135-
    142, 1972.

14. Assimacopoulos-Jeannet, F. and Jeanrenaud, B.   Clinics in
    Endocrinology and Metabolism 5: 337-365, 1976

15. Coleman, D.L.   Diabetologia 9: 294-298, 1973.

16. Mahler, R.J. and Szabo, O.   Amer. J. of Physiol. 221: 980-983,
    1971.

17. Cuendet, G.S., Loten, E.G., Jeanrenaud, B. and Renold, A.E.
    J. Clin. Invest. 58: 1078-1088, 1976.

Health and Sugar Substitutes
Proc. ERGOB Conf., Geneva 1978, pp. 22-26 (Karger, Basel 1978)

THE POSSIBLE ROLE OF POLYHYDRIC ALCOHOLS IN THE PATHOGENESIS OF VASCULAR

DISEASE AND NEUROPATHY IN DIABETES MELLITUS

R. S. Clements, Jr.

Department of Medicine and Diabetes Research and Training Center, University

of Alabama in Birmingham, University Station, Birmingham, Alabama 35294, USA

INTRODUCTION

In recent years, evidence has accumulated to suggest that alterations in the intracellular concentrations of certain polyhydric alcohols may be involved in the pathogenesis of certain of the late complications associated with diabetes mellitus. It has been observed that exposure of the lens, the peripheral nerve and the arterial wall to elevated concentrations of glucose leads to the intracellular accumulation of sorbitol, a linear six-carbon polyhydric alcohol. This phenomenon is associated with an increase in intracellular water in the lens and arterial wall, a decrease in the rate of nerve impulse conduction in the peripheral nerve, and impairment of the oxidative metabolism of the arterial wall. In those tissues in which exposure to hyperglycemia results in elevated intracellular sorbitol concentrations, a concomitant decrease in the intracellular concentration of myo-inositol consistently is observed. Since this six-carbon cyclic polyhydric alcohol is thought to play a role in a number of essential membrane functions, abnormalities in its metabolism could be involved in the mechanisms through which hyperglycemia leads to cell damage. The relative roles of increased intracellular sorbitol and decreased intra-cellular myo-inositol concentrations in the pathogenesis of diabetic neuropathy and vascular disease will be considered in this discussion.

HYPERGLYCEMIA AND THE ACCUMULATION OF SORBITOL IN ARTERIAL WALL AND NERVE

By analogy to studies of "sugar" cataracts[1], a number of investigators have postulated that sorbitol accumulation could have pathogenetic potential in such tissues as the nerve and the large blood vessels[2,3]. The presence of the polyol pathway in mammalian peripheral nerve has been unequivocally established, and its activity has been found to be exquisitely sensitive to the ambient glucose concentration[4]. The induction of experimental diabetes consistently leads to elevated concentrations of polyol pathway intermediates (sorbitol and fructose) as well as decreased myo-inositol concentrations and decreased nerve conduction velocities in the sciatic nerve of the rat[5,6]. In these studies, careful treatment with insulin was found to correct all of these abnormalities. Of particular interest was the observation that the functional abnormalities could only be corrected when complete normalization of the blood glucose concentrations was achieved and maintained.

In contrast to previous observations in the lens, no increase in the water content of the peripheral nerve of the diabetic rat could be detected and there appeared to be little relationship between polyol accumulation and the water content of this tissue[7]. The more recent observation by Greene et al. that the decreased motor nerve conduction velocity could be corrected by oral myo-inositol supplementation (a maneuver which had no effect upon the nerve glucose or sorbitol concentrations) suggests that the observed increase in the activity of the polyol pathway in the peripheral nerve of the diabetic may be only tangentially related to the pathogenesis of diabetic neuropathy[6].

Polyol pathway activity has also been demonstrated in the media of the arterial wall[8]. When incubated with elevated extracellular glucose concentrations, the arterial wall accumulates sorbitol intracellularly and the water content of this tissue increases[3]. The increase in water content impairs the diffusion of oxygen into and accelerates the release of lactate

from this tissue. That polyol pathway activity is responsible for these
abnormalities is suggested by the observation that they can be prevented by
the use of inhibitors of the enzyme aldose reductase. However, the fact that
elevation of the extracellular myo-inositol concentrations can also obviate
these derangements suggest that disordered myo-inositol metabolism may well
be involved in their pathogenesis.

ABNORMALITIES IN MYO-INOSITOL METABOLISM

Myo-inositol is a constituent of a class of membrane phospholipids whose
turnover has been speculated to be involved in numerous cellular processes
including electrolyte transport and nerve impulse conduction[9,10]. Since
the active intracellular transport of this material is inhibited by elevated
extracellular glucose concentrations, it is not surprising that its intracellular concentration is decreased in certain tissues of the diabetic
animal. In the human diabetic, it has been recently observed that a
substantial portion of the dietary myo-inositol intake is lost in the urine
and that the volume of distribution of myo-inositol is decreased[11]. Furthermore, preliminary evidence has suggested that (as in the rat) increased
dietary myo-inositol intake may have a salutory effect upon the nerve conduction velocities of patients with established diabetic polyneuropathy[12].

To determine whether the effect of hyperglycemia upon nerve myo-inositol
metabolism is due to impaired intracellular transport of this material or
to decreased rates of its incorporation into membrane phosphoinositides,
we have evaluated these phenomena in the rat nerve. The uptake of water-
soluble $2-^3$H-myo-inositol by the nerve of the streptozotocin-diabetic rat
was found to be decreased by only 20%. In contrast, the incorporation of
$2-^3$H-myo-inositol into nerve phospholipids was decreased by 85% in the
diabetic rat and did not return to normal following careful insulin therapy.
Whether this decrease in incorporation of myo-inositol into phospholipids

is due to limited substrate availability within the axon, or to alterations
in the nerve CDP-diglyceride:inositol phosphotransferase activity must await
direct enzymatic analysis. In any event, these observations suggest that
hyperglycemia results in a profound alteration in the phosphoinositide
metabolism of the peripheral nerve and raise the possibility that this
metabolic abnormality may be related to the reversible functional defects
in the diabetic human and rat nerve. Whether a similar defect exists in
the arterial wall of the diabetic animal has, as yet, not been studied.

SUMMARY

Defects in the metabolism of six-carbon linear and cyclic polyhydric
alcohols have been described in the nerve and the arterial wall of the
animal with experimental diabetes. While a direct relationship between
these abnormalities and the pathogenesis of nerve and large blood vessel
disease has not been demonstrated, it is tempting to speculate that such
relationships may exist. If so, manipulation of the intracellular
concentrations of these polyhydric alcohols might have therapeutic potential
in delaying the development of or decreasing the rate of progression of
certain of the late complications associated with human diabetes mellitus.

REFERENCES

1. van Heyningen, R. Nature 184: 194-195, 1959.

2. Gabbay, K.H., Merola, L.O. and Field, R.A. Science 151: 209-210, 1966.

3. Morrison, A.D., Clements, R.S.,Jr. and Winegrad, A.I. J. Clin. Invest.
    51: 3114-3123, 1973.

4. Stewart, M.A., Sherman, W.R., Kurien, M.M., Moonsammy, G.I. and
    Wisgerhof, M. J. Neurochem. 14: 1057-1066, 1967.

5. Gabbay, K.H. in Vascular and Neurologic Changes in Early Diabetes,
    edited by Camerini-Davolos, R.A. and Cole, H.S. pp. 417-424, Academic
    Press, New York, 1973.

6. Greene, D.A., DeJesus, P.V. and Winegrad, A.I. J. Clin. Invest. <u>55</u>:
    1326-1336, 1975.

7. Stewart, M.A., Kurien, M.M., Sherman, W.R. and Cotlier, E.V. J.
    Neurochem. <u>15</u>: 941-946, 1968.

8. Clements, R.S.,Jr., Morrison, A.D. and Winegrad, A.I. Science <u>166</u>:
    1007-1008, 1969.

9. Hendrickson, H.S. and Reynerten, J.L. Biochem. Biophys. Res. Commun.
    <u>44</u>: 1258-1264, 1971.

10. Pumphrey, A.M. Biochem. J. <u>112</u>: 61-70, 1969.

11. Clements, R.S.,Jr. and Reynertson, R. Diabetes <u>26</u>: 215-221, 1977.

12. Clements, R.S.,Jr., Vourganti, B., Darnell, B. and Oh, S. Diabetes <u>27</u>:
    436, 1978.

Health and Sugar Substitutes
Proc. ERGOB Conf., Geneva 1978, pp. 27-34 (Karger, Basel 1978)

SUGAR AND ORAL HEALTH: EPIDEMIOLOGY IN HUMANS

T.M. Marthaler

Div. of Applied Prevention, Dept. of Cariology, Periodontology
and Preventive Dentistry, Dental Institute, University of Zurich,
Switzerland

INTRODUCTION

Dental caries and periodontitis are the most widespread diseases. This does not mean that the destructive oral processes are
active at all periods of life, but their consequences can be seen
in virtually all adults above the age of forty since there is no
restitution of the damage produced during active phases of the
two diseases.

Periodontitis is not related to sugar consumption although a
few short term results suggest that sucrose may promote the formation of dental plaque[1,2]. Periodontitis was widespread already
in prehistoric periods. Studies on ancient and medieval skulls
revealed extremely low prevalence of caries. Only part of the
individuals were afflicted, and the fraction of teeth involved
was very low. Incisors and canines remained unattacked. The few
lesions which developed were found in molars[3].

In highly developed countries industrial production of sugar
started after 1850, and caries began to increase very rapidly.
Modern statistics demonstrate an extremely high caries activity.
Norwegian schoolchildren examined in 1940 may be taken as an
example. At age 13, three-quarters of the upper incisors were
attacked by caries. Only one in 20 molars had remained unattacked seven years after its eruption[4].

WORLD-WIDE EPIDEMIOLOGY OF DENTAL CARIES AND SUGAR CONSUMPTION

For a scientific study of the epidemiology of dental caries in
modern man, the number of decayed, missing and filled teeth (DMFT)

in children is most frequently used. World-wide mapping of sugar
consumption and DMF-levels has not yet been made on an international cooperative basis. FAO-data on sugar consumption (average per
year and head) and average numbers of DMF-teeth of children at age
11 to 12 have been compiled from 19 countries[5]. The relation between these data is shown in Figure 1.

Figure 1, based on data of 1959

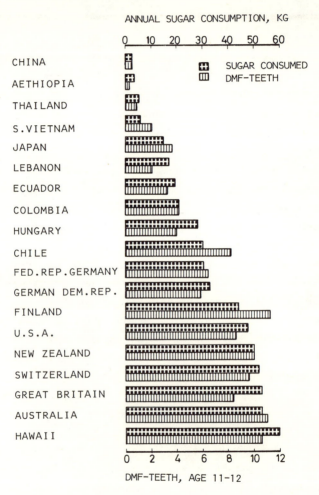

ANNUAL SUGAR CONSUMPTION, KG

DMF-TEETH, AGE 11-12

Obviously, there is a very strong correlation between sugar consumption and dental caries levels. This is in agreement with the results of many decades of research which have been summarized by several authors[6,7,8,9].

STUDIES IN DEVELOPING NATIONS AND REGIONS

In Nigeria, importation of sugar, sugar confectionery and other refined foods started in about 1946. Extremely low caries prevalence was still found in 1963-65 in malnourished village peasants living on starchy diets deficient in high quality proteins. On the other hand, Nigerians of high socio-economic background having consumed high amounts of imported sweets for years showed DMF averages approaching the level observed in Caucasian residents[10]. Several references in that paper indicate a similar trend in other African countries.

A particularly rapid increase of caries was seen in Canadian Eskimos. In Eskimos under 16, 3.3 DMF teeth were present in 1969, while 6.1 were found in 1973. In the age group 16 to 40, the increase was from 4.3 to 7.6. In 1969, most Eskimos were still subsisting on caribou, seal, fish flour and tea. By 1973, the majority had shifted to diets rich in refined carbohydrates including large amounts of candy bars, snack foods and soft drinks[11]. A rapid increase of carbohydrate consumption and dental caries was also described in Alaskan Eskimos. In this case, however, an increase in the consumption of sucrose-containing sweets was not explicitly stated[12].

Rising caries activity is also possible in countries which must be regarded as developed, but where sugar consumption has been low until recently. To cite an example, Hungarian children aged 3 to 6 years showed 3.8 carious deciduous teeth in 1955, and 5.3 in 1975. The author cites other data indicating a rise of caries activity in Hungary where the average annual sugar consumption of 24 kg per head in 1955 rose to 37 kg in 1975[13].

A large number of similar reports have attracted the interest of the WHO. In a Technical Report[14] it was stated that "There is convincing epidemiological evidence that, in many large population groups, the prevalence of dental caries rises and falls with changes in the total consumption of sugar. This is a matter of serious concern especially in those countries where traditional dietary habits are being abandoned in favour of an increased consumption of fermentable carbohydrates." Since more than half of the world's population is living in areas with extremely low caries prevalence as yet (southern and eastern Asia, Africa and the Pacific), the outlook for the near future is appalling.

HIGH CARIES LEVELS IN REMOTE AREAS

In isolated areas of New Guinea, averages of up to 5.6 DMF teeth at age 12-24 were found in the absence of sucrose consumption[15]. Some authors suggested that under severe conditions of malnutrition, rapid decay of teeth is possible due to specific structural defects[10].

It must be kept in mind, however, that in most areas where populations live on monotonous, primitive and inadequate diets, caries levels are extremely low[7].

Southern Morocco has had little contact with modern civilisation. Averages of 8.3 and 10.0 DMF teeth were found at ages 16-20 and 20-24. In this case, high caries activity is easily explained by the frequent consumption of dates which are the most important food item. Very sweet tea has been consumed for centuries[16].

LOW CARIES LEVELS IN COUNTRIES WITH HIGH SUGAR CONSUMPTION

Even in countries with high sugar consumption there may still be a very small part of the population showing few or no decayed teeth. Research in such individuals has not been able to isolate a single factor which could explain the unusual situation. It must be kept in mind that the severity of carious destruction depends on a large number of minor influences viz saliva, tooth morphology, eating habits etc. The effect of these factors levels out in populations but may produce considerable variations in individuals.

It is pertinent to note that it is the frequency of sugar in-

take or the time during which sugar is available to bacteria of
dental plaque which is the main determinant of caries activity.
The amount of sugar consumed is unimportant and the correlation
of sugar intake and extent of decay exists only on an epidemiological basis. This important aspect has recently been reviewed[17].

A special situation is represented by individuals with hereditary fructose intolerance. These individuals do not eat food
containing fructose and sucrose, but they frequently eat starchy
food, especially bread. They show very little or no decay[7], although their eating frequency is in the usual range[18].

DENTAL CARIES AND TOOTH LOSS

The ultimate consequences of high caries activity are quite
different in developing and in developed countries.

Developing countries usually have few dentists, less than 1
per 10'000 people and often less than 1 in 100'000. Teeth affected by caries are progressively destroyed. The majority of sound
teeth and those with arrested lesions remain in the oral cavity
up to the age of 40 to 60. In this age range, the chronic inflammatory processes of periodontitis start to be a frequent reason
for tooth loss.

In developed countries, loss of teeth is often enhanced due to
the failure of traditional, treatment-oriented dentistry which
can not cope effectively with rapidly progressing carious destruction. Since high-quality dental restorative treatment is expensive, extractions of teeth in young adults of lower economic
layers are sometimes very frequent. To cite an example, 12 percent
of the 16 to 34 year-old Scots of the lowest social classes are
estimated to be already edentulous. At age 35-54, 56 percent of
the population have no natural teeth left[19]. Similar percentages
of edentulous adults have been reported from several other countries. Early tooth loss is due to the combined effect of dental
caries and social conditions coupled with the tacit agreement of
patients and dentists that teeth are not important enough to be
saved or cared for. Tooth loss is also enhanced by insertion of
partial dentures.

LOW CARIES INSPITE OF HIGH SUGAR CONSUMPTION: EFFECT OF PREVENTION

Caries prevention on an individual or collective basis creates the most important deviation from the rule that high sugar intake is associated with high caries activity. Fluoridation of drinking water is the classical example. Artificial water fluoridation was first introduced in 1945. It now reaches over a hundred million inhabitants of the USA and many millions in other countries including Eastern Europe[20]. Other preventive methods are being developed. Salt fluoridation may have a considerable impact in countries with centralized production of salt for human consumption[21].

Programs at school based on information regarding prevention, supervised application of fluorides at least 6 times per year and regular instructions in toothbrushing have produced marked reductions of dental caries. The number of carious surfaces fell by about 50 percent after 4 years[22] or even by more than 60 percent after 12 years[23].

Such results show that caries prevention can be very effective. By very strict application of oral hygiene programs, it has even been possible to reduce dental caries by 50 to 90 percent in children[24] and by more than 90 percent in adults[25]. The main result in the study on adults was a total arrest of periodontal destruction.

In developed countries prevention of caries and periodontitis will make considerable progress in the near future. However, for the vast majority of mankind, dental decay is a growing problem.

REFERENCES

1. Ainamo, J., Sjöblom, M., Ainamo, A. and Tiainen, L.
    J. Clin. Periodontol. 4: 151-160, 1977.
2. Plüss, E.M. J. Clin. Periodontol. 5: 35-40, 1978.
3. Corbett, M.E. and Moore, W.J. Caries Res. 10: 401-414,
    1976.
4. Toverud, G. Milbank Memorial Fund Quarterly 35: 127-196,
    1957.
5. Büttner, W. in Grundfragen der Ernährungswissenschaft,
    edited by Cremer, H.-D. pp. 175-191, Rombach, Freiburg i.Br.
    1971.
6. Newbrun, E. Odont. Revy 18: 373-386, 1967.
7. Marthaler, T.M. Caries Res. 1: 222-238, 1967.
8. Bibby, B.G. editor J. dent. Res. 49: 1191-1352, 1970.
9. Caldwell, R.C. and Stallard, R.E. A textbook of preventive
    dentistry. W.B. Saunders, Philadelphia, 1977.
10. Enwonwu, C.O. Caries Res. 8: 155-171, 1974.
11. Mayhall, J.T. J. dent. Res. 56: 55-61, 1977.
12. Bang, G. and Kristoffersen, T. Scand. J. dent. Res. 80:
    440-444, 1972.
13. Bruszt, P., Banoczy, J., Esztary, I., Hadas, E., Marosi, I.,
    Nemes, J. and Albrecht, M. Community Dent. Oral Epidemiol.
    5: 136-139, 1977.
14. Wld. Hlth. Org. Techn. Rep. Ser. 1972, No. 494.
15. Schamschula, R.G., Adkins, B.L., Barmes, D.E., Charlton, G.
    and Davey, B.G.: J. dent. Res. 56: 62-70, 1977.
16. Ahrens, G., Augustin, B. and Völcker, S. Dtsch. zahnärztl.
    Z. 31: 848-854, 1976.
17. Newbrun, E. and Frostell, G. Caries Res. 12(Suppl.1):
    65-73, 1978.
18. Grünig, F. In preparation.
19. Todd, J.E. and Whitworth, A. Adult Dental Health in Scot-
    land. Her Majesty's Stationery Office, London, 1974.
20. Backer Dirks, O., Künzel, W. and Carlos, J.P. Caries Res.
    12(Suppl.1): 7-14, 1978.

21.   Marthaler, T.M., Mejia, R., Toth, K. and Vines, J.J.   Ca-
      ries Res. 12(Suppl.1): 15-21, 1978.

22.   Poulsen, S. and Risager, J.   Community Dent. Oral Epidemiol.
      3: 161-165, 1975.

23.   Marthaler, T.M.   Helv. odont. Acta 21: 63-68. In Schweiz.
      Mschr. Zahnheilk. 87: 823-828, 1977.

24.   Hamp, S.E., Lindhe, J., Fornell, J., Johansson, L.-Å. and
      Karlsson, R.   Community Dent. Oral Epidemiol. 6: 17-23, 1978.

25.   Axelsson, P. and Lindhe, J.   J. Clin. Periodontol. 5:
      133-151, 1978.

II. Absorbtion, metabolism and safety of sugar substitutes

a) Non-nutritive sweeteners

Moderator: P. Shubik, Omaha
Co-Moderator: G. Zbinden, Zurich

Health and Sugar Substitutes
Proc. ERGOB Conf., Geneva 1978, pp. 36-40 (Karger, Basel 1978)

MUTAGENICITY OF SACCHARIN IMPURITIES

D.R. Stoltz, B. Stavric and R. Klassen

Health & Welfare Canada, Health Protection Branch, Food
Directorate, Toxicology Research Division, Ottawa, Ontario,
K1A 0L2, Canada.

INTRODUCTION

In 1975 Kramers[1] reviewed a total of 17 mutagenicity studies
on saccharin. Equivocal results in a variety of assay systems
were tentatively attributed to the occurrence of varying
amounts of mutagenic impurities in commercial saccharins. Two
years later, mutagenic activity was demonstrated in organic
solvent soluble impurities concentrated from one of two lots
of saccharin fed to rats in the positive Canadian cancer study.
Mutagenic activity, detected with the Ames Salmonella test, was
subsequently found in impurities extracted from many but not
all lots of saccharin examined[2].

CONCENTRATION OF IMPURITIES

One kg of sodium saccharin, dissolved in 1.5L distilled H_2O,
was mixed with 1L methanol and 1L chloroform, shaken and the
lower layer collected. The aqueous solution was extracted once
more with 1L of chloroform. The chloroform extracts were
pooled, evaporated to dryness and the residue assayed for
mutagenicity.

MUTAGENICITY ASSAYS

The mutagenicity of concentrated impurities, dissolved in
DMSO or ethanol, was determine according to established

TABLE I

MUTAGENICITY OF ORGANIC SOLVENT EXTRACTS OF SACCHARIN

PROCESS	LOT NO.	IMPURITIES[c]	MUTAGENICITY[a]	TIMES TESTED
	S-1022	13	+[b]	16
	6368	13	+	1
MAUMEE	GS-1233	5	−	2
	S-1469	20	+	3
	GSC-0129	16	+	1
	F,G,H,I,J	1-5	−	2 each
	1648	18	+	8
	QA-80	86	−	1
REMSEN-	QB-125	305	−	1
FAHLBERG	191010	51	+	2
	"RF-HICKS"	212	?[d]	1

[a] Mutagenicity for TA98 in the presence of fortified liver homogenate.

[b] A 100% increase over the number of spontaneous revertants was taken to indicate a positive (+) response; a negative response is indicated by (−).

[c] Milligrams of organic solvent soluble impurities extracted from 1 kg of saccharin.

[d] Toxicity of the extract prevented assessment of mutagenic activity.

procedures with strains of <u>Salmonella typhimurium</u>[3] obtained
from Dr. Bruce Ames (Berkeley, California).

Results of mutagenicity testing of the organic solvent
soluble impurities from saccharin samples are summarized in
Table I. Although several of the saccharins from which these
impurities were extracted have been used in cancer studies, it
is not possible to correlate the carcinogenicity of any
sample of saccharin with the presence of mutagenic impurities
for the reasons listed below[2]:

1. The design and thoroughness of the cancer studies varies
    considerably, eg. one and two generation studies.

2. In several cancer studies, more than one lot of saccharin
    was used.

3. The extent of mutagenicity testing of impurities varies
    from lot to lot since it was not possible to obtain
    sufficient quantities of saccharin to confirm initial
    results with certain samples.

Thus, determination of the relevance of the mutagenic
impurity to the carcinogenicity of saccharin will depend upon
isolation, identification, synthesis and biological testing of
the mutagen.

ISOLATION OF INDIVIDUAL IMPURITIES

Since supplies of the saccharin (containing mutagenic
impurities) used in the recent Canadian cancer study are
limited, the approach taken was to identify another large sample
of saccharin with mutagenic impurities. Once the mutagen has
been identified in this sample, analytical methods will be
employed to check previous samples of saccharin for the
presence of this mutagen and to determine whether the same

compound is responsible for the mutagenic activity observed in concentrated impurities from different lots of saccharin.

Isolation of individual impurities is in progress, using high performance liquid chromatography coupled to the Salmonella mutagenicity assay.

CONCLUSION

Speculation regarding the mechanism of action of saccharin in biological systems must take into account all relevant observations. Although correlations between mutagenicity and carcinogenicity[4] suggest that the mutagenic impurity may be a carcinogen, the mutagen may not be present in sufficient quantity to influence cancer studies on saccharin. Recent reports that saccharin is nucleophilic[5], does not bind to DNA[6], is not metabolized[7], and is negative in most validated short-term tests for carcinogens[8] indicate that saccharin per se is not a classical electrophilic carcinogen. It is suggested that saccharin per se or saccharin-induced urine composition alterations exert a promoter effect on bladder carcinogenesis. Initiation may be due to the mutagenic impurity or endogenous chemicals such as tryptophan metabolites or exogenous carcinogens such as nitrosamines in water supplies or mycotoxins in animal feed.

QUESTIONS

1. What progress has been made in the isolation and identification of the mutagenic saccharin impurity?

2. What is the level of mutagen in saccharin?

3. What are potential origins of impurities?

4. Are there any particular problems associated with mutagenicity testing of complex mixtures?

REFERENCES

1. Kramers, P.G.N. Mutation Res. 32:81-92, 1975.

2. Stoltz, D.R., Stavric, B., Klassen, R., Bendall, R.D. and Craig, J. J. Envir. Path. Toxicol. 1:139-146, 1977.

3. Ames, B.N., McCann, J. and Yamasaki, E. Mutation Res. 31:347-364, 1975.

4. McCann, J., Choi, E., Yamasaki, E. and Ames, B.N. Proc. Nat. Acad. Sci. USA 72:5135-5139, 1975.

5. Ashby, J., Styles, J.A., Anderson, D. and Paton, D. Fd. Cosmet. Toxicol. 16:95-103, 1978.

6. Lutz, W.K. and Schlatter, Ch. Chem.-Biol. Interactions 19:253-257, 1977.

7. Ball, L.M., Renwick, A.G. and Williams, R.T. Xenobiotica 7:189-203, 1977.

8. Office of Technology Assessment, Congress of the United States, in Cancer Testing Technology and Saccharin, pp. 91-108, 1977.

Health and Sugar Substitutes
Proc. ERGOB Conf., Geneva 1978, pp. 41-47 (Karger, Basel 1978)

THE METABOLISM, DISTRIBUTION AND ELIMINATION OF NON-NUTRITIVE SWEETENERS

A. G. Renwick

Clinical Pharmacology, Faculty of Medicine, University of Southampton, Medical and Biological Sciences Building, Bassett Crescent East, Southampton SO9 3TU, U. K.

INTRODUCTION

Two non-nutritive sweeteners, saccharin and cyclamate, have been widely used in human food although both are currently the subject of considerable debate concerning their safety. Both saccharin and cyclamate are strong acids with pKa values of 2.2 and 1.9 respectively[1], and are normally used as the water soluble sodium salts. Highly ionised organic acids usually show incomplete absorption from the gut and are excreted in the urine unchanged. Early studies reviewed in 1959[2] suggested that saccharin and cyclamate exhibited both of these characteristics. However, with the advent of sophisticated analytical techniques, reports appeared suggesting that cyclamate[3] and saccharin[4,5] underwent slight metabolism in the body (<1% of the dose) to cyclohexylamine and 2-sulphamoylbenzoic acid respectively.

METABOLISM

Since the initial discovery that cyclohexylamine, an indirectly acting sympathomimetic amine, was a metabolite of cyclamate in dog and man[3], a large number of studies have attempted to define the site and extent of this metabolic reaction.

Sodium Cyclamate — $NHSO_3Na$ Cyclohexylamine — NH_2

In man, a single oral dose of cyclamate was only partly absorbed, about 40% was excreted in the urine and the remainder in the faeces[6], with negligible metabolism to cyclohexylamine. However, if cyclamate was given in regular daily doses the ability to convert it to cyclohexylamine increased, in some individuals, until the urinary elimination reached a plateau after a period of about one week of continued intake[6, 7, 8]. The extent of the reaction showed extreme inter-individual differences (from undetectable to 30% of the dose or more[6, 7, 8]) with about 20% of an induced population metabolising 2% or more of the dose[6, 7, 8, 9, 10]. The ability to metabolise cyclamate was rapidly lost on giving a cyclamate free diet[6], and the induction and loss of activity in vivo was mirrored by similar changes in the ability of faecal organisms to effect this reaction in vitro[11]. Induction of cyclamate metabolism in other animal species was similar to man[6, 9], although the time taken for induction in the rat showed very large differences from one study to another[6, 12, 13]. The site of the reaction was shown to be the gut flora in the rat, rabbit, guinea pig[6] and pig[9], although different micro-organisms were probably responsible in each host species. Different micro-organisms may also have been responsible in the same host species since clostridia able to metabolise cyclamate were isolated from converter rat faeces[11] and cyclamate pre-treatment caused an increase in the numbers of clostridia in this study and a follow-up[13]. However, other workers found no such increase in numbers[12] and also showed that neomycin administration, which does not greatly affect clostridia, caused suppression of cyclamate metabolism[12, 14].

Since the host tissues were not able to metabolise cyclamate[9], only the unabsorbed material is a potential source of cyclohexylamine. In view of the wide inter-individual differences it is possible that some subjects may be able to convert all of the unabsorbed material, i.e. up to 60% of the dose, to the more toxic metabolite. However, in any attempt to define an acceptable daily intake for cyclamate based on a no-effect level for cyclohexylamine, a figure of 25% is a realistic value to use, since this is the average value for good converters (>5% of dose as cyclohexylamine) during periods of continued intake. Using this conversion figure and applying a safety factor of 100 would give an adequate safeguard for good converters taking cyclamate, whilst non-converters would not be at risk.

Detailed studies designed to further investigate the slight metabolism of saccharin to 2-sulphamoylbenzoic acid reported by some workers[4, 5] have yielded largely equivocal results.

Sodium Saccharin

2-Sulphamoylbenzoic Acid

Studies using radiolabelled saccharin showed that artefactual "metabolites" could be caused by either the choice of an inappropriate solvent for chromatography[15] or the presence of an impurity in the radiolabelled saccharin[16]. Of the two most recent studies, one confirmed earlier reports that 2-sulphamoylbenzoic acid was a metabolite of radiolabelled saccharin (up to 1% of dose)[17] while the other study found no metabolism (<0.2% of dose)[18]. The positive study[17] also found labelled CO_2 in the expired air and $CO_3^=$ in the urine (up to 1% of dose) but these were not detected (<0.04% of dose) by the other workers[18]. Metabolism of saccharin was not induced by feeding rats diets containing up to 5% saccharin[18]. Thus although saccharin, like cyclamate, is incompletely absorbed from the gut (about 10-20% of the dose is eliminated in the faeces), the microflora cannot be induced to metabolise the compound by pre-treatment. Saccharin was not a substrate for the enzyme system induced in rat faeces by chronic cyclamate administration which hydrolysed the N-S bond of cyclamate[18].

Recent studies on the metabolism of the common impurities of saccharin have shown that the polar impurities (2-sulphamoylbenzoic acid[18], 4-sulphamoylbenzoic acid[19] and 5-chlorosaccharin[20]) were rapidly excreted without significant metabolism, whereas the less polar impurities (toluene-2-sulphonamide[21], toluene-4-sulphonamide[19] and benz[d]isothiazoline-1, 1-dioxide[22]) underwent extensive metabolism and rapid excretion. Studies on the fates of the 2-alkylbenzenesulphonamide impurities have provided a possible explanation for the contradictory reports of saccharin metabolism.

Benz[d]isothiazoline-1, 1-dioxide

Toluene-2-sulphonamide

Oxidation of the alkyl side chain was accompanied by ring closure (for toluene-2-sulphonamide) or ring opening (for benz[d]isothiazoline-1,1-dioxide). The oxidation intermediate probably involved (3-hydroxybenz[d]isothiazoline-1, 1-dioxide) had chromatographic properties similar to saccharin and underwent further oxidation to both saccharin and 2-sulphamoylbenzoic acid. Thus if the radiolabelled dose of saccharin used by earlier workers[4, 5, 17] contained a small amount of labelled 3-hydroxybenz[d]isothiazoline-1,1-dioxide this would not be readily detected in the dose material, but would appear in the urine as 2-sulphamoylbenzoic acid. Thus, within the limits of detectability set by recent studies[16, 18], saccharin is not significantly metabolised in either normal or pre-treated rats or human subjects.

DISTRIBUTION AND ELIMINATION

There have been few studies on the distribution and kinetics of elimination of the sweeteners. Investigations of the distribution of radiolabelled cyclamate in rats[23], and dog[24] showed that the highest levels were found in tissues with a good blood supply, i.e. kidney, liver, lungs and spleen. The levels in the urinary bladder were not measured in these studies. The sweetener crossed the placenta of the rat[23] and monkey[25] but less readily than did the metabolite, cyclohexylamine[25]. The tissue distribution of radiolabelled saccharin was similar to cyclamate[15, 16, 18] except that the urinary bladder was analysed and found to contain higher levels of radio-activity than any other organ. The compound crossed the placenta of rat[18] and monkey[26] to give a distribution in the foetus similar to the adult with the urinary bladder containing the highest amounts[18].

Cyclamate[27] and saccharin[28] are eliminated from the blood by glomerular filtration and renal tubular secretion, the latter process being saturated by saccharin at plasma concentrations greater than 200µg/ml[29]. This concentration was found in rats given 5% saccharin diet, although the level showed a diurnal variation with the maximum at about 6a.m. (200µg/ml) and the minimum at about 6p.m. (90µg/ml)[30]. Studies on the excretion of [^{3}H] saccharin after intravenous administration[31] showed that the compound was very rapidly cleared from the plasma at doses up to 600mg/kg. Such high doses produced plasma concentrations well in excess of 200µg/ml but gave a half-life (30min) only slightly higher than lower non-saturating doses (t$\frac{1}{2}$ about 20min). This suggests that renal tubular secretion is not the main mechanism by which the compound is cleared from plasma. However, high doses were accompanied by a decrease in the apparent volume of distribution which may have opposed the increase in $t\frac{1}{2}$ resulting from saturation of renal tubular secretion. Studies are currently underway to investigate further the pharmacokinetic validity of the high dose 2-generation bioassay, in an attempt to answer the following questions:-

1) Does a slower clearance of saccharin from foetal tissues, particularly the bladder[18], result in very high exposure in utero during chronic saccharin intake?

2) Is the weaning stage of a 2-generation study accompanied by plasma saccharin levels very much higher than found in adults given the same diet?

3) How is the compound handled in man, what plasma levels are found in humans receiving a fixed dose (1g) and a normal saccharin containing diet?

REFERENCES

1. Kojima, S., Ichibagase, H. and Iguchi, S. Chem. Pharm. Bull. (Tokyo) 14: 965-971, 1966.

2. Williams, R. T. in "Detoxication Mechanisms", 2nd Ed., pp. 500-501, Chapman & Hall, London, 1959.

3. Kojima, S. and Ichibagase, H. Chem. Pharm. Bull. (Tokyo), 14: 971-974, 1966.

4. Pitkin, R. M., Anderson, D. W., Reynolds, W. A. and Filer, L. J. Proc. Soc. Exp. Biol. Med. 137: 803-806, 1971.

5. Kennedy, G., Fancher, O. E., Calandra, J. C. and Keller, R. E. Fd. Cosmet. Toxicol. 10: 143-149, 1972.

6. Renwick, A. G. and Williams, R. T. Biochem. J. 129: 869-879, 1972.

7. Leahy, J. S., Taylor T. and Rudd, C. J. Fd. Cosmet. Toxicol. 5: 595-596, 1967.

8. Davis, T. R. A., Adler, N. and Opsahl, J. C. Toxicol. Appl. Pharmacol. 15: 106-116, 1969.

9. Collings, A. J. in Sweetness and Sweeteners, edited by Birch, G. C., Green, L. F. and Coulson, C. B. pp. 51-68, Applied Science Publishers Ltd., London, 1971.

10. Wills, J. H., Jameson, E., Stoewsand, G. and Coulston, F. Toxicol. Appl. Pharmacol. 12: 292, 1968.

11. Drasar, B. S., Renwick, A. G. and Williams, R. T. Biochem. J. 129: 881-890, 1972.

12. Bickel, M. H., Burkard, B., Meier-Strasser, E. and Van Den Broek-Boot, M. Xenobiotica 4: 425-439, 1974.

13. Renwick, A. G. in Drug Metabolism - from Microbe to Man, edited by Parke, D. V. and Smith, R. L. pp.169-189, Taylor & Francis, London, 1977.

14. Sonders, R. C., Netwal, J. C. and Wiegand, R. G. Pharmacologist, 11, 241, 1969.

15. Matthews, H. B., Fields, M. and Fishbein, L. J. Agr. Food. Chem. 21: 916-919, 1973.

16. Byard, J. L. and Golberg, L. Fd. Cosmet. Toxicol. 11: 391-402, 1973.

17. Lethco, E. J. and Wallace, W. C. Toxicology 3: 287-300, 1975.

18. Ball, L. M., Renwick, A. G. and Williams, R. T. Xenobiotica 7: 189-203, 1977.

19. Ball, L. M., Williams, R. T. and Renwick, A. G. Xenobiotica, 8: 183-190, 1978.

20. Renwick, A. G. Xenobiotica, in press.

21. Renwick, A. G., Ball, L. M., Corina, D. L. and Williams, R. T. Xenobiotica, in press.

22. Renwick, A. G. and Williams, R. T. Xenobiotica, in press.

23. Taylor J. D., Richards, R. K. and Davin, J. C. Proc. Soc. Exp. Biol. Med. 78: 530-533, 1951.

24. Miller, J. P., Crawford, L. E. M., Sonders, R. C. and Cardinal, E. V. Biochem. Biophys. Res. Comm. 25: 153-157, 1966.

25. Pitkin, R. M., Reynolds W. A. and Filer, L. J. Proc. Soc. Exp. Biol. Med. 132: 993-999, 1969.

26. Pitkin, R. M., Reynolds, W. A., Filer, L. J. and Kling, T. G. Am. J. Obstet. Gynecol. 111: 280-286, 1971.

27. Klaverkamp, J. F. and Dixon, R. L. Proc. Western Pharmacol. Soc. 12: 75-77, 1969.

28. Goldstein, R. S., Hook, J. B. and Bond, J. T. J. Pharmacol. Exp. Therap. 204: 690-695, 1978.

29. Bourgoignie, J., Hwang, K. H. and Bricker, N. S. Abstract presented
     to the 10th Annual Meeting of the American Society of Nephrology, 1977.
30. Renwick, A. G. unpublished results.
31. Sweatman, T. W. and Renwick, A. G. unpublished results.

Health and Sugar Substitutes
Proc. ERGOB Conf., Geneva 1978, pp. 48-53 (Karger, Basel 1978)

REPLICATION AND PERMEABILITY IN THE ANIMAL MODEL

T.A. Lawson

Eppley Institute for Research in Cancer and Allied Diseases,
University of Nebraska Medical Center, 42nd & Dewey, Omaha,
Nebraska, 68105, U.S.A.

INTRODUCTION

The mammalian urinary bladder consists of an outer muscle wall
which is separated from the transitional epithelium by a capil-
lary bed, connective tissue and a basement membrane. The transitional epithelium, which is two to three cell layers thick, constitutes the inner (luminal) tissue of the bladder. The epithelium exhibits polyploidy, i.e., cells with more than the normal
amount of nuclear DNA. The functional behavior and properties of
the transitional epithelium will be considered here. The transitional epithelium is the site of most of the bladder tumors which
occur in man and animals.

REPLICATION

The most prominent feature of cellular replication in the
bladder epithelium is the very low rate of cell division. Cell
replication can be quantitated by observing the number of cells
in mitosis in any given population. In mice, only about one
bladder epithelial cell in ten thousand is in division at any
one time[1,2]. Farsund[3] could detect only five epithelial cells
in mitosis from eight mice in which about ten thousand cells
were counted in each bladder.

The other parameter which gives a measure of cell replication
is DNA synthesis, which precedes mitosis. It can be determined
qualitatively and quantitatively by utilizing radioactive (tri-
tium or carbon-14) thymidine. Thymidine is the 2'-deoxyriboside
of the base thymine and incorporates specifically into DNA[4].
Quantitatively, DNA synthesis can be measured by the technique of
autoradiography, or by the extraction of the DNA from the tissue[5]

and measurement of radioactivity per unit of DNA. In most instances, when the rate of mitosis is low, so is the rate of DNA
synthesis.

Only 0.1% to 0.5% of the epithelial cells in mouse[2,3,8] and
rat bladder epithelium[9] are normally engaged in DNA synthesis
at one time. This means that these epithelial cells have a mean
lifespan of up to 200 days. One might speculate that the reason
for the extreme stability of the epithelium is to reduce the
chance of errors in replication which could upset the physical
integrity of the bladder and reduce its efficiency in performing
its specialized functions of storage and excretion of urine.

The very low level of DNA synthesis precludes accurate
measurements of any inhibition of DNA synthesis or thymidine incorporation. This type of measurement has assumed new significance with the demonstrations that chemical carcinogens inhibit
the incorporation of thymidine into DNA[10,11,12,13,14,15]. Lawson
et al. showed that single doses of bladder carcinogens produced
an inhibition of bladder epithelial DNA synthesis which was followed by a wave of enhanced DNA synthesis[6,16]. In a similar,
though unrelated, study, bladder carcinogens were shown to produce
hyperplasia and enhanced cell proliferation on sub-chronic
feeding, whereas non-carcinogens did not[17]. Chronic feeding of
sodium saccharin (7.5%; w/w) in the diet inhibited epithelial
DNA synthesis for at least six weeks, after which time the DNA
synthesis in the saccharin-treated animals returned to the control levels. Saccharin does not appear to induce this inhibition
in the same way as chemical carcinogens as it is not metabolically activated and does not interact with DNA.

Studies of DNA synthesis provide information on the proli-
ferative status of the tissue and can give an indication of
the carcinogenic potency of a chemical[10,11,12,13,14,15]. As yet,
there is no explanation for the correlation between the inhibition of DNA synthesis and carcinogenicity, but the correlations
are very strong. Establishing the finer details of the mechanism
by which chemical carcinogens inhibit the incorporation of thymidine into DNA could yield valuable information on the mode of
action of chemical carcinogens.

The other feature of the bladder epithelium to be considered
in this section is the polyploid nature of the tissue. The basal

and intermediate layers of the epithelium consist of diploid and
tetraploid cells (cells with two or four sets of chromosomes).
The surface cells have higher ploidies, especially in mice where
binucleate cells are often present[2].

In a study of the variation of ploidy levels in the mouse
bladder epithelium with age, the proportion of diploid cells
decreases by 25% during the first six months, with a corresponding increase in tetra- and hexaploid cells[20]. In related
studies with chemicals that are carcinogenic or necrogenic to
the bladder epithelium, Farsund showed that cells at different
ploidy levels reacted differently to the various agents[21,22,23].

Cells that synthesize considerable amounts of tissue-specific
proteins usually undergo polyploidization[24]. The mechanism by
which polyploid cells are formed in the bladder epithelium is
related to the formation of binucleate cells which on subsequent division, yield polyploid cells[2,25]. However, multinu-
cleate cells in the bladder may be formed by fusion of cells[26].

The functional significance of polyploidy is equally unclear.
In the liver, there are considerable differences in the ploidy
of the parenchymal cells, but they behave essentially the same.
Tissues stimulated to abnormal and excessive growth in response
to a stimulus show increased levels of polyploidy, e.g., hyper-
tropic myocardium[27]. It is difficult to see how this mechanism
applies to the bladder, but one of the consequences of polyploidy
is enlargement of the cells, which has been observed in the surface layer of epithelial cells[19]. It is these surface cells
which undergo the greatest changes in size with the repeated
distension and emptying of the bladder.

PERMEABILITY

The mammalian bladder is considered to be a unique structure
among vertebrates[28]. Its primary function is to retain urine
until it can be voluntarily voided. The mammalian urothelium
acts as a permeability barrier and prevents dilution of the urine
by osmotic pressure. The structure and chemical composition of
the urothelium have been reviewed[28,29]. The permeability of
the urothelium to water, ions and a variety of other solutes
has been studied in a number of species in vivo and in vitro. Although there is no major flow of any material across the membrane,

there is some very limited exchange of materials by a passive
diffusion. There is no active transport as found in toad bladders[29]. Water[30] and a variety of small ions have been shown to
pass in this way[31]. Water passes more easily than ions. Lipo-
philic materials cross the luminal membrane much more easily than
ions or water. In utero, the transport process in the bladder is
an active one, but becomes passive by parturition. These differences may be of significance in considering the greater carcinogenicity of saccharin in F_1 generation, compared to the F_o
generation.

The permeability of the bladder can be drastically altered if
the cell junctions are broken or the luminal membrane breached.
This can be achieved experimentally with necrogenic agents like
cyclophosphamide, which strip the epithelium[32] or agents which
destroy the luminal integrity[32]. Measurements of permeability
can be used to indicate that alterations, such as damage to the
luminal membrane and cell junctions or the presence of tumors,
have occurred in the epithelium[32,33,35]

REFERENCES

1. Clayson, D.B. and Pringle, J.A.S. Brit. J. Cancer 20:564-568, 1966.

2. Levi, P.E., Cowen, D.M. and Cooper, E.H. Cell Tissue Kinet. 2:249-262, 1969.

3. Farsund, T. Virchows Arch. B. Cell Path. 18:35-49, 1975.

4. Cleaver, J.E. in Thymidine Metabolism and Cell Kinetics, North Holland, Amsterdam, 1967.

5. Parish, J.H. in Principles and Practice of Experiments with Nucleic Acids, Longman, London, 1972.

6. Lawson, T.A., Dawson, K.M. and Clayson, D.B. Cancer Res. 30:1586-1592, 1970.

7. Baserga, R. in Methods in Cancer Research, Volume 1, edited by H. Busch, Academic Press, New York and London, pp. 45-116, 1967.

8. Dzhioev, F.K., Wood, M., Cowen, D.M., Campobasso, O. and Clayson, D.B. Brit. J. Cancer 23:772-780, 1969.

9. Hiramatsu, T. J. Nara. Med. Assn. 25:101-105, 1974.

10. Friedman, M.A. and Staub, J. Mutat. Res. 37:67-76, 1976.

11. Seiler, J.P. Mutat Res. 46:305-310, 1977.

12. Slaga, T.J., Bowden, G.T., Shapas, B.G. and Boutwell, R.K. Cancer Res. 33:769-776, 1973.

13. Slaga, T.J., Bowden, G.T., Shapas, B.G. and Boutwell, R.K. Cancer Res. 34:771-777, 1974.

14. Zedeck, M.S., Grab, D.J. and Stemberg, S.S. Cancer Res. 37:32-36, 1977.

15. Mirvish, S.S., Chu, C. and Clayson, D.B. Cancer Res. 38:458-466, 1978.

16. Lawson, T.A., Dzhioev, F.K., Lewis, F.A. and Clayson, D.B. Biochem. J. 111:12P, 1969.

17. Clayson, D.B., Lawson, T.A., Santana, S. and Bonser, G.M. Brit. J. Cancer 19:297-310, 1965.

18. Bresciani, F. Europ. J. Cancer 4:343-350, 1968.

19. Fulker, M.J., Cooper, E.H. and Tanaka, T. Cancer 27:71-82, 1971.

20. Farsund, T. Virchows Arch. B. Cell Path. 18:35-49, 1975.

21. Farsund, T. Virchows Arch. B. Cell Path. 21:279-298, 1976.

22. Farsund, T. Virchows Arch. B. Cell Path. 25:179-189, 1977.

23. Farsund, T. Virchows Arch. B. Cell Path. 27:1-6, 1978.
24. Brodsky, W.Y. and Uryvaeva, I.V. in Int. Rev. Cytol. 50, edited by Boume, G.H. and Danielli, J.F., Acad. Press, New York and London, pp. 275-332, 1977.
25. Nadal, C. and Zaidela, F. Expt. Cell Res. 42:99-116, 1966.
26. Martin, B.F. J. Anat. 112:433-445, 1972.
27. Sandritter, W. and Scomazzoni, G. Nature (London) 202:100-101, 1964.
28. Hicks, R.M. Biol. Rev. 50:215-246, 1975.
29. Carruthers, J.S. and Bonneville, M.A. J. Cell Biol. 73: 382-399, 1977.
30. Manicci, H.D., Shoemaker, W.C., Wase, A., Strauss, H.D. and Geyer, S.V. Proc. Soc. Exptl. Biol. Med. 87:569-571, 1954.
31. Johnson, J.A., Cavert, H.M., Lifson, N. and Visscher, M.B. Am. J. Physiol. 165:87-92, 1951.
32. Fellows, G.J. and Turnbull, G.J. Rev. Europ. Etudes Clin. et Biol. 16:303-310, 1971.
33. Turnbull, G.J. Ph.D. Thesis, University of Leeds, 1971.
34. Hicks, R.M. J. Cell Biol. 28:21-31, 1966.
35. Cooper, E.H. in The Biology and Management of Bladder Cancer, Blackwell Scientific Publications, Oxford, England, pp. 37-64, 1975.

Health and Sugar Substitutes
Proc. ERGOB Conf., Geneva 1978, pp. 54-57 (Karger, Basel 1978)

END POINTS IN BLADDER CARCINOGENESIS

D.B. Clayson

Eppley Institute for Research in Cancer and Allied Diseases,
University of Nebraska Medical Center, 42nd & Dewey, Omaha,
Nebraska, 68105, U.S.A.

The questions to be considered are: (i) whether the induction
of bladder tumors as a result of administration of chemicals to
experimental animals is always indicative of a common mechanism,
and (ii) whether such results are of probable direct relevance
to man. Answers to these questions will provide a background
against which the significance of bladder tumors induced by
commercial saccharin may be judged.

Most classic chemical carcinogens exert their effect through
a triphasic mechanism. Carcinogens, such as polycyclic aromatic
hydrocarbons, aromatic amines, nitrosamines and aflatoxins, must
first be activated by host tissue enzymes to highly reactive,
positively charged intermediates (electrophiles). In the second
phase, the electrophiles interact with electron-rich receptor
sites in the tissue, including thiols, phosphates, nitrogen and
oxygen functional groups, etc. These abound in all biological
macromolecules. The critical interaction, if it exists, is
probably with specific receptor sites in DNA, although other
interactions may be equally important. The DNA lesions or carcinogen complexes may be restored to normal by the DNA repair
systems or may be "locked in" by cell replication to form tumor
progenitor cells which in the third phase develop into frank
clinical tumors.

Aromatic amine, nitrosamine and nitrofuran-containing bladder
carcinogens, such as 2-naphthylamine, 4-aminobiphenyl, dibutyl-
nitrosamine, and FANFT almost certainly exert their effect in
this way, although there are still large areas of ignorance as

far as the detailed mechanism is concerned. Radomski and his
associates[1,2] have, for example, demonstrated the presence of
4-aminobiphenyl and proposed it as an active intermediate in
carcinogenesis by this agent. It is difficult to avoid the conclusion that agents acting in this fashion may be carcinogens in
man.

A number of other agents, such as diethyleneglycol,[3,4,5]
diethylstilbestrol[6], 4-ethylsulfonylnaphthalene-1-sulfonamide,[7,8]
xylitol and terephthalic acid, when administered at high dose
levels also lead to rodent bladder cancer. In each case, tumorigenesis is accompanied by stone and it is likely that the
bladder stone plays a critical part in tumorigenesis. With diethyleneglycol, for example, female rats and mice do not develop
stone or bladder tumors, whereas both stone and bladder tumors
are induced in males of both species. This has been explained
as reflecting the anatomical differences in the male and female
urethra, the latter shorter organ being more easily able to
void micro-stones or other niduses on which calculi might form.
Further evidence to support the concept that stone may play a
critical role in rodent bladder cancer development comes from
the study of mouse bladder implantation. In this technique,
pellets are surgically implanted into the lumen of the mouse
bladder and the mice killed and the bladders examined for tumors some 40-50 weeks later[9]. A wide variety of agents led to
low yields of tumors under these conditions[10] - Table VII, suggesting that it is the physical nature of the implant rather
than carcinogenic impurities in it which led to tumors. Mobley
and his associates[11] showed that different materials, when implanted into rat bladder, likewise led to tumors. The late Dr.
J.W. Jull[12] found that if mice carrying bladder pellets were
allowed to live beyond 40-50 weeks, the tumor yield and malignancy was greatly increased.

The role of stone in bladder tumor formation in rodents is
probably at least due partially to increasing the rate of proliferation in the bladder epithelium from its normally very low
level[13] to appreciably higher levels[14]. Thus, it is envisaged

that stone affects the developmental rather than the inductive phase of bladder cancer formation. In man, it is generally accepted by urological surgeons that stone is not associated with bladder cancer. The only exception occurs in a few cases in which the stone is trapped in a bladder diverticulum. In this case, it might be expected to exert its effect more intensively on the epithelium within the diverticulum in contrast to a free-floating stone, which would affect specific areas of the whole bladder to a much lesser extent.

Bladder epithelial infestation or bilharzia, appears to be associated with cancer in man[15, 16], although bladder threadworm (Trichosomoides crassicauda) in rats has a much less definite effect[17]. This, again, could be the result of stimulation of epithelial proliferation by the parasites[13]. Bacterial infections, however, have not been associated with bladder tumorigenesis and are more common in women, who develop lower incidences of bladder cancer, than in men.

The question has been asked, especially in connection with the rat bladder tumors induced by sodium saccharin, whether microcrystalluria might act as a tumor developing agent at the very high levels used (5% and 7.5% in the diet). There is presently no evidence to support this speculation.

There is an urgent need for the further study of factors which may affect the development rather than the initiation of bladder tumors, if we are to distinguish tumor-inducing chemicals in experimental animals which pose a real threat to human health, from those which may affect only the development of experimental bladder tumors and may be relatively safer contaminants of man's environment.

REFERENCES

1. Radomski, J.F. et al. Cancer Res. 37:1757, 1977.
2. Moreno, H.R. and Radomski, J.F. Cancer Lett. 4:85, 1978.
3. Weil, C.S. et al. Arch. Environm. Hlth. 11:569, 1965.
4. Hueper, W.C. and Payne, W.W. Arch. Environm. Hlth. 6:484, 1963.
5. Fitzhugh, O.G. and Nelson, A.A. J. Ind. Hyg. 28:40, 1946.
6. Dunning, W.F. et al. Cancer Res. 7:511, 1947.
7. Clayson, D.B. and Bonser, G.M. Brit. J. Cancer 10:311, 1965.
8. Clayson, D.B. et al. Biochem. Pharmacol. 16:619, 1967.
9. Jull, J.W. Brit. J. Cancer 5:327, 1951.
10. Clayson, D.B. and Cooper, E.H. Adv. Cancer Res. 13:271, 1970.
11. Mobley, T.L. et al. Invest. Urol. 3:325, 1966.
12. Jull, J.W. Unpublished observations.
13. Schreiber, H. et al. Virchows Arch. B. Zellpath. 4:30, 1969.
14. Clayson, D.B. and Pringle, J.A.S. Brit. J. Cancer 20: 564, 1966.
15. Ferguson, R.R. J. Pathol. Bacteriol. 16:76, 1911.
16. Clayson, D.B. in Biology and Clinical Management of Bladder Cancer, edited by Cooper, E.H. and Williams, R.E. Chapter 3. Blackwell: Oxford, England, 1975.
17. Chapman, W.H. Invest. Urol. 7:154, 1964.

Health and Sugar Substitutes
Proc. ERGOB Conf., Geneva 1978, pp. 58-63 (Karger, Basel 1978)

SHORT-TERM PRESCREENING TESTS FOR CARCINOGENICITY

Ch. Schlatter

Institute of Toxicology, Swiss Federal Institute of Technology and
University of Zurich, CH-8603 Schwerzenbach, Switzerland

INTRODUCTION

After several years of much controversy about the usefulness of the famous
Ames-test it is nowadays almost generally accepted that the mutation tests on
micro-organisms are well suited to detect a certain property of a chemical to
induce mutations, and also tumours, if the conditions in man are similar to
those in the microbial systems[1]. The important role of activation, deactiva-
tion, translocation and elimination as processes determining the local concentration of the chemical in question has been recognized and there is agreement
on the enormous difficulties to simulate these reactions in simple in vitro
systems. Nevertheless, excellent correlations with more than 90 % concordant
results between mutagenicity in the Ames-system and carcinogenicity in animals
have been found for that group of carcinogens which are believed to act by
highly reactive electrophilic intermediates which may become covalently bound
to DNA. However, there is increasing evidence that not every carcinogen
operates by this so called 'genotypic' mechanism[2]. Compounds such as pheno-
barbitone, DDT, dieldrin, chloroform or sex hormones are some examples of
tumorigenic compounds probably not fitting into the theory of electrophilic
attack to DNA. Especially, the controversial case of saccharin has greatly
stimulated these discussions.

It seems that the 2-stage-concept of tumour-initiation and promotion developed in the early days of chemical carcinogenesis[3] will encounter a renais-
sance and will show to be important not only for skin-tumorigenesis but also
for the formation of tumours in other organs. The importance of the class of
'genotypic' carcinogens, presumably responsible for tumour initiation, may
well be exceeded by this second class of so called 'epigenetic' carcinogens[2]
probably acting mainly on promotion. Some of the speculative characteristics
of these epigenetic carcinogens could be listed as follows:

- mechanism of action unknown, probably many different ways
- dose-response relationship unknown,
   BUT - no arguments for one-hit theory
        - existence of threshold levels very likely
- role in human carcinogenesis unknown, probably important (only a small part
  of human tumours explicable by action of 'genotypic' carcinogens alone)

SACCHARIN

1. Short-term test detecting interaction with DNA

a) Microbial Mutagenicity

Ames-tests were performed by several authors and were found to be essentially negative[2, 4, 5, 6, 7, 8, 9]. Upon re-examination of those rare preparations exhibiting a weakly positive result it was found that impurities were
responsible for the mutagenicity[6]. The finding[10] that mouse urine after receiving a high dose of saccharin was much more mutagenic than one expected
from its content of saccharin is hard to explain and needs confirmation. The
formation of mutagenic metabolites can be ruled out since saccharin is not
metabolised at all[11]. It was shown that some impurities, of yet unknown structure, which could be extracted with organic solvents from saccharin in
amounts of some 10 mg/kg, are sometimes weakly positive in the Ames-test
especially with the salmonella strain TA 98, a detector of frame-shift
mutagens[6].

It seems unlikely that these mutagenic compounds are responsible for the
bladder tumours in long-term studies on rats, since the concentration in a
diet of 5 % saccharin was generally lower than 1 ppm. Only very strong carcinogens induce tumours at such low concentrations. However, the weak mutagenicity in the Ames system (less than 100 revertants/plate containing 100 μg of
extract) is not suggestive for a strong carcinogenic potency of these
impurities.

b) DNA Repair

Saccharin was negative in two DNA-repair assays[4].

c) Binding to DNA

We tested the interaction of saccharin with DNA by determining the radioactivity in highly purified DNA of liver and bladder tissues after oral administration of ca. 400 mg/kg ^{35}S-labelled saccharin[12]. No radioactivity on DNA
was found. Since the binding even of weak carcinogens to DNA is easily detec-

table, this negative result strongly supports the negative Ames-tests and demonstrates the absence of genotypic carcinogenicity of saccharin. Some examples of covalent binding indexes (CBI) for rat liver DNA of some selected chemicals from our laboratory are presented below.

	CBI
Aflatoxin B_1	10200
Aflatoxin M_1	830
Benzo(a)pyrene	3.6-19.1
Benzene	1.7
Ethinylestradiol	1.5
Estrone	1.1
Toluene	<0.04
Saccharin liver	<0.005
bladder	<0.5

The lack of a metabolic breakdown of saccharin and its low lipophilicity are further arguments against a direct interaction with DNA[11].

d) Point Mutation in Drosophila

Conflicting results were obtained by different authors[8], most probably, impurities being responsible for the discrepancies[13]. Drosophila seems to be very susceptible for these still unknown substances. Purified saccharin was not mutagenic in drosophila[13].

2. Short-term tests with complicated mechanism of action not necessarily related directly to DNA

a) Dominant Lethal Tests

4 dominant lethal studies were performed in mice and rats (reviewed in[8]). It is difficult or even impossible to draw any firm conclusions since in one study on mice where high amounts (5000 mg/kg orally for 5 days) were administered, no effects were found whereas in another work with consistently lower dose levels significantly increased pre- and post-implantation losses were noted. Remarkably, these effects were distributed over several weeks after the administration. In a study on rats with dose levels up to 5000 mg/kg no consistent differences to the control group were seen.

b) Mutation in Mammalian Cells

A very weak mutagenic activity was recently found by Clive in cultured mouse lymphoma cells[4]. The system used in rather new, the end-points detected

are not yet defined, the examples studied are so far few and the results with
saccharin were only reported in summarized form. In addition the high concentrations used were markedly cytotoxic. Therefore an assessment of the results
is not yet feasible.

c) Sister Chromatid Exchange

Because mutations that are the results of large chromosomal changes cannot
be induced in bacteria, tests with mammalian cells have to be used for the
detection of such alterations. One of these tests is the determination of
sister chromatid exchange in cell culture, where by different staining properties of chromatides treated with bromodeoxyuridine, an exchange of chromatid
strands becomes visible. These exchanges occur especially during the S-phase
of cell replication[14].

It has been shown that a wide variety of chemical mutagens and carcinogens
may increase the normal level of sister chromatid exchange. Simultaneously
chromosomal aberrations are induced. Although many mutagens known to damage
DNA predominantly by covalent binding induce sister chromatid exchange the
possibility of other mechanisms of action cannot be ruled out. The high level
of occurrence in untreated cells supports the existence of other ways for
induction of these effects. The value of the test for identification of
chemical mutagens is not yet established and much work is still needed for
validation of the test[1]. Commercial and purified saccharin gave no convincing
results in one study[15] but was found to induce some increase of sister chromatid exchange in another [16]. The concentrations used were rather high (30 -
60 mMol/1) and the increase of exchange was only 40 - 60 % above the background level, while most of the tested mutagens exhibited increases of up to
tenfold at much lower concentrations of 10^{-5} - 1 mMol/1[14].

d) Cell Transformation

Saccharin was negativ in Styles cell-transformation assay[2]. This test was
shown to have a capacity for detecting genotypic carcinogens at least as good
as the Ames-test. Recently the oncogenic transforming activity of saccharin
was tested in cultures of the C3H/10T1/2 mouse embryo cell line[17]. Saccharin
in concentrations of 2 mg/ml did not induce cell transformation in contrast
to 3-methyl-cholanthren (MCA; 1 μg/ml). Likewise it did not act as an initiator when followed by a treatment with the known promoting agent tetra-
decanoyl-phorbol-13-acetate (TPA). However in a third set of experiments
where MCA (0.1 μg/ml) was used as initiator, the number of transformed cell

foci was similar when commercial and purified saccharin at 100 μg/ml, or TPA at 0.1 μg/ml were used as promotors. These most recent and exciting findings of a weak but significant co-carcinogenic action of the saccharin system are in agreement with the results of experiments on rats where the incidence of bladder tumours after a single administration of N-methyl-nitrosourea was enhanced by continuous feeding with saccharin[18].

CYCLAMATE

Although not so extensively studied as saccharin no positive effects were found with cyclamate or its main metabolite cyclohexylamine in microbial muta-genicity tests, in studies with drosophila and in dominant lethal tests. The data have been reviewed[19]. Direct binding to DNA was not examined. Cyclamate does not seem to belong to the class of genotypic carcinogens. Until now a test for sister chromatid exchanges has not been done, nor have the compounds been examined in the cell culture assay for their possible promoting capabil-ity. The cytogenetic effects are contradictory[19]. However, the alterations from positive in vivo studies are weak and genetically not very relevant[19]. The existing data do not allow firm conclusions to be drawn on possible epi-genetic carcinogenic properties from short-term tests. However, the need for more comprehensive studies is not too great since the results from long-term studies with cyclamate are not so conflicting as with saccharin[20].

SUMMARY

Both saccharin and cyclamate are inactive in short-term tests which are suitable for detecting a direct interaction with DNA. Both compounds are therefore not 'genotypic' carcinogens. Saccharin, however, is weakly active in the test for sister chromatid exchange and acts as weak co-carcinogen in a cell transformation assay. Thus, a weak 'epigenetic' carcinogenic activity of saccharin is likely. Cyclamate has not been examined in these test systems.

REFERENCES

1.   European Environmental Mutagen Society
     Mutation Res. 53: 361-367, 1978.

2.   Ashby, J., Styles, J.A., Anderson, D. and Paton D. Fd. Cosmet.
     Toxicol. 16: 95-103, 1978.

3.   Berenblum, I. and Shubik, P. Br. J. Cancer 1: 383-391, 1947.

4.   Office of Technology Assessment, Congress of the United States,
     in Cancer Testing Technology and Saccharin, pp. 91-108, 1977.

5.   Pool, B. Toxicology 11: 95-97, 1978.

6.   Stoltz, D.R., Stavric, B., Klassen, R., Bendall, R.D. and Craig,J.
     J. Envir. Path. Toxicol. 1: 139-146, 1977.

7.   Levitt, M.J. and Bon, C. Chem. & Eng. News 55: No. 18, 4, 1977.

8.   Kramers, P.G.N. Mutation Res. 32: 81-92, 1975.

9.   Brusick, D. in Report of the Toxicology Forum on Saccharin, held in
     Omaha, NE, USA, 1977.

10. Batzinger, R.P., Ou, S.-Y.L. and Bueding, E. Science 198: 944-946,
     1977.

11. Ball, L.M., Renwick, A.G. and Williams, R.T. Xenobiotica 7:
     189-203, 1977.

12. Lutz, W.K. and Schlatter, Ch. Chem.-Biol. Interactions 19:
     253-257, 1977.

13. Kramers, P.G.N. Mutation Res. 56: 163-167, 1977.

14. Evans, H.J. in Progress in Genetic Toxicology, edited by
     Scott, D., Bridges, B.A. and Sobels, F.H., pp. 57-74,
     Elsevier / North Holland, Amsterdam / New York / Oxford, 1977.

15. Abe, S. and Sasaki, M. J. Natl. Cancer Inst. 58: 1635-1641, 1977.

16. Wolff, S. and Rodin, B. Science 200: 543-545, 1978.

17. Mondal, S., Brankow, D.W. and Heidelberger, C. Science 201:
     1141-1142, 1978.

18. Hicks, R.M. and Chowaniec, J. Cancer Res. 37: 2943-2949, 1977.

19. Cattanach, B.M. Mutation Res. 39: 1-28, 1976.

20. National Cancer Institute, Report of the Temporary Committee for
     the Review of Data on Carcinogenicity of Cyclamate, NCI,
     Bethesda, MA, USA, 1977.

Health and Sugar Substitutes
Proc. ERGOB Conf., Geneva 1978, pp. 64-69 (Karger, Basel 1978)

SYNCARCINOGENIC ACTION OF SACCHARIN AND SODIUM-CYCLAMATE IN THE
INDUCTION OF BLADDER TUMOURS IN MNU-PRETREATED RATS

U. Mohr, U. Green, J. Althoff and P. Schneider

Department of Experimental Pathology, Medical School Hannover,
Karl-Wiechert-Allee 9, 3000 Hannover 61, Federal Republic of
Germany

INTRODUCTION

Following the concept of initiation and promotion, it was
apparently the idea of Marion Hicks to examine the interference
of artificial sweeteners in the urinary tract of animals primed
for urinary bladder carcinogenesis by a locally active carcinogen,
methylnitrosourea[1,2]. As is usual in science, methods are
repeated either to establish confirmation or dissapproval. Thus
the first description was closely followed, i.e. 2mg MNU were
instilled into the urinary bladder. After 20 weeks, it was clear
that 2mg of MNU did not correspond to the reportedly subcarcinogenic dose[1]. Nevertheless, the experiment was continued for the
life of the animals to elucidate parameters such as tumour
latency, type and location, and comparative patterns of the effect
of saccharin, sodium cyclamate and calcium carbonate.

MATERIALS AND METHODS

Chemicals: N-methyl-n-nitrosourea (NMU) was supplied by
Deutsches Krebsforschungszentrum, Heidelberg, FRG (purity 99.6%).
Saccharin (Sherwin Williams Company, Chemical Toledo Laboratories,
Ohio, USA: Lot S1469, 1022, 3022) and sodium-cyclamate (Abbott
Laboratories, North Chicago, USA: List No. 5683-04-PMED), as
well as calcium-carbonate (Merck, Darmstadt, FRG) were used.
Animal diet preparation with saccharin, cyclamate and calcium-
carbonate was comercially pelleted (Altromin, Lage/Lippe, FRG).

Animals: Female Wistar/AF-Han rats of an initial average
body weight of 195g were kept under standard laboratory conditions (Makrolon cages, type III; room temperature $22°\pm2°C$;
relative humidity $55\pm5\%$; air change 20 times per hour).

2mg NMU, freshly prepared in 0.5 ml distilled water and not

more than 15 minutes old, was instilled into the urinary bladder
(catheter: 0.66 mm diameter). Thereafter 50 rats per group were
given saccharin (2%) and sodium-cyclamate (2%) in their diet
(after 10 weeks, the level was increased to 4%); calcium-
carbonate was administered at 3%.   Normal diet (Altromin Standard
Diät tpf 1320, Lage/Lippe, FRG) was given to untreated controls
(100 rats), the H_2O group and the group treated with NMU only.

Upon spontaneous death, complete autopsies were performed;
moribund animals were sacrificed; organs were fixed in 10%
buffered formalin; graded sections were cut from each kidney,
ureter and urinary bladder, and were stained with hematoxylin
and eosin.

RESULTS

There was no significant difference in survival times between the
6 groups (Table 1); also average weight development did not vary
significantly and neither did the food intake and drinking water
consumption.   The mean daily intake of sweeteners ranged from
1.4 to 2.5g per kg body weight.   The administration of 2 mg MNU
instilled only once into the urinary bladder led to necrosis of
the urothelium (renal pelvis, ureter and urinary bladder).   Neoplasms occurred not only in the urinary bladder, but also in
the ureter and renal pelvis (Table 2).   The histological
evaluation is not entirely completed in terms of the multiplicity
of tumour origin.   The preliminary data shows clearly that there
is no marked difference in the tumour incidence between the
groups receiving MNU alone or with saccharin, calcium-carbonate
or cyclamate; the incidence is about the same in all groups
receiving MNU with or without further treatment (Table 1).
There were 15 -20% multiple benign tumours in all groups, i.e.
transitional cell papillomas and about 20% multifocal malignant
tumours in all groups, i.e. transitional cell carcinomas.
Occasionally, a less differentiated sarcoma was found.   No
difference was discovered in the incidence of urinary bladder
neoplasms, which would indicate a promoting or syncarcinogenic
effect in these sets of experiments.   This is supported by the
observations that average tumour latencies were similar in the
NMU groups, as was average survival time, and that tumour types
and morphology were identical.

Table 1   Urinary Tract Neoplasms in Rats Treated with MNU and Artificial Sweeteners

Treatment	Effective № of Rats	Survival (weeks)	Urinary Tract %	Neoplasms of		
				Renal pelvis %	Ureter %	Urinary Bladder %
Untreated Control	100	98 ±15	1	–	–	0
H$_2$O– Instillation	50	93 ±20	2	–	–	2
MNU only	49	76 ±29	57	28	17	39
MNU + Ca CO$_3$	49	86 ±23	65	43	11	39
MNU + Saccharin	50	78 ±25	65	57	12	31
MNU + Na – Cyclamate	50	81 ±27	70	43	6	40

Table 2   Body weight, food and additive intake

Treatment	No. of animals	Week	Average weight (g) mean	s.d.x	Food daily intake (g)/kg b.w.	Artificial Sweetener daily intake (g)/kg b.w.
Untreated Controls	100	0	204.8	11.5	68.02	
	99	52	301.8	31.9	52.88	
	59	104	323.0	48.9	51.98	
H₂O - Instillation	50	0	203.4	19.4	66.85	
	47	52	298.4	36.3	50.64	
	28	104	322.5	51.2	50.42	
MNU only	50	0	194.2	13.6	69.67	
	38	52	281.1	28.9	58.38	
	13	104	319.2	42.9	51.50	
MNU + Ca CO₃	50	0	194.6	16.5	70.63	2.12
	43	52	292.8	32.9	55.70	Ca CO₃ 1.67
	15	104	315.7	37.6	58.82	1.76
MNU + Saccharin	50	0	192.1	17.8	69.68	1.39
	43	52	270.4	22.8	60.98	2.44
	14	104	292.1	45.6	63.68	2.55
MNU + Na-cyclamate	50	0	193.1	19.8	70.28	1.41
	43	52	257.0	22.6	63.50	2.54
	14	104	291.1	31.6	59.70	2.39

x = standard deviation

Furthermore, the urothelium of the ureter was affected; transitional cell papillomas and carcinomas developed, often simultaneously with the neoplasms found in the urinary bladder. The same holds true for the renal pelvis. This portion of the urinary tract was in fact the most affected.

However, before coming to any premature conclusions, the role and interference of toxic effect, renal changes, papillary necroses, stone formation, regeneration and reflux caused by changes in the distal segments, have to be investigated. Pathological changes of kidney tubules were frequent, as were necroses, haemorrhages, calcium deposits, degenerative and regenerative lesions, as well as hyperplasia and dysplasia of the urothelium on both the papillary and contralateral sides of the renal pelvis. In addition, if one interprets the comparatively higher incidence of renal pelvis neoplasms as a trend suggesting some effect of saccharin or cyclamate, then this effect is non-specific, since it was also found by chronic administration of calcium-carbonate. From this observation, it is possible that for a severely damaged and primed urinary tract and urothelium, any additional burden may be extremely harmful, and if survival is long enough, may lead to pathological changes, including tumour development is some cases.

A whole range of alterations was observed in the urothelium of the renal pelvis, ureter and urinary bladder. These ranged from the focal hyperplastic lesions to generalised papillary hyperplasia and dysplasia, to papillomas, papillary exophytic malignant growth and invasive transitional cell carcinomas. The latter tumours showed varying degrees of differentiation. Focally, squamous cell metaplasia with mild or extensive keratinization were found as well as areas of almost sarcomatous patterns which showed less differentiation and anaplasia.

CONCLUSION

Comparing the results with those previously reported[1], the doses of MNU used in these parallel experiments were not subcarcinogenic. These findings were also confirmed in other recent publications [2,3]. So, it is difficult to comment on the validity of the previously described model. The reasons why 2 mg MNU should be more effective in the hands of one

experimentor might be related to storage, age of the compound,
purity, time lapse between the preparation of solutions and the
treatment of animals, and strain-specific sensitivities and
reactions.

It appears that the above-mentioned model led to results
which require much additional work for interpretation. Therefore,
this model should not be used at present as a basis for drawing
legislative conclusions on the biological effects of a particular
food additive. A complete catalogue of information from different
experimental approaches would seem to be required, which could
provide the necessary background for relating such data to man.

REFERENCES

1.   Hicks, R.M., Wakefield, J.St.J., Chowaniec, J. Nature 243:
     347-349, 1973.
2.   Hicks, R.M., Wakefield, J.St.J., Chowaniec, J. Chem.-Biol.
     Interactions 11: 225-233. 1975.
3.   Hicks, R.M., Wakefield, J.St.J., Chowaniec, J. Nature 243:
     424, 1973.

Health and Sugar Substitutes
Proc. ERGOB Conf., Geneva 1978, pp. 70-75 (Karger, Basel 1978)

CO-CARCINOGENICITY TESTING OF SACCHARIN AND DL-TRYPTOPHAN FOLLOWING ORAL
INITIATION WITH N-[4-(5-Nitro-2-furyl)-2-thiazolyl]formamide

S.M. Cohen, J.B. Jacobs*, M. Arai and G.H. Friedell

Department of Pathology, St. Vincent Hospital, Worcester, MA 01604, USA

Increasingly, the process of carcinogenesis is being considered a multi-stage process with a different mechanism of action for each of the various stages. The best studied multi-stage theory is the 2-stage theory initially described for murine skin carcinogenesis involving initiation and promotion.[1] [2] A similar process has subsequently been demonstrated in other tissues including the liver[3] and urinary bladder.[4] For the bladder, it has been shown[4] that injection into the rat bladder of a subcarcinogenic dose of N-methyl N-nitrosourea (MNU) followed by oral administration of either cyclamate of saccharin resulted in a high incidence of bladder cancer. Cyclamate or saccharin alone induced a very low incidence of bladder cancer. Cyclophospha-mide following MNU did not result in bladder tumors. Our experiment was designed to determine whether the presence of at least 2 stages exist in bladder carcinogenesis using an initiating chemical fed in the diet[5] rather than injected into the bladder.

As our initiating chemical we used a known bladder carcinogen, the nitro-furan FANFT, which was fed to rats for 6 weeks at a level in the diet of 0.2%. This feeding period was chosen on the basis of data obtained from a previous experiment performed in male weanling Fischer rats.[6] When FANFT was administered in these initial experiments for 8 or more weeks followed by control diet until 84 weeks, most of the rats had bladder lesions. Six weeks or less of FANFT followed by control diet resulted in reversible hyperplastic lesions. The bladder returned to normal within 2-6 weeks after FANFT was discontinued and all of these rats had normal bladders at 84 weeks.

The design of the present experiment is shown in Fig. 1. In contrast to the previous experiment, this experiment involved a total of 104 weeks rather than 84 weeks. Most of the groups had 20 rats at the beginning of the

*Presenter

experiment. FANFT at a level of 0.2% of the diet or control diet was fed to appropriate groups for 6 weeks. DL-tryptophan was fed in the diet at a level of 2% and sodium saccharin at a dose of 5% of the diet. Tryptophan was chosen as a possible promoting agent because of the suggested relationship between abnormal urinary tryptophan metabolite levels and bladder cancer in humans and experimental animals. Saccharin was used because of its weak carcinogenicity in various experimental systems when fed alone and since it previously gave positive results in the MNU experimental system.[4] These chemicals were fed either immediately after FANFT administration or after a delay of six weeks when the rats were fed control diet only. The groups with this delay period were used to determine the irreversibility of the initiation phase by FANFT and to avoid overlap between the presence of FANFT in the body and the feeding of the promoting chemical. As in previous experiments, rats fed FANFT for 6 weeks had normal appearing bladders after 6 weeks on control diet. Groups not prefed FANFT were fed tryptophan or saccharin beginning after the sixth week of the experiment. Tryptophan was fed until the end of the experiment at 104 weeks. Saccharin was discontinued after the 83rd week in Groups 1-3 because some of the rats in the 2 groups prefed FANFT had developed hematuria. They were fed control diet until the end of the experiment. Other groups received only control diet, FANFT for 6 weeks (Group 8), or various longer intervals of FANFT (Group 9-11).

Tumors that were benign by histologic criteria were designated as papillomas. A diagnosis of malignancy was based on the presence of nuclear pleomorphism, loss of differentiation to the surface, and the presence of mitoses. The presence or absence of invasion was determined microscopically and if questionable the lesion was considered as non-invasive. The papillomas and cancers were usually transitional cell, frequently with areas of squamous differentiation or undifferentiated cells. The distribution of bladder lesions in the present experiment is shown in Table 1. Long term FANFT administration again induced a 100% incidence (Groups 9-11). These rats all died before the end of the 80th week from bladder cancer. FANFT fed for only 6 weeks, however, followed by control diet resulted in 4 of 20 rats with cancer and 1 papilloma at the end of 104 weeks. This is in contrast to the results we previously found at 84 weeks when the bladders of rats fed FANFT for 6 weeks were normal.

Rats prefed FANFT and then fed tryptophan significantly increased the incidence of bladder cancer compared to rats fed 6 weeks of FANFT. Tryptophan

alone and the rats fed only control diet did not have any bladder papillomas
or cancers. The incidences of cancer in rats fed saccharin after prefeeding
by FANFT were very high whether saccharin was administered immediately after
FANFT or after a 6 week delay. As with tryptophan, saccharin alone did not
induce papillomas or cancer.

The lesions induced in the group fed FANFT for 6 weeks were single, small
masses protruding into the lumen of the bladder, even though one of the
cancers showed microscopic submucosal invasion. In contrast, the tumors
induced by tryptophan and saccharin after FANFT prefeeding were frequently
multiple and were large lesions often distending the bladder and filling the
lumen. Also, the number of invasive lesions with tryptophan was somewhat
more common than with 6 weeks of FANFT alone, and invasiveness was even more
common in rats fed saccharin, including 1 with invasion into the adjoining
prostate. Also, saccharin-induced cancers appeared earlier than tryptophan-
induced lesions with several of the rats dying before the end of the experiment
due to hematuria and marked weight loss (Table 1). The average survival was
less, but even more significant was the number of rats surviving to the end
of the experiment. Saccharin showed greater activity even though it was not
fed after the 83rd week while tryptophan was fed until the end of the experiment at week 104. The control group shows a decreased survival due to some
of the rats being sacrificed periodically for electron microscopic examination.

Bladders from rats in appropriate groups were also examined by scanning
and transmission electron microscopy at the end of weeks 6 and 12 and at the
end of the experiment in an attempt to identify early changes. Unlike in our
previous experiment, one of 2 rats fed FANFT for 6 weeks and examined at 6
weeks had pleomorphic microvilli on the luminal surface of epithelial cells,
a marker of irreversibility in the FANFT-Fischer rat model. The 2 rats
examined after 6 weeks of FANFT plus 6 weeks of control diet had normal
appearing bladders. The finding of pleomorphic microvilli in 6 week FANFT-
fed rats might explain the appearance of a low incidence of bladder cancers
in the rats fed FANFT for 6 weeks in the present experiment and not in our
previous one.[6] Rats prefed FANFT and then fed saccharin also had pleomorphic
microvilli present at the end of week 12 of the experiment (6 weeks of FANFT
plus 6 weeks of saccharin), but they were not present after 12 weeks in the
rats prefed FANFT and then fed tryptophan. Pleomorphic microvilli were
present on bladder tumors induced by FANFT, FANFT plus saccharin, and FANFT

plus tryptophan, but pleomorphic microvilli were not present in control rats
or rats fed only tryptophan or saccharin.

The present results confirm the enhancing capacity of saccharin on bladder
carcinogenesis, but in this experiment the initiating agent, FANFT, was fed
to the rats in contrast to injecting the carcinogen directly into the bladder
as in the MNU experiment.[4] Tryptophan also showed activity although to a
lesser extent. Saccharin and tryptophan alone did not induce bladder tumors,
but the number of rats in each group was insufficient to detect the low
incidences reported by others, and feeding of tryptophan and saccharin was
not begun until the end of the sixth week of the experiment when the rats
were 10 weeks old. If one considers the present experiment in the perspective
of the 2 stage model of carcinogenesis, saccharin and tryptophan are acting
as promoting agents.

Topics for discussion:
  Length of time of initiating dose; presence of stones and calcification;
  dose of saccharin; presence of other tumors; growth of rats; purity of
  saccharin; specific chemical effect versus secondary effect on urine composition.

REFERENCES

1. Berenblum, I. and Shubik, P. Brit. J. Cancer 1: 383-391, 1947.

2. Boutwell, R.K. CRC Critical Rev. Toxicol. 2: 419-443, 1974.

3. Pitot, H.C. Amer. J. Pathol. 89: 401-412, 1977.

4. Hicks, R.M. and Chowaniec, J. Cancer Res. 37: 2943-2949, 1977.

5. Cohen, S.M., Arai, M. and Friedell G.H. Proc. Amer. Assoc. Cancer Res.
   19: 4, 1978.

6. Jacobs, J.B., Arai, M., Cohen, S.M. and Friedell, G.H. Cancer Res., 37:
   2817-2821, 1977.

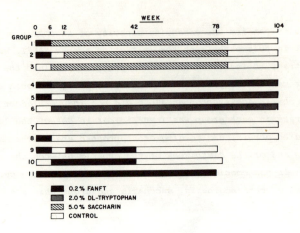

Fig. 1. Experimental design.

Table 1. Results of the Experiment.

Group	Effective # of Rats	Average Survival (Weeks)	# Alive At End of Experiment (%)	Urinary Bladder				
				Normal	Simple Hyperplasia	Nodular or Papillary Hyperplasia	Papillomas	Cancer
1. FANFT→Saccharin	19	94±10	6 (32)	0	0	1	0	18
2. FANFT→Control+→ Saccharin	18	93±16	9 (50)	0	1	4	0	13
3. Control→Saccharin	20	102±8	19 (95)	18	2	0	0	0
4. FANFT→Tryptophan	19	102±5	18 (95)	0	5	3	1	10
5. FANFT→Control→ Tryptophan	20	102±7	17 (85)	0	3	3	4	10
6. Control→Tryptophan	19	102±10	17 (89)	16	3	0	0	0
7. Control	42	99±12	27 (64)	37	4	1	0	0
8. FANFT→Control	20	101±6	16 (80)	5	9	1	1	4
9. FANFT→Control→ FANFT*→Control	16	66±8	0	0	0	0	0	16
10. Control→FANFT*→ Control	19	71±6	0	0	0	0	0	19
11. FANFT*	40	60±6	0	0	0	0	0	40

+ Control diet.

* Long term administration of FANFT; the other FANFT designations in the table refer to 6 weeks of FANFT administration at a level of 0.2% of the diet.

Health and Sugar Substitutes
Proc. ERGOB Conf., Geneva 1978, pp. 76-81 (Karger, Basel 1978)

CHRONIC BIOASSAY REVIEW

Ian C. Munro and Douglas L. Arnold

Toxicology Research Division, Food Directorate, Health Protection
Branch, Health and Welfare Canada, Tunney's Pasture, Ottawa,
Ontario, K1A 0L2   Canada.

Introduction

The safety of saccharin (S) for human consumption controversy
is almost as old as S itself[8]. Two major aspects of this controversy concern the method by which S is synthesized and whether
rodents are the appropriate species when bladder tumors are the
most significant pathological finding[10,16].

The following is a brief summary of the chronic studies which
examined the toxicological effects of S per se. These studies
have all been criticized, but this matter will be left for the
panel discussion.

A) Rats - One Generation Feeding Studies

Fitzhugh, et al.[3] fed diets containing 0 (7M, 9F), 1.0 (10 M,
10F) or 5.0% S (9M, 9F) for 2 years. The only significant pathological change was in the 5% rats, where 7 had abdominal lymphosarcomas and 4 of these animals also had thoracic lymphosarcomas.
Since the strain of rat used had a variable spontaneous incidence
of lymphosarcomas, it was concluded that S was relatively nontoxic.

Lessel[6] fed groups of 20 male and 20 female rats diets containing 0, 0.005, 0.05, 0.5 or 5% S for 2 years. One female and 4
male rats in the 5% S group had bladder calculi and another male
had kidney calculi. The female rat with calculi had an extensive
transitional cell papilloma (TCP) of the bladder, while another 5%

female without calculi had hyperplasia and papillomata. This
study is often cited by advocates of the bladder calculus
hypothesis for bladder tumors[17] to illustrate the possible mechanism by which S elicits bladder tumors.

The results of the following three studies have not been published, but some data are found in the National Research Council
(NRC)[9] and Office of Technology Assessment (OTA)[10] reports.

A Nat. Inst. of Hygienic Sciences (Toyko) study used 54 control
and 54 S treated rats. The S level was increased from 2 to 5%
during the first 150 days on test. No bladder tumors were
reported.

The Litton Bionetics Study consisted of 2 experiments run in
parallel; a single control group had 20 males and 20 females while
the 1 and 5% S groups in each replicate had 26 males and 26
females each. The female was the more sensitive sex; but the
incidence of spontaneous tumors, bladder hyperplasia and chronic
glomerulonephritis was quite variable between the 2 replicates.
One bladder papilloma was reported for a 5% female.

Bio-Research Consultants fed groups of 25 male rats diets
containing either 0, 1 or 5% S for 104 weeks. One control group
and duplicate groups of S treated animals were used. The S was
from 2 sources. A a slight increase in the incidence of malignant
tumors in the 1% group of the 2nd replicate was reported but S did
not affect the number of bladder lesions.

Schmahl[11] fed groups of 52 male and 52 female rats diets
containing 0, 100 or 250 mg/kg of saccharin. Examination of the
bladder was emphasized, but the author concluded that S had no
detectable oncogenic effect.

Groups of 54-56 male rats were fed diets containing either 0.0
or 2.5 g of S/kg b.w./day for 28 months with iterim kills at 12

and 24 months. No pathological changes due to treatment were
reported[4].

Munro, et al.,[7] fed diets providing 0, 90, 270, 810 or 2430 mg
S/kg b.w./day to groups of 50 male and 50 male rats for 26 months.
Grossly visible calculi as well as ones small enough to pass
through the urethrum were reported for 67 animals of the 600 on
test. The calculi were not associated with S treatment nor with
the bladder tumors (TCP) which were found in a male control, 1 in
a 90 mg/kg female and 2 in males dosed with 810 mg/kg.

B) Mouse - One Generation Feeding Studies

The results of two studies have not been published, but some
data are found in the NRC[9] and OTA[10] reports.

The Nat. Inst. of Hygienic Sciences (Toyko) fed groups of 50
male and 50 female mice diets containing 0, 0.2, 1.0 or 5.0% S for
21 months, with interim kills at 12 and 18 months. The treated
animals had a slight but not statistically significant increase in
ovarian tumors.

Bio-Research Consultants fed groups of 26 male and 26 female
mice diets with 0, 10,000 ppm or 50,000 ppm S. Two experiments
were run in parallel with S from 2 sources. The only significant
pathology in treated animals concerned a non statistical increase
in vascular tumors.

Kroes, et al.,[5] fed diets with 0, 0.2 of 0.5% S in a 6 generation study; 50 male and 50 female mice from the Fo, F_{3b} and F_{6a}
generations were fed the test diets for 20 months. No significant
treatment-related pathological effects were observed.

C) Hamster - One Generation Feeding Study

Groups of 30 male and 30 female hamsters received S produced by
the Maumee procedure in their drinking water, at levels of: 0.0%,
0.156%, 0.312%, 0.625%, 1.25%. No urinary or treatment related
neoplasms were reported[1].

D) Rat - Two Generation Feeding Studies

Tisdel, et al.,[15] fed groups of 20 male and 20 female rats
diets containing 0, 0.05, 0.5 or 5.0% S for 90 days prior to
mating. After weaning, the Fo portion of the study was terminated
and 20 F_1 males and 20 F_1 females from each group were kept on
test for 100 weeks. Transitional cell carcinomas (TCC) were found
in 7/20 bladders from the 5.0% male S group and five squameous
cell carcinomas were seen only in the S females.

In a combination three-generation-chronic-feeding study (24-28
months)[14], groups of 10 male and 20 female animals were fed a diet
containing 0, 0.01, 0.1, 1.0, 5.0, or 7.5% S. For the F_{1a} generation, 48 males and 48 females were selected with interim kills
at 14 and 18 months. The incidence of bladder tumors were: 1 in
a male control; 1 in male fed 5% S and 7 in males and 2 in females
fed 7.5% S. All the tumors were diagnosed as TCC except one tumor
in a male fed 7.5% S, which was diagnosed as a TCP.

In an attempt to rationalize these findings with the negative
one generation results, the Health Protection Branch (HPB)
examined the purity of the various S samples used. Stavric, et
al.,[13] reported that orthotoluenesulphonamide (o-TS) was a major
impurity in S synthesized by the Remsen-Fahlberg procedure.
Consequently, a two generation study was undertaken at HPB to
determine the carcinogenic potential of o-TS. Arnold, et al.,[2]
fed groups of 50 male and 50 female rats one of the following
diets with tap water ad lib, except where noted: control; 2.5,
25 or 250 mg o-TS/kg b.w.; 250 mg 0-TS/kg b.w. with 1% NH_4Cl in
the drinking water; or 5% S produced by the Maumee procedure.
Both generations received their respective diets for lifetime.
The incidence of TCP in the Fo generation were: 1 in a male
control; 1 in a 2.5 mg o-TS male; 1 in 250 mg o-TS male; 4 in S

males and 1 in a 2.5 mg o-TS female. TCC were found in 3 Fo male

S animals. In the F_1 generation, TCP were observed in 4 S males

and 2 in 2.5 mg o-TS females. TCC were found in 8 S males and 2 S

females.

Recently, Schmahl[12] has reported that o-TS produced bladder

tumors in a lifetime feeding study where groups of 75 male and 76

female rats received dosages of 0, 20 or 200 mg o-TS/kg b.w./day.

QUESTIONS

1.   What is the mechanism by which S elicits bladder tumors?

2.   What, if any, role do the impurities in S have regarding the

     observed bladder tumors?

3.   Are the results with a two generation study interpretable in

     view of the uncontrolled levels of S that the fetus is

     exposed to?

4.   Why are the bladder tumors only observed in male rats?

REFERENCES

1.   Althoff, J., Cardesa, A., Pour, P. & Shubik, P. Cancer Lett.
     1:21-24, 1975.

2.   Arnold, D.L., Charbonneau, S.M., Moodie, C.A. & Munro, I.C.
     Toxicol. Appl. Pharmacol. 4: 164 (Abstract #78), 1977.

3.   Fitzhugh, P.G., Nelson, A.A. & Frawley, J.P. J. Am. Pharm.
     Ass. 40:583, 1951.

4.   Furuya, T., Kawamata, K., Kaneko, T., Uchida, O., Horuichi,
     S. & Ikeda, Y. Jap. J. Pharmacol. 25:5556 (Suppl.) (abstract
     #60), 1975.

5.   Kroes, R., Peters, P.W.J., Berkvens, J.M., Verschuuren, H.G.,
     De Vries, Th. & Van Esch, G.J. Toxicol. 8:285-300, 1977.

6.   Lessel, B. Third International Congress, Food Science and
     Technology. SOS/70 Proceedings, pp. 764-770, Washington,
     D.C., August 9-14, 1970.

7. Munro, I.C., Moodie, C.A., Krewski, D. & Grice, H.C.
    Toxicol. Appl. Pharmacol. $\underline{32}$:513-526, 1975a.

8. Munro, I.C., Stavric, B. & Lacombe, R. Toxicol. Ann. 1974,
    ed. C.L. Winek, pp. 71-89, 1975.

9. National Research Council Publication no. 238-137, 1974.

10. Office of Technology Assessment, OTA Congress of the United
    States, October 1977.

11. Schmahl, V.D. Arzneim. Forsch. $\underline{23}$:1466-1470, 1973.

12. Schmahl, D. Z. Krebsforsch $\underline{91}$:19-22, 1978.

13. Stavric, B., Lacombe, R., Watson, J.R. and Munro, I.C. J.
    Assoc. Off. Anal. Chem $\underline{57}$:678-681, 1974.

14. Taylor, J.M. & Friedman, L. Toxicol. Appl. Pharmacol. $\underline{29}$:154
    (abstract #200), 1974.

15. Tisdel, M.O., Nees, P.O., Harris, D.L., Derse, P.H. in
    Symposium: Sweeteners (Inglett, G.E., Ed.), pp. 145-158.
    Avi Publishing Company, Inc., Westport, Conn., 1974.

16. Toxicology Forum on Saccharin Omaha, Nebraska, May 9-11,
    1977.

17. Weil, C.S., Carpenter, C.P. & Symth, H.F., Jr. Arch.
    Environ. Health $\underline{11}$:569-581, 1965.

Health and Sugar Substitutes
Proc. ERGOB Conf., Geneva 1978, pp. 82-84 (Karger, Basel 1978)

EXPERIMENTS IN RATS ON THE QUESTION OF A POSSIBLE CARCINOGENIC
EFFECT OF CYCLAMATE, CYCLOHEXYLAMINE, SACCHARINE AND ORTHO-
TOLUOLSULPHONAMIDE (OTS)

D. Schmähl

Institute of Toxicology and Chemotherapy, German Cancer Research
Center, 6900 Heidelberg, Im Neuenheimer Feld 280, Germany

In the Institute of Toxicology and Chemotherapy of the German
Cancer Research Center, investigations in rats on the question
of a possible carcinogenicity of the above mentioned compounds
have been carried out since 1970. In a long-term study[1], sodium-
cyclamate (daily dose 1,000 and 2,500 mg/kg), cyclohexylamine
(daily dose 200 mg/kg), sodiumsaccharine (daily dose 100 and
250 mg/kg) and combinations of cyclamate and saccharine (10:1)
were administered orally over the whole lifespan of the animals.
The maximum total doses applied were up to 2,188 g/kg of
cyclamate, 177 g/kg of cyclohexylamine and 210 g/kg of saccharine. In spite of the high doses and the lifetime duration
of the experiments, neither a chronically toxic nor a carcinogenic effect of the substances could be found. It is remarkable
that the blood pressures of the animals treated with cyclohexylamine corresponded to those of the control group.

In another experimental setup[2], we examined whether a syncarcinogenic effect of cyclamate can be found when it is applied
to rats in combination with the bladder carcinogenic agent
butyl-butanol-nitrosamine. This substance was applied to 40
male Sprague-Dawley rats in daily doses of 10 mg/kg in the
drinking water. After a median induction time of 400 ± 45 days,
all test animals died of squamous cell carcinomas of the urinary
bladder. Additional application of the high dose of 2,500 mg/kg/
day of sodiumcyclamate did not intensify the bladder carcinogenic
effect of the nitrosamine.

Studies that were started in March 1976 and that are still
unpublished deal with the question of a transplacentary effect
of cyclamate or saccharine; this report is based on the status
of June 1, 1978. Female Sprague-Dawley rats were applied
0.2, 1.0 or 5.0 g/kg of sodiumcyclamate or sodiumsaccharine
orally in the 14th, 17th and 20th day of pregnancy by gavage.
An untreated control group of pregnant rats was given water
at the same time. In the control, 25 male and 33 female animals
were brought up. Up to now, 21 of them have died. In no case
did we observe a malignant tumor. The group that was applied
the lowest dose of cyclamate consisted of 29 male and 25 female
rats, 28 of which have died up to now. In these animals, we
observed one leiomyosarkoma and one adenocarcinoma of the
uterus. In the group that was applied 1.0 g/kg of cyclamate,
41 male and 39 female animals were brought up; 41 of them
have died. Here, one myeloic leukemia and one neurogenous
sarkoma were found. The group with the highest dose of cyclamate
consisted of 22 male and 31 female animals, 31 of which have
died; one of them showed a Theka cell tumor. In the medium dose
group, 35 male and 23 female rats were brought up; 35 animals
died without a malignant tumor. The highest dose group consisted
of 32 male and 25 female animals. 26 animals have died, one
animal showed a neurogenous sarkoma. In no case did the bladders
show signs of malignancy. Although the experiments have been
running for 27 months, we have not yet found an indication for
a carcinogenic effect after prenatal application of high doses
of saccharine or cyclamate in the critical phase of pregnancy.
A final evaluation will, however, only be possible after termi-
nation of the experiment (observation of the animals until their
natural death).

We also examined the essential impurity of saccharine, ortho-
toluolsulphonamide (OTS) for carcinogenic effects[3]. Orthotoluol-
sulphonamide was applied to male and female Sprague-Dawley rats
in daily doses of 200 mg/kg and 20 mg/kg bodyweight respectively.
The maximum dose applied amounted to 17 g/kg. A shortening of

the average life expectation was not observed in comparison
to the control animals. The incidence of malignant tumors in
the animals treated with OTS was identical with the one of
the control animals.

We did, however, find one animal in the test groups that had a
carcinoma of the urinary bladder and seven animals with
papillomas of the bladder.

The results obtained in our institute up to now do not give
any indication for a carcinogenic effect of the artificial
sweeteners examined in various experimental designs. Nevertheless, we are planning a two-generation experiment for the
future; it will be started before the end of 1978.

REFERENCES

1. Schmähl, D., Arzneimittelforsch. (Drug Research) 23,
   1466-1470 (1973)

2. Schmähl, D., Krüger, F.W., Arzneimittelforsch. 22,
   999-1000 (1972)

3. Schmähl, D., Z. Krebsforsch. 91, 19-22 (1978)

Health and Sugar Substitutes
Proc. ERGOB Conf., Geneva 1978, pp. 85-90 (Karger, Basel 1978)

NON—NUTRITIVE SWEETENERS AND HUMAN BLADDER CANCER

I.I. Kessler

Department of Epidemiology & Preventive Medicine
University of Maryland School of Medicine
655 W. Baltimore Street, Baltimore, Md. 21201 U.S.A.

INTRODUCTION

On the basis of presumed carcinogenic effects in laboratory animals, cyclamates were banned by the Secretary of Health, Education, and Welfare in 1970.[1] On similar grounds, saccharin, the other major nonnutritive sweetener (NNS), was removed from the list of food products generally regarded as safe in 1972 and was proposed for an outright ban by the Food and Drug Administration in April 1977.[2]

The relevance of animal tests to the problem of human cancer etiology is unclear. Species and strains within species differ widely in their response to the same environmental agents.[3] Whether carcinogenic risks to moderately exposed humans can be inferred from massively exposed animals is also moot. In addition to variations in dosage, consideration must also be given to duration of exposure, route of administration, and other details of the experimental conditions.

Evidence on the possible role of NNS in human cancer, particularly that of the urinary bladder, is not abundant. Correlational analyses fail to show any changes in bladder cancer mortality trends that might be attributed to saccharin[4] and cyclamate.[5] Three studies[6-8] among diabetics whose exposure to NNS is likely to be increased also failed to demonstrate an attributable cancer risk.

The normal findings in these investigations must be interpreted with caution. Correlations, positive or negative, can result from the temporal coincidence of entirely unrelated events. Mortality studies require the often unjustified assumption that death rates reflect disease incidence rather than variations in treatment, state of disease at detection, or death certification practices.

Case-control studies offer a potentially more powerful method for evaluating the carcinogenicity of NNS in man. In the first two of such investigations,[9,10] the relative risks of bladder cancer were not increased among artificial-sweetener users. However, the sample sizes were rather small, sweetener exposures were not intensively explored, and mailed questionnaires rather than personal interviews were employed.

In a considerably larger and hospital-based study,[11] similar normal findings were reported. It should be noted that attention was directed primarily at the effects of smoking and occupational factors, with NNS exposure histories elicited only among 163 of the most recent subjects. A large study[12] using hospitalized bladder cancer patients and neighborhood controls has recently been completed in Canada. Bladder cancer risks were increased 60 percent among men who used saccharin tablets, but not among those who drank dietetic beverages or ate dietetic foods that contain saccharin. Risk ratios were also not increased among women in any of these categories. Our hospital-based case-control study, on which a preliminary report was published in 1976,[13] is described.

MATERIALS AND METHODS

All Baltimore-area residents with bladder cancer, discharged from 19 participating hospitals between 1972 and 1975, were identified. The only other general hospital in the region, a small one, has no urologic service. Out of a total of 634 surviving patients with histopathologically confirmed bladder malignant neoplasms who were processed, 519 (82 percent) agreed to participate in the study. Those excluded comprised refusers as well as senile, dying, or other uninterviewable patients. Five hundred nine others died, while 157 cases identified late during the study, remained unprocessed.

Control subjects were chosen in random fashion from hospital registration lists of cancer-free patients without bladder conditions who were hospitalized at the same institutions and at approximately the same time as the bladder cancer patients and who were of the same sex, race, age (±3 years), and current marital status. Of the 519 controls sought, 390 (75 percent) were selected at first sampling. In less than 7 percent of the cases, refusals made it necessary to select more than two controls before a willing and eligible participant was found.

All patients and controls were then subjected to intensive personal interview with respect to smoking habits, occupational history, and use of NNS. The latter was probed in terms of table sweeteners, diet beverages, diet foods, and total intake in all forms. For each specific NNS-containing substance, information was obtained on the frequency, quantity, and duration of use by type and brand name. To reduce the likelihood of including cancers unrelated to sweeteners, ingestion of saccharin or cyclamate from one year before the date of cancer diagnosis and thereafter was ignored for each patient and matched control. The interviewers were not aware of the case or control status of their subjects at the time of the interview.

Relative frequencies, quantities, and duration of NNS use among patients and controls were calculated, and the statistical significance of differences was compared. Comparisons were also made in terms of relative risk with and without simultaneous adjustment for potential confounding factors. In addition, the data were examined for evidence of dose-response relationships, which might shed some light on the nature of the association between NNS use and human bladder cancer.

Findings with respect to total artificial-sweetener ingestion are presented in detail. Data specific to saccharin and cyclamate, to be discussed more fully in a subsequent article, are also described.

RESULTS

The proportions of patients and controls who ever used NNS in any form were essentially the same. As to NNS powders, tablets, or drops, there were no substantial differences in mean servings per day, mean days per week, or mean years of use among men. Women tended to use somewhat more NNS tablets, though over a shorter duration, than their controls. On the other hand, mean years of NNS use was significantly greater among the female controls (p < 0.01).

Exposure to artificially sweetened beverages of all kinds was equivalent in patients and controls of each sex. With a few exceptions, the same applied for NNS-containing diet foods. Use of diet ice cream was reported more often by bladder cancer patients, but there were no significant quantitative differences in exposure. Diet pastry and salad dressings were eaten for significantly fewer years by the patients (p < 0.05).

In general, the relative risks of bladder cancer were not significantly increased by NNS use, whether matching of case-control pairs was taken into consideration or not. The only exception was diet ice cream, for which the relative risk among women alone was 3.50.

An overall relative risk of bladder cancer among NNS users, simultaneously adjusted for smoking habit, occupation, age, race, sex, diabetes mellitus, and several other potentially confounding factors, was calculated, using a multiple logistic method.[14] The value of 1.04 was insignificantly different from the null value 1.00. Comparable figures specific for men and women were 1.11 and 0.80 respectively, also not significantly different from 1.00.

To examine the relationship between bladder cancer and NNS dose, study subjects were divided into three equal groups according to level of lifetime

NNS exposure. Patients, both men and women, tended to report relatively more NNS use at low levels, but relatively less at medium and high levels, than controls. Use of table sweeteners was somewhat exceptional in that use in male patients exceeded that in controls, though insignificantly, in prevalence of high exposure levels. The only significant difference was among women drinking low levels of diet beverages ($p < 0.05$). When these figures were adjusted for possible confounding factors and transformed into risk ratios, no evidence of an increase in relative risk with increasing exposure level was apparent.

Patients and controls did not differ significantly in the proportions who ate or drank foods containing either saccharin or cyclamate. The relative risks of bladder cancer in saccharin and cyclamate users were 1.01 and 0.97, respectively, for both sexes combined. (Table 1) Male patients had somewhat higher, but still insignificant, odds ratios compared with female patients. On the average, saccharin was consumed for significantly shorter periods by patients than controls ($p < .05$). The same was true for cyclamate. In mean serving-years, there were also no significant differences between patients and controls for either of these sweeteners.

Relative risks of bladder cancer by specific sweetener use did not significantly differ from 1.00 in either men or women. (Table 2) However, odds ratios tended to be somewhat higher than null value in men and somewhat lower in women. When relative risks of bladder cancer were calculated separately for smoking and nonsmoking NNS users, these were found to be 0.84 among smokers and 1.36 among nonsmokers, neither significantly different from 1.00. The highest relative risk (1.69), which was observed in male non-smokers, did not differ significantly from 1.00. However, when this figure was adjusted for possible confounding factors by the multiple logistic method,[14] the calculated relative risk of 2.61 had a 95 percent confidence interval of 1.20 to 5.67.

Exposure histories of the subjects to cigarettes and other tobacco products were specifically elicited. Patients were significantly more likely than controls to use tobacco and to smoke cigarettes ($p < 0.01$). Men smoked cigarettes for approximately five years longer, on the average, than their controls ($p < .01$). Relative risks for bladder cancer among smokers were 1.78 and 1.57 in men and women, respectively.

Patients were somewhat more likely than controls to have graduated from high school and to be widowed or divorced. Diabetes mellitus was slightly less prevalent among them, and relatively fewer were of the Jewish faith. Otherwise, the bladder cancer patients were demographically similar to the controls, both in toto and by sex.

The relative risks for bladder cancer among NNS users, which were detectable at varying   β levels in this investigation, were estimated by the arc sine transformation method.   A 37 percent increase in bladder cancer risk could have been detected among NNS users with a power of 80 percent, assuming that population prevalences of NNS use approximate those of the control patients.

Table 1

NNS Use Among Bladder Cancer Patients and Controls

By Type and Measure of NNS Use

Type/Measure	Males		Females		Both Sexes Combined	
	Cases n=365	Controls n=365	Cases n=154	Controls n=154	Cases n=519	Controls n=519
Saccharin						
Ever used, percent	31.8	30.1	39.6	42.9	34.1	33.9
Mean person-yrs. used†	9.8	12.1	10.0	15.2√	9.9	13.3√
Mean serving-yrs. used†*	40.5	51.7	45.3	31.0	42.1	43.9
Relative risk	1.08		0.87		1.01	
(95% confidence limits)	(0.79–1.48)		(0.55–1.37)		(0.78–1.31)	
Cyclamate						
Ever used, percent	23.6	21.6	29.2	35.7	25.2	25.8
Mean person-yrs. used†	7.4	11.1	8.3	11.6	7.7	11.3√
Mean serving-yrs. used†*	39.4	32.7	59.0	43.0	46.0	36.9
Relative risk	1.12		0.74		0.97	
(95% confidence limits)	(0.79–1.58)		(0.46–1.19)		(0.73–1.28)	

†Excluding non-users

*Serving-years = servings per day x years of use summed overall brands used
  which contained the given artificial sweetener.

√$p < 0.05$

Table 2

Relative Risk* of Bladder Cancer in Saccharin and Cyclamate Users**

Adjusted† For Possible Confounding Factors‡

Sweetener	Sex	Relative Risk	95% Confidence Limits‡		
Saccharin	Male	1.13	0.80	–	1.62
	Female	0.82	0.48	–	1.43
	Both Sexes	1.06	0.79	–	1.42
Cyclamate	Male	1.15	0.78	–	1.70
	Female	0.61	0.34	–	1.14
	Both Sexes	0.97	0.71	–	1.32
Saccharin and/or	Male	1.11	0.78	–	1.58
Cyclamate	Female	0.77	0.44	–	1.33
	Both Sexes	1.03	0.77	–	1.38
Saccharin and	Male	1.18	0.80	–	1.76
Cyclamate	Female	0.63	0.35	–	1.12
	Both Sexes	1.00	0.73	–	1.37

*Approximated by odds ratio
**Excluding those using sweetener < 6 months
†By multiple logistic methods of Prentice[14]
‡Smoking habit, occupation, age, race, sex, diabetes mellitus, marital status, education, overweight, dieting and memory
‡By maximum likelihood method of Cox[15]

REFERENCES

1.   Egeberg, R.O. et al: JAMA 211:1358-1361, 1970

2.   Federal Register 42:19996-20010   (April 15) 1977

3.   Kessler, I.I.: Publication Series No. PS 7705, Center for the Study of Drug Development, University of Rochester Medical Center, October 1977

4.   Armstrong, B. and Doll, R.: Br J. Prev Soc Med 28:233-240, 1974

5.   Burbank, F. and Fraumeni, J.F., Jr.: Nature 227:296-297, 1970

6.   Kessler, I.I.: J Natl Cancer Inst 44:673-686, 1970

7.   Armstrong, B. and Doll, R.: Br J Prev Soc Med 29:73-81, 1975

8.   Armstrong, B. et al.: Br J Prev Soc Med 30:151-157, 1976

9.   Morgan, R.W. and Jain, M.G.: Can Med Assoc J 111:1067-1070, 1974

10. Simon, D. et al.: J Natl Cancer Inst 54:587-591, 1975

11. Wynder, E.L. and Goldsmith, R.: Cancer 40:1246-1268, 1977

12. Howe, G.R. et al.: Lancet 2:578-581, 1977

13. Kessler, I.I.: J Urology 115:143-146, 1976

14. Prentice, R.L.: Biometrics 32:599-606, 1976

15. Cox, D.R.: in Analysis of Binary Data, Methuen & Co. Ltd. New York, 1970

II. Absorbtion, metabolism and safety of sugar substitutes

b) Nutritive sweeteners

Moderator: H. Mehnert, Munich
Co-Moderator: R.E. Froesch, Zurich

Health and Sugar Substitutes
Proc. ERGOB Conf., Geneva 1978, pp. 92-97 (Karger, Basel 1978)

SAFETY OF NUTRITIVE SWEETENERS : FRUCTOSE AND SORBITOL

G. Van den Berghe[*]

Laboratoire de Chimie Physiologique, Université de Louvain and International
Institute of Cellular and Molecular Pathology, U.C.L. 75.39 - Avenue Hippocrate
75, B-1200 Brussels, Belgium.

Fructose constitutes one of the main natural sweetening agents : it is
present in fruit, where it can account for up to 40 % of the dry weight, in
honey, in numerous vegetables and, in the form of sucrose, in many carbohydrate
nutrients. Although less abundant, sorbitol, its corresponding polyol, is also
widely distributed in fruits and vegetables. Both substances have been
extensively used as substitutes for sucrose in the diet of patients with
diabetes mellitus, as a source of calories in parenteral nutrition, and are
now being advocated as general purpose sweetening additives. The evaluation
of their safety in this respect requires a description of their metabolism and
a discussion of the findings observed upon parenteral as well as dietary
administration of high doses of fructose.

METABOLISM OF FRUCTOSE AND SORBITOL

Fructose is metabolized mainly in the liver, the kidney and the small
intestine due to the presence in these tissues of a specialized pathway[1]. The
first reaction of this pathway is the phosphorylation of fructose into fructose
1-phosphate by ketohexokinase, which utilizes ATP as the phosphoryl-donor.
Ketohexokinase has a low K_m for fructose (approxim. 0.5 mM) and a V_{max} of
10 U/g at 37°C. The phosphorylation of fructose occurs therefore much faster
than that of glucose. Fructose 1-phosphate is split by aldolase into D-
glyceraldehyde and dihydroxyaceton phosphate. D-glyceraldehyde is
phosphorylated into D-glyceraldehyde 3-phosphate by triokinase. The
preferential phosphoryl-donor is ATP but GTP can also be utilized at 10 % of
the rate of utilization of the adenine nucleotide[2]. Since both triose
phosphates are intermediates of the glycolytic-gluconeogenic pathway, fructose
is in part broken down to lactate plus pyruvate and in part converted into
glucose and glycogen. Small amounts of fructose are metabolized to sorbitol,

[*] Onderzoeksleider N.F.W.O.

α-glycerophosphate and glycerol, and to CO_2, ketone bodies and triglycerides.

The utilization of fructose by peripheral tissues, with the possible exception of adipocytes[3], seems to be negligible because these tissues do not possess the specialized enzymes ketohexokinase and triokinase. Sorbitol is converted to fructose in the liver by sorbitol dehydrogenase; its further metabolism is therefore identical to that of the ketose.

EFFECTS OF PARENTERAL ADMINISTRATION OF FRUCTOSE

Although in 1957, the discovery of hereditary fructose intolerance[4] provided a first indication of the potential toxicity of the ketose, it did not become apparent until the late 1960's that high doses of intravenous fructose could also be deleterious to normal organisms, catabolism of adenine nucleotides and lactic acidosis being the prominent findings.

a. Catabolism of adenine nucleotides

In 1967, Perheentupa and Raivio[5] reported that the oral or intravenous administration of fructose at the dose of 0.5 g/kg body weight, provoked hyperuricaemia and hyperuricosuria in normal children as well as in those with hereditary fructose intolerance. Animal experiments by Mäenpää et al.[6], that were later confirmed in man[7], showed that the parenteral administration of fructose provoked within minutes a dramatic depletion of liver ATP. This phenomenon is explained by the rapid phosphorylation of fructose at the expense of ATP. The elevation of uric acid can be accounted for by a deinhibition of AMP deaminase. This enzyme, which constitutes the limiting step in the catabolism of adenine nucleotides, is 95 % inhibited by the physiological concentrations of P_i and GTP prevailing in the liver cell[8]. The utilization of inorganic phosphate to rephosphorylate ADP in the mitochondria and of GTP, presumably at the triokinase step, decreases this inhibition and results in a loss of adenine nucleotides under the form of uric acid.

The fructose-induced hyperuricaemia should thus not be considered as a harmless phenomenon, but as a symptom of the loss of ATP in fructose-metabolizing tissues. As shown in experimental animals, the depletion of ATP, the energy currency of the cell, results in series of disturbances, most notably inhibition of protein synthesis[6].

b. Lactic acidosis

Due to (1) the higher activity of ketohexokinase as compared with the glucose-phosphorylating capacity of hexokinase plus glucokinase, (2) the fact that fructolysis bypasses the regulatory phosphofructokinase step of glycolysis, and (3) the stimulation of pyruvate kinase by fructose 1-phosphate, lactate formation from fructose is severalfold faster than from glucose. Bergström et al.[9] have called attention to the considerable increase in blood lactate, accompanied by a fall in pH and in standard bicarbonate, observed upon parenteral nutrition with fructose in human subjects. This phenomenon appears life-threatening in liver failure and has led to the recommendation of great caution in the clinical use of intravenous fructose[10]

EFFECTS OF DIETARY ADMINISTRATION OF FRUCTOSE

Human and animal observations, indicating that the serum lipid levels are not only influenced by the intake of fat, but also by the amount and type of carbohydrate, have led to numerous studies of the effect of high-fructose regimens on this parameter (for a review, see [11]). In man, diets rich in fructose have repeatedly been shown to induce higher levels of serum tri-glycerides than diets containing complex carbohydrates such as starch, although wide individual variations and also negative findings have been reported. In rats, high-fructose regimens consistently elevate the level of plasma tri-glycerides 2- to 3-fold above the basal values observed with chow, as compared with 0-60 % increases with a high-glucose diet.

Numerous investigations have been devoted to the mechanisms whereby fructose influences the metabolism of lipids (for a review see [12]). From these studies it appears that the hypertriglyceridaemic effect of the ketose is caused by an increase in the hepatic synthesis and release of triglyceride molecules and by a decrease in their removal from the circulation, the latter process occuring mainly in adipose tissue.

a. Influence of fructose on lipid metabolism in the liver

Up to twofold increases in the output of triglycerides in very low-density lipoproteins by the perfused liver have been described when the donor animal has been fed a high-fructose diet [13], as well as when the ketose is added to the perfusion medium [14]. A dual mechanism is apparently responsible for this effect :

(1) An enhanced esterification of fatty acids into triglycerides. This may be explained by the 3- to 8-fold increase in the concentration of α-glycero-phosphate [15], which is considered the primary factor influencing the esterification process. There is, however, no general agreement with respect to this explanation because an increase in the hepatic concentration of α-glycerophosphate has not been observed in rats fed a high-fructose diet [16] In accordance with experiments that have shown a reciprocal relationship between the oxidation and esterification of fatty acids, fructose has been

reported to inhibit the oxidation of labeled fatty acids in isolated liver preparations [14]. (2) An increased rate of synthesis of fatty acids. This results in an enhanced release of triglycerides according to the general correlation which has been demonstrated between both processes [17]. The nearly 2-fold stimulation of the rate of synthesis of fatty acids, which has been reported in rats fed fructose as compared with glucose [18], can be explained by an increase in the supply of both acetyl-CoA and α-glycerophosphate.

Two mechanisms have been postulated for the 40-60 % increase in the hepatic concentration of acetyl-CoA, observed upon administration of high-fructose diets [16] : (a) the already mentioned higher rate of fructolysis as compared to glycolysis, increasing the supply of pyruvate; (b) the activation of pyruvate dehydrogenase, enhancing the formation of acetyl-CoA. The 2- to 3-fold increase in the proportion of pyruvate dehydrogenase in the active form which has been reported upon administration of a load of fructose [19], is, however, not found with more physiological amounts of the ketose [20].

The stimulatory effect of α-glycerophosphate on the synthesis of fatty acids has been explained by a decrease in the concentration of long-chain fatty acyl-CoA, resulting from the esterification process. Long-chain fatty acyl-CoA have indeed been shown to exert a feed-back inhibition on acetyl-CoA carboxylase [21], the first committed enzyme of fatty acid synthesis, and their concentration is lowered in conditions associated with elevated lipogenesis [22].

b. Influence of fructose on lipid metabolism in adipose tissue

An impairment of the removal of triglycerides from the circulation, which is believed to depend on the adipose tissue clearing-factor lipase, has also been reported in animals fed fructose [23]. The increase in the activity of this enzyme, which is observed after the feeding of glucose, has indeed not been duplicated by giving fructose. This finding has been attributed to the inability of the ketose to raise the level of plasma insulin [24].

CONCLUSIONS

Although most of the noxious effects of fructose have been observed with high, pharmacological doses of the ketose, we feel that there is sufficient reason to restrain the consumption of fructose to its level found in a normal, well-balanced diet. One may wonder why the ketose is an easily tolerated ingredient, except in the unusual case of hereditary fructose intolerance. This may be explained by the fact that fructose does not enter the liver freely but requires a carrier-mediated transport with an apparent K_m which is about 2 orders of magnitude higher than the K_m of ketohexokinase [25]. This carrier-mediated transport limits the phosphorylation of post-prandial concentrations of fructose and accordingly a lowering of ATP is not observed in these conditions [20]. The oral administration of high doses of fructose (1 g/kg body weight and more) has, nevertheless, been reported to induce a hyperuricaemia [26] which is more pronounced in patients with gout and in their healthy children [27]. This probably reflects small increases in the catabolic rate of adenine nucleotides. Restriction of fructose intake may thus be indicated in patients with gout and other forms of hyperuricaemia such as glycogenosis type I.

Although the hypertriglyceridaemic effect of diets rich in fructose has not been demonstrated unequivocally in man, animal experiments provide strong indications that this ketose favors triglyceride synthesis. In view of the potential importance of hypertriglyceridaemia in the pathogenesis of athero-sclerosis, this finding constitutes the principal reason against the promotion of an increase in the consumption of fructose.

REFERENCES

1. Hers, H.G. "Le Metabolisme du Fructose",Editions Arscia, Brussels, 1957.
2. Frandsen, E.K. and Grunnet, N. Eur. J. Biochem. 23: 588-592, 1971.
3. Froesch, E.R. and Ginsberg, J.L. J. Biol. Chem. 237: 3317-3324, 1962.
4. Froesch, E.R., Prader, A., Labhart, A., Stuber, H.W. and Wolf, H.P. Schweiz. Med. Wochenschr. 87: 1168-1171, 1957.
5. Perheentupa, J. and Raivio, K. Lancet 2: 528-531, 1967.
6. Mäenpää,P.H., Raivio, K.O. and Kekomäki, M.P. Science 161: 1253-1254, 1968.
7. Bode, J.C., Zelder, O., Rumpelt, H.J. and Wittkamp, U. Eur. J. Clin. Invest. 3: 436-441, 1973.
8. Van den Berghe, G., Bronfman, M., Vanneste, R. and Hers, H.G. Biochem. J. 162: 601-609, 1977.
9. Bergström, J., Hultman, E. and Roch-Norlund, A.E. Acta Med. Scand. 184: 359-364, 1968.
10. Woods, H.F. and Alberti, K.G.M.M. Lancet 2: 1354-1357, 1972.
11. Nikkilä, E.A. Adv. Lipid Res. 7: 63-134, 1969.
12. Van den Berghe, G. Curr. Top. Cell. Regul. 13: 97-135, 1978.
13. Schonfeld, G. and Pfleger, B. J. Lipid Res. 12: 614-621, 1971.
14. Topping, D.L. and Mayes, P.A. Biochem. J. 126: 295-311, 1972.
15. Wieland, O. and Matschinsky, F. Life Sci. 2, 49-54, 1962.
16. Zakim, D., Pardini, R.S., Herman, R.H. and Sauberlich, H.E. Biochim. Biophys. Acta 144 : 242-251, 1967.
17. Windmueller, H.G. and Spaeth, A.E. Arch. Biochem. Biophys. 122: 362-369, 1967.

18. Romsos, D.R. and Leveille, G.A. Biochim. Biophys. Acta 360: 1-11, 1974.

19. Söling, H.D. and Bernhard, G. FEBS Lett. 13: 201-203, 1971.

20. Topping, D.L. and Mayes, P.A. Biochem. Soc. Trans. 5: 1001-1002, 1977.

21. Bortz, W.M. and Lynen, F. Biochem. Z. 339: 77-82, 1963.

22. Tubbs, P.K. and Garland, P.B. Biochem. J. 93:550-557, 1964.

23. Bar-On, H. and Stein, Y. J. Nutr. 94: 95-105, 1968.

24. Cryer, A., Riley, S.E., Williams, E.R. and Robinson, D.S. Biochem. J. 140, 561-563, 1974.

25. Sestoft, L. and Fleron, P. Biochim. Biophys. Acta 345, 27-38, 1974.

26. Emmerson, B.T. Ann. Rheum. Dis. 33: 276-280, 1974.

27. Stirpe, F., Della Corte, E., Bonetti, E., Abbondanza, A., Abbati, A. and De Stefano, F. Lancet 2: 1310-1311, 1970.

Health and Sugar Substitutes
Proc. ERGOB Conf., Geneva 1978, pp. 98-102 (Karger, Basel 1978)

HEPATIC METABOLISM OF XYLITOL

A. Jakob

Metabolic Unit, Department of Medicine, University Hospital,
8091 Zurich, Switzerland

INTRODUCTION

Xylitol is added to foods as a nutritive sweetener to substitute sucrose.
Together with fructose and glucose it is also infused intravenously during
parenteral nutrition. Most of the xylitol administred to man and laboratory
animals is metabolized by the liver. Some of its pronounced metabolic
effects may be compared with those of fructose and of ethanol. The evaluation
of the safety of xylitol administration has to take these effects into consideration.

XYLITOL METABOLISM IN THE PERFUSED RAT LIVER

The conversion of xylitol to intermediates of hepatic glycolysis and gluconeogenesis is schematically shown in fig. 1. One equivalent of NADH is
produced and one ATP is consumed per mole of xylitol metabolized. In livers
from starved rats 60 - 80 % of the xylitol taken up is converted to glucose,
lactate production is low (1, 2, 3). In livers from fed rats lactate production
is also increased (2). Lactate uptake and glucose formation from lactate is
inhibited by xylitol. The same effect is observed if ethanol is added instead
of xylitol (fig. 2 and 3). Since, as in the case of ethanol oxidation the first
step of xylitol metabolism is an oxidation by a cytosolic dehydrogenase,
it is not surprising that this cellular compartment is strongly reduced by
xylitol (1, 2). The inhibitory effect of xylitol on lactate uptake is explained
by the observation that xylitol dehydrogenase competes with other dehydrogenases for NAD. Xylitol uptake and metabolism is itself controlled by the
rate of reoxidation of NADH (fig. 4) and thus the competition between
different dehydrogenases for NAD is defined by their midpotential. Since
the midpotential of xylitol dehydrogenase is lower than that of lactate

dehydrogenase, xylitol is an effective inhibitor of lactate uptake (1).

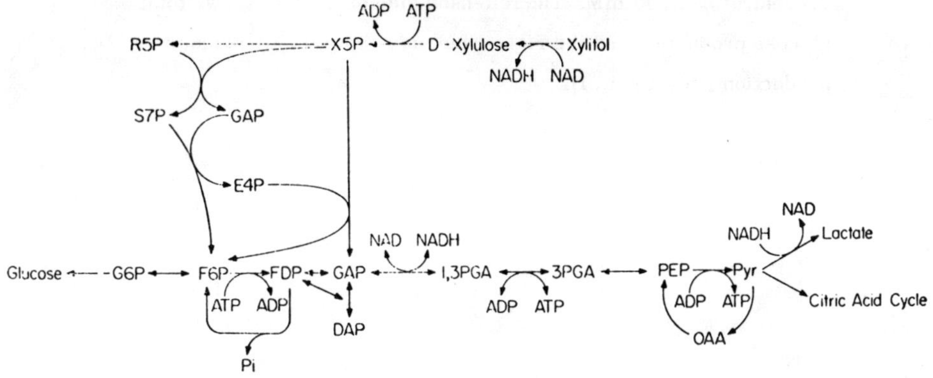

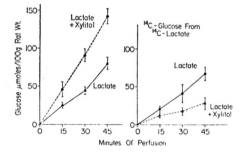

Fig. 1 Scheme of xylitol metabolism in liver. R5P, ribose-5-P; X5P,
D-xylulose-5-P; S7P, Sedoheptulose-7-P; GAP, glyceraldehyde-3-P;
E4P, erythrose-4-P; G6P, glucose-6-P; F6P, fructose-6-P; FDP,
fructose-di-P; 1,3PGA, 1,3-di-P-glycerate; 3PGA, 3-P-glycerate;
PEP, P-enolpyruvate; Pyr, pyruvate; DAP, dihydroxyacetone-P;
OAA, oxalacetate. (from reference 1).

Fig. 2 Effect of xylitol on glucose production from (^{14}C)-lactate in perfused
livers. Livers from starved rats were perfused in a recirculating
system with bicarbonate buffer containing initially 12 mM lactate.
(U-^{14}C)-lactate was added to give a specific activity of about 6000 cpm/mol.

When present, xylitol was added from the start of perfusion at a
concentration of 10 mM. The left–hand side of the fig. shows total
glucose production and the right–hand side shows (^{14}C)–glucose
production (from ref. 1).

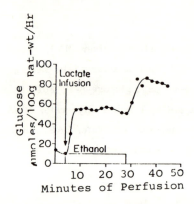

Fig. 3 Effect of 2 mM ethanol on glucose production from lactate (1.5 mM)
         by a liver perfused in a non–recirculating system. The infusion of
         lactate started at the time indicated by the arrow and continued to
         the end of the experiment. Ethanol was infused as indicated by the
         bar (from ref. 4).

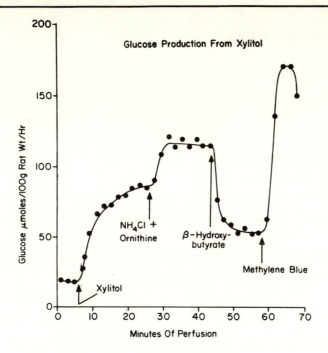

Fig. 4 Regulation of glucose production from xylitol. NH$_4$Cl+ornithine was
used to stimulate the utilisation of ATP (urea synthesis) resulting in
an enhanced rate of reoxidation of NADH. β-Hydroxybutyrate was
used to produce the opposite effect and the artificial electron
acceptor methylene blue was finally added as an oxidant (from ref. 4).

At high concentrations xylitol can affect the hepatic adenine nucleotide and
phosphate (P$_i$) contents in the liver in the same way as fructose because it is
also rapidly phosphorylated. It causes a depletion of ATP, total adenine nucleotides and P$_i$. As a consequence the production of uric acid increases (2).

CONCLUSION

The metabolic effects of xylitol in the perfused rat liver are the consequence
of the introduction of carbon skeletons into the gluconeogenetic pathway and
of the generation of reducing equivalents in the cytosol.

QUESTIONS TO BE DISCUSSED

The knowledge of these biochemical facts is a prerequisite for the evaluation of benefits and risks of the use of xylitol as a sugar substitute. However they are not the only criteria to be considered and the question how relevant these findings are for human physiology and pathophysiology has to be asked and answered.

What are the risks or the benefits of:

1) glucose production from xylitol,

2) the reduction of the cytosolic cell compartment (short-and longterm effects),

3) the depletion of total adenine nucleotides (especially ATP) and P_i and of an enhanced production of uric acid?

Which are additional physiological and pathophysiological considerations (e. g. resorption from the gut, accumulation of lactate in the blood) ?

REFERENCES

1.   Jakob, A. , Williamson J.R. and Asakura, T.J. Biol. Chem.
     246. 2623 - 7631 (1971).

2.   Blair, J.B. , Cook, D.E. and Lardy H.A.   J. Biol. Chem.
     248. 3601 - 3607 (1973).

3.   Woods, H.F. and Krebs H.A.   Biochem. J.
     134. 437 - 443 (1973).

4.   Williamson J.R. , Jakob A. and Refino, C.   J. Biol. Chem.
     246. 7632 - 7641 (1971).

Health and Sugar Substitutes
Proc. ERGOB Conf., Geneva 1978, pp. 103-108 (Karger, Basel 1978)

SUGAR ALCOHOLS IN ANIMAL AND HUMAN NUTRITION

K.K. Mäkinen

Section of Biochemistry, Institute of Dentistry, University
of Turku, SF-20520 Turku 52, Finland

INTRODUCTION

The chemical bases for the nutritional interest certain acyclic sugar alcohols include the following:

a. Combustion values which are similar to those of the corresponding aldoses or ketoses;

b. Absence of reducing carbonyl groups. Open chain structure;

c. The similarities to common sugars in the configuration at various C-atoms;

d. Evidence of high metabolic capacity in man;

e. Absence of evidence of toxicity in man;

f. First-step metabolic independence of insulin and metabolism principally in the liver;

g. Technological suitability for various food manufacturing purposes;

h. Pleasant or appealing organoleptic properties;

i. Wide occurrence in Nature.

These reasons underlie the present growing interest in the use of many sugar alcohols in experimental research, as well as in several practical applications of which the following have current utility value:

a. Use of xylitol, sorbitol and mannitol as low- or noncariogenic sweeteners.

b. Use of xylitol and sorbitol as substitutes for sucrose or glucose in the diabetic diet.

c. Use of polyol mixtures in feeding of domestic animals for facilitation of fat-soluble vitamin absorption.

d. Use of xylitol and sorbitol as energy sources in parenteral nutrition.

This situation is based on systemic toxicological, nutritional
and clinical research particularly on xylitol and sorbitol. For
xylitol, the following estimated safe daily doses for adult
humans have been suggested: orally, 50-100 g; parenterally:
0.125-0.250 g/(hr x kg body weight); adult diabetics: oral dose,
up to 70 g/ day (diabetic children have received 30 g of xylitol/
day without adverse effects[1]). Suggested sorbitol doses are lower
because of poorer absorption. For similar reasons peroral
sorbitol is better tolerated than peroral mannitol. The administration of combinations of xylitol, glucose and fructose in
total parenteral nutrition is considered justified in patients in
whom hyperglycemia during infusion of glucose alone is difficult
to control with insulin[2]. In domestic animals (cattle and calves,
sows, pigs, sheep) the tolerability of polyol mixtures chiefly
consisting of xylitol, sorbitol, mannitol, arabinitol, galactitol
and rhamnitol is clearly greater than 100 g per 100 kg body
weight (unpublished results).

PRESENT STATE OF KNOWLEDGE
The present state of knowledge of sugar alcohols in animal and
human nutrition is directly or indirectly based on about three
hundred original publications which have mainly appeared during
the sixties and seventies and are reviewed elsewhere[3]. This information has also been touched upon several symposia and
congresses of which the following can be regarded as most
important:
1. "Metabolism, Physiology, and Clinical Use of Pentoses and
   Pentitols", Hakone, Japan, August 1967[4].
2. "Sugars in Nutrition", Nashville, Tennessee, U.S.A., October
   1969[5].
3. "Zucker-Symposiums I and II", Würzburg, W. Germany, May 1971
   and May 1976[6,7].
4. "Sugars and Sugar Substitutes", München, W. Germany, October
   1974[8].
5. "Monosaccharides and Polyalcohols in Nutrition, Therapy and
   Dietetics", Basle, June 1975[9].
6. Meeting of the International Society of Parenteral Nutrition,
   Kyoto, August 1975[10].
7. "Sweeteners and Dental Caries", Durham, New Hampshire, October
   1977[11].

The present state of sugar alcohol research is suitably illustrated by the re-examination of the Turku sugar study[12] (1972-1974) subjects in March-February 1978 (Fig. 1). The approx. 50 volunteers who consumed a xylitol diet (with small amounts of sorbitol) for two years were examined with regard to several parameters (Table 1). A small group of chronic users of xylitol (and sorbitol) was separated from this group in 1974. These subjects have regularly consumed these polyols for more than 5 years (Fig. 2). These follow-up medical examinations revealed both the chronic users and the 1972-1974 subjects all to be healthy with no acute or delayed pathological changes in urine and blood chemistry.

The information to date suggests that the consumption of a xylitol (and possibly sorbitol) diet is associated with increased activity levels of the salivary lactoperoxidase (LPO)[13,14]. The biochemical mechanism of this phenomenon is not yet exactly known, but the increased activity levels have been explained as physiological responses. There is so far no firm evidence that other exocrine glands, such as the mammary and lacrimal glands, would react in this way. The elevated LPO concentrations after xylitol have been suggested to increase the innate defence mechanisms of exocrine secretions, as LPO is part of a physio-logical antimicrobial system.

PERTINENT QUESTIONS

1. Does exogenous xylitol have any effect on the speed or efficacy of the glucuronate cycle, with a possible effect on the biosynthesis of certain glycoproteins?
2. Will xylitol act as a therapeutic agent in a glucose 6-phosphate dehydrogenase deficiency?
3. Will certain sugar alcohols be of practical value in enhancing the absorption of vitamins and trace elements?
4. Does the oral administration of mixtures of sugar alcohols have a positive effect on the growth rate of the offspring of domestic animals, and the production of meat, milk and fur?
5. To what extent would certain sugar alcohols exert a positive influence on the antimicrobial qualities of specific exocrine secretions?

TABLE 1. List of parameters determined in connection with the re-examination of the Turku sugar study subjects 5.5 years after the commencement of the trial, and the formula diet study on chronic xylitol users (cf. Figs. 1 and 2). All examinations resulted in values which fell within the physiological range.

BLOOD	URINE
Aspartate aminotransferase	Catecholamines
Alanine aminotransferase	Metanephrines
Alkaline phosphatase	3-Methoxy-4-OH-mandelic acid
γ-Glutamyltranspeptidase	Urea, uric acid, creatinine
α-Amylase, lipase	Na, K, Ca, Mg, P, Cl, pH
Leucine aminopeptidase	α-Amylase, leucine aminopeptidase
Arginine aminopeptidase	Protein, bilirubin
Lactic acid, triglycerides	Acid excretion
Uric acid, urea, creatinine	Specific gravity, volume
Glucose, xylitol, insulin	Leucocytes, erythrocytes
Protein, bilirubin	Epithelial cells, crystals
Na, K, Ca, Mg, P, Cl	Blood, albumin, urobilinogen
Cholesterol (free and total)	Bodies precipitated by HAc
Lipoprotein fractionation	Glucose, xylitol
pH, P_{CO_2}, P_{O_2}, HCO_3^-	Oxalic acid
Base excess, total CO_2	UV and visible spectrum
Sedimentation of erythrocytes	OTHERS
Leucocytes, hemoglobin	Blood pressure
	Lens opacity

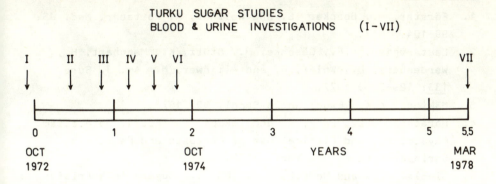

FIG. 1. Overall schedule of the Turku feeding studies[12] (1972-1974) and re-examination (1978).

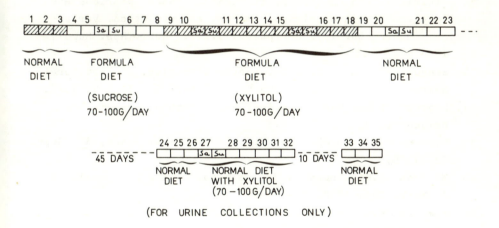

FIG. 2. Overall schedule of the formula diet study on nine chronic xylitol users. The subjects have consumed xylitol almost regularly over five years (1972-1978). In January-March 1978 the subjects were examined during the 4-week consumption of a defined formula diet for parameters shown in Table 1.

REFERENCES

1. Förster, H., Boecker, S. and Walther, A. Fortschr. Med. 95: 99-104, 1977.
2. Leutenegger, A.F., Göschke, H., Stutz, K., Mannhart, H., Werdenberg, D., Wolff, G. and Allgöwer, M.   Am. J. Surg. 133: 199-205, 1977.
3. Mäkinen, K.K.   Experientia Suppl. 30, 1978.
4. Horecker, B.L., Lang, K. and Takagi, Y. (Eds.). Metabolism, Physiology, and Clinical Use of Pentoses and Pentitols, Springer-Verlag, New York, 1969.
5. Sipple, H.L. and McNutt, K.W. (Eds.).   Sugars in Nutrition, Academic Press, New York, 1974.
6. Zucker-Symposium-Würzburg. Dtsch. zahnärztl. Z. 26: No. 11, 1971.
7. Zuckersymposium II-Würzburg. Dtsch. zahnärztl. Z. 32: Suppl. 1, 1977.
8. Zöllner, N. and Henckenkamp, I.-U. (Eds.).   Sugars and Sugar Substitutes.   Nutr. Metab. 18: Suppl. 1, 1975.
9. Ritzel, G. and Brubacher, G. (Eds.).   Monosaccharides and Polyalcohols in Nutrition, Therapy and Dietetics, Verlag Hans Huber, Bern, 1976 (Intern. J. Vit. Nutr. Res. Suppl. 15, 1976).
10. Schuberth, O.O. (Ed.). International Society of Parenteral Nutrition Proceedings, Acta Chir. Scand. Suppl. 466, 1976.
11. Sweeteners and Dental Caries, NIH Workshop, Durham, New Hampshire, October, 1977.
12. Scheinin, A. and Mäkinen, K.K.   Acta Odont. Scand. 33: Suppl. 70, 1975.
13. Mäkinen, K.K., Bowen, W.H., Dalgard, D. and Fitzgerald, G. J. Nutr. 108: 1978. In press.
14. Mäkinen, K.K., Tenovuo, J. and Scheinin, A.   J. Dent. Res. 55: 652-660, 1976.

Health and Sugar Substitutes
Proc. ERGOB Conf., Geneva 1978, pp. 109-113 (Karger, Basel 1978)

α-D-GLUCOPYRANOSIDO-1,6-SORBITOL AND α-D-GLUCOPYRANOSIDO-1,6-MANNITOL (PALATINIT®)

G. Siebert and U. Grupp

Department of Biological Chemistry, University of Hohenheim, Postfach 106, D-7000 Stuttgart-70, Germany

INTRODUCTION

When the saccharose molecule is modified in two different aspects, i) by transglycosidation into a 1→6 glycosidic bond, and ii) by reduction of the fructose moiety into sorbitol and mannitol, respectively, hydrogenated palatinose is obtained (Palatinit[R]) which represents a 1:1 mixture of α-D-glucopyrano-sido-1,6-sorbitol (GPS) and α-D-glucopyranosido-1,6-mannitol (GPM). Its building stones, glucose as well as sorbitol and mannitol, are well documented in regard to their intermediary metabolism and should not create, therefore, any problem concerning compatibility, wholesomeness, etc.

One might expect, however, from experiences with isomaltose and palatinose (isomaltulose) as well as with maltitol that enzymatic cleavage in the intestinal tract may be slow when compared with natural disaccharides like saccharose or maltose; therefore the question arises whether the metabolic fate of Palatinit may depend on its substrate properties for digestive carbohydrases, and the subsequent rate of absorption from the intestine.

As described elsewhere, Palatinit is well characterized by derivatization and a number of chemical and physical methods (1); quantitative determination of the two disaccharide alcohols GPS and GPM is performed either by gas chromatography after silylation, or by an enzymatic procedure which produces three reduced pyridine nucleotides per mol of GPS and one per mol of GPM (1) in a highly specific manner.

DIGESTION AND ABSORPTION

Palatinit is cleaved by homogenates from human jejunal mucosa at a rate of 35 nmoles/min x mg protein, with a k_M of 5.5 mM; relative rates are for maltose:saccharose:palatinose: Palatinit = 100:25:11:2, and quite similar also for the corresponding rat tissue. Pure α-glucosidase (maltase) from yeast has been unequivocally identified as being responsible for the cleavage of Palatinit whereas invertase (saccharase) is completely inactive; inhibition studies on human intestinal mucosa also indicate α-glucosidase as being responsible for the cleavage of Palatinit (2).

Digestion of Palatinit in the small intestine is incomplete, both in man and rat (2). This is demonstrated e.g. in the rat by caecal enlargement (+200-300 % of total weight and tissue mass as well) which is a very reliable indicator of bacterial fermentation below the small intestine. A significant increase of fecal nitrogen excretion, due to enhanced bacterial mass, the occurence of diarrhoea after too high initial doses (more than 2 g per young rat or around 100 g per adult humans) also point to incomplete digestion. However, if foregoing adaptation has taken place young rats tolerate 5 g per day easily whereas 100 g per adult men as a single dose do not even cause flatulence.

Incomplete digestion, resulting naturally then in incomplete absorption, in the small intestine is also demonstrated by analyses of the contents of rat intestinal tract for Palatinit and its components (2); at different times after a test-meal of 1.7 g given to adapted rats, 120-150 mg of GPS + GPM + sorbitol + mannitol are found in the caecum, but only one tenth of that amount in the large intestine. Such data are corroborated by observations on caecectomized rats where now the large intestine is the site where Palatinit is recovered.

All available data point to the caecum in the rat, and probably to the upper colon in men, where undigested Palatinit is cleaved and the split products are degraded by bacterial fermentation. In both species fecal excretion is very small, and

lies in the range of about 1 % of the amount ingested (2). In
consequence, utilization of Palatinit given per os is nearly
complete, but, the slow digestion in the small intestine rele-
ases glucose only in such small amounts that its metabolic
removal compensates for a possible rise of blood sugar (2).
Even after 100 g, taken at once by fasting human volunteers,
no significant rise of blood sugar is observed. The absence of
an increase of plasma insulin under such conditions is in agreement with all other data (2).

ENERGY METABOLISM

In contrast to free sorbitol which provides as much energy
as regular monosaccharides in the rat (3), when compared to
free mannitol which according to literature (references in (2))
is said to be almost non-caloric after oral uptake, GPS and
GPM do not differ in their caloric utilization when energy-
dependent growth of young rats was the assay system. However,
Palatinit demonstrates reduced energy yield in the rat between
53 and 75 %, depending on the type of diet and experiment (2);
in weight maintenance as well as in growth of young rats,
energy requirement was much higher with diets containing 34.5 %
Palatinit instead of either corn starch or saccharose. The
above-stated caloric reduction holds if it is true that feeding
Palatinit does not cause any diminished energetic utilization
of the remaining carbohydrate, fat, and protein of the diet
given to the rats.

In man, caloric reduction is well below 50 % as shown by
indirect calorimetry in a respiratory chamber in a 12 hour
experiment in which saccharose and Palatinit were compared with
the same group of volunteers. Under conditions where 4 male
persons of 292 kg total weight received 60 g per person of
either saccharose or Palatinit, CO_2 production increases to
43.6 l excess CO_2 after saccharose and 15.2 l excess CO_2 after
Palatinit, thus indicating less than 50 % utilization of the
disaccharide alcohol in man.

Experiments of this kind are somewhat difficult to inter-
prete since total yield of excess CO_2 is only 23 and 8 % of
ingested carbon; one is led to the assumption that the difference is due to a shift - in fasting subjects - from glycogen
and protein breakdown and some fatty acid oxidation towards
oxidation of saccharose or Palatinit, thus sparing body
reserves.

In addition, saccharose in doses of 60 g per person certainly leads to an insulin secretion whereas Palatinit does not.
The importance of the lack of a stimulus for insulin secretion
is seen in feeding experiments for 5 weeks in rats: fat content
is significantly reduced, and lean body mass increased, with
34.5 % Palatinit in a casein-starch and in a casein-saccharose
diet (2).

We have shown (4) elsewhere that prolonged feeding of either
sorbose or sorbitol leads to significantly lower levels of
plasma insulin in rats, and in the case of sorbitol also to a
reduced fat content, concomitant with increased lean body mass.
Thus, the assumption is justified that reduced body fat after
Palatinit should also be due to a diminished action of insulin,
thus preventing a higher energy flow from carbohydrates into
triglycerides in adipose tissue.

GENERAL OBSERVATIONS

Like a great number of oligosaccharides, disaccharide alcohols as Palatinit are excreted, after oral uptake, in small
amounts of about 0.1 % of the dose in urine. Handling of
Palatinit, GPM and GPS in the kidney leads to clearance values
of 0.5 - 1.0 ml/min, thus demonstrating that intravenous infusion of several grams in 3 hours is tolerated quite well
while plasma and urinary concentrations of above 800 mg/100 ml
and around 10 % respectively are found. Palatinit remains under
these condition confined to the extracellular space of the
rat (2).

Cultures of mouse fibroblasts (L-929) tolerate Palatinit
in concentrations up to 200 mM without any sign of damage;
glucose metabolism of such cells progresses unimpaired,
Palatinit is not used at all.

CONCLUSIONS

Palatinit is shown, in this paper, to represent a degree of modification of saccharose that metabolic utilization requires the symbiotic cooperation between mammalian tissues and intestinal bacteria. In the light of a much reduced cariogenicity, shown elsewhere (5), metabolic compatibility and safety, demonstrated in this paper, Palatinit qualifies as a serious candidate for sugar substitution.

References:

1) Gau, W., Grupp, U., Kurz, J., Müller, L., Siebert, G. and Steinle, G.: Z. Lebm. Unters. Forsch., in the press.

2) Grupp, U. and Siebert, G.: Res. exp. Med., in the press.

3) Schnell-Dompert, E. and Siebert, G., Hoppe-Seyler's Z. physiol. Chem., in the press.

4) Schnell-Dompert, E., Hannover, R. and Siebert, G., unpublished observations.

5) Karle, E.J. and Gehring, F.: Dt. zahnärztl. Z., 31: 189-191, 1978.

Health and Sugar Substitutes
Proc. ERGOB Conf., Geneva 1978, pp. 114-119 (Karger, Basel 1978)

HYDROGENATED STARCH HYDROLYSATES

P. LEROY

ROQUETTE FRERES
62136 - LESTREM , FRANCE

The greater part of the daily carbohydrate intake is brought
in the food in the form of starches, which, after digestion, are
absorbed in glucose form. For many years, starch hydrolysis products are manufactured and used for manufacture of food products :
- glucose syrups in confectionery products
- malto dextrins, atomized glucoses : infantile food, ice creams,
  delicatessen.
These products can be considered as a starch more or less predigested according to the starch hydrolysis degree.
The use of hydrogenation derivatives of glucids in food products
is more recent : the sorbitol is probably the most generally
used. The sugar reduction is not only applied to simple molecules
(ex. hexoses, pentoses) but also to starch hydrolysates (ex. Lycasin, Malbit) : the disappearing of the reducing power makes that
these products have a certain interest from a technological point
of view for the control of browning reactions, from a biological
point of view by the reduction of fermentability (dental decay)
or blood glucose response.
The use of these hydrogenation derivatives will be accordingly to
the requested properties, depending on the composition which differ
well from a product to another according to its manufacturing
process.

The starch is a polymer of D-glucose where the molecules are
bound essentially between them by a α-1-4 link introducing the
reducing function of the basis element, the glucose.
This polymer hydrolysis can be worked out in different ways and
at more or less high degrees. If at all events, the hydrolysates

are always composed of less or more polymerised glucose, their
composition differs greatly and consequently it will be the same
with their hydrogenation derivative ; that's the reason for it's
essential to precise, when speaking of hydrogenated starch hydrolysates, some characteristics of these products and their raw
materials, the starch hydrolysates.
Concerning these last, the analytical basis element is the reducing power that we express in Dextrose Equivalent (DE) and which
gives the importance of the released reducing functions, that is
to say the advance of hydrolysis. If this characteristic keeps its
whole value in a certain hydrolysis system, it is of insufficient
meaning by the fact that several hydrolysis systems of starch
are used :
- acide hydrolysis
- enzyme hydrolysis carrying with :

αamylase (E.C. 3-2-1-1) : α-1-4-glucan-4 glucanohydrolase
βamylase (E.C. 3-2-1-2) : α-1-4-glucan - maltohydrolase
  amyloglucosidase (E.C. 3-2-1-3) : α-1-4 glucanohydrolase

The hydrolysis products arising from the application of these
agents are going to be of different composition (Tab.1), and to
a same DE, the compositions can be very different :

DE	DP glucose	DP2	DP3	DP4	DP5	DP6	DP7	DP 8to10	DP > 10
20	2	6,2	8,3	6,2	6,2	12	10	9,4	39,7
25	10,4	7,7	7,8	7,8	7,5	7,2	6,7	17,5	27,4
33	6,5	24	17	13	4	2,5	2,1	5,3	25,6
40	20	8	6,8	6,4	6,2	5,7	5,5		
40	6,5	38	22	9	2	1,9	2,5	2,5	15,6
50	4	47	24	2,5	2,5	3,5	3		
59	6,5	51	17	0,7	1,5	2,0	2,0	4,7	14,6

Tab. 1 indicative composition of starch hydrolysates of different
      DE.

The hydrogenation of reducing functions set free by hydrolysis of
α-1-4 link leads to the formation of the corresponding polyol

glucose ⎯⎯⎯⎯⎯⎯→ sorbitol

maltose ⎯⎯⎯⎯⎯→ maltitol (glucosyl sorbitol)

maltotriose ⎯⎯⎯⎯→ maltotriitol (gluco-gluco-sorbitol)

tetraose ⎯⎯⎯⎯→ tetraitol

a.s.o...

The hydrogenated starch derivatives compose therefore a range of
products having many varieties, as much as the starch hydrolysates
from which they are issued. It must be meanwhile noted that the
total hydrolysis of the hydrogenated derivatives' components leads
to sorbitol and glucose : the relation between both components is
directly bound with the DE of the non-hydrogenated product.

The hydrogenation of the reducing group placed at the end of the
chain of a dextrose polymere changes the spatial configuration at
this extremity. What are the consequences of this structural modification on the ability to the enzyme saccharification with regard
to the non-hydrogenated product ?

By using enzymes such as pancreatin, the amyloglucosidase, it's
possible to study in vitro the digestibility of the hydrogenated
starch hydrolysates with regard to the hydrolysates from which
they are issued.

The enzyme conversion can be followed in bulk by the evolution
of the appeared reducing sugars ' rate and more finely by the
chromatographic analysis of products arising from the enzymes
effect.

a) composition of the tested products in vitro

DE	:DP1	:DP2	:DP3	:DP4	:DP5	:DP6	:DP7	:DP8	:DP9	:DP10	>DP10
34	5,8	23,5	20,5	15,0	7,5	6,4	2,2	1,2	1,2	1,0	15,7
48	6,2	51,5	19,0	0,5	1,5	2,7	3,0	1,5	1,1	0,2	12,8
59	4,5	71	20	1	2	0,5	-	-	-	-	-

b) enzym saccharification with pancreatin

The substrates in solution to 30% have been incubated in presence of pancreatin with pH 6,5 and at 37°C.

The pancreatin affects the polysaccharides in setting free essentially maltose. Thereby, the rate of reducing sugars appearing on the hydrolysis of a non hydrogenated product with faint DE, is situated at about 55%.

The pancreatin action on the hydrogenated polysaccharides effects a reducing power insofar it affects a hydrogenation product of a hydrolysate with a faint DE, the products composed are a few glucose, maltose.

	reduc. sugars	glucose	maltose	sorbitol	maltitol
34M	→ 15,5	:0 →10	:0 →10	:62 →62	:24 →32 :
48M	→ 4,8	:0 →30	:0 →35	: 8 →8	:52 →50
59M	→ 1				

c) enzym saccharification with amyloglucosidase

The substrates in solution to 30% have been incubated in presence of amyloglucosidase with pH 4,5 and at 60°C.

The amyloglucosidase affects the starch in setting free essentially glucose. The enzym digestion of starch hydrolysates is almost total with obviously appearance of glucose as a reaction product. Meanwhile, the conversion of hydrogenated polysaccharides makes appear on the one hand glucose and on the other hand maltitol : it appears all the more glucose as the DE before hydrogenation is faint.

	reduc. sugars	glucose	sorbitol	maltitol
34M	→ 46	:0 →47	:62 →11	: 24 →43 :
48M	→ 24	:0 →24	:80 →15	: 52 →64
59M	→ 84	:0 →84	:75 →11	: 71 →80 :

In vitro, we state that the hydrogenated starch hydrolysates are all the better hydrolysed with release of glucose because the

initial DE is not very high. We result essentially in a mixture
of saccharides (glucose or maltose according to the specificity
of the used enzym) of sorbitol and maltitol.
But in vivo what is the digestibility of these products ?
The hydrogenation of starch hydrolysates making disappear the
reducing groups could lead to think that the blood glucose response to their ingestion was comparable to the one of sorbitol,
that's to say there would not be significant increase of the
blood glucose rate.
The scanning of the carbohydrates absorption is classically performed by charge tests and it could have been established that
the ingestion of the starch hydrolysates produced, by the healthy
persons, blood glucose responses which differed not significantly of these induced by the glucose (Dodds and coll ; Butterfield;
Kearsley and Col).
In studying the blood glucose response to the charge of product
6563, hydrogenated derivative of a moderately hydrolysed starch,
Björling and Coll have established a blood glucose response comparable to that of an identical charge of saccharose after 30 and
60 minutes and a little higher glycemia to 90-120 mn with the
hydrogenated derivative than with the saccharose.
Blood glucose responses comparable to those effected by the glucose have been found by Kearsley-Birch with on the one hand derivative products of the hydrolysates reduction to 21,43 DE and on
the other hand of a syrup with a high content in maltose.
Meanwhile, the maltitol has caused a fainter hyperglycemia but
however higher to the one noticed with the hydrogenation derivative of an hydrolysate to 65 DE. An increase response of the glycemia and the insulinemia with the maltitol have also been established by Kamoï.
Fossati and Coll have studied, by obeses subjects, the behaviour
of glycemia and insulinemia without oral overweight of an hydrogenated starch hydrolysate with following composition : sorbitol
6%, maltitol 66%, higher hydrogenated polysaccharides 28%. It is
noticed that this product effects a blood glucose increase comparable but fainter that the one got with the glucose only, the
blood glucose surfaces being without significant difference ;
meanwhile the insulinic response is significantly fainter.

The whole of these remarks show that the blood glucose responses are comparable to those obtained with the non hydrogenated derivatives if we apply to products coming from moderately hydrolysed starch.

In order to note a decrease of the peak of hyperglycemia, products strongly hydrolysed and hydrogenated are used.

Nevertheless, blood glucose reponses are still obtained, they prove that the dextrose is free and consequently the hydrolysis either digestive or at the time of absorption on the intestinal level of components in their basis units : glucose and sorbitol.

REFERENCES

1.   Dodds - Fairweather - Miller - Rose
      Lancet i, 485 (1959)

2.   Butterfield, Proc. R. Soc. Med. 57 196 (1964)

3.   Kearsley - Fairmurst - Green
      Proc. nutr. soc. 34-60A (1975)

4.   Björling - Frostell - Dahlquist
      Acta odont. Scand. p. 31 (1971)

5.   Kearsley - Birch, IRCS. Med. Sci. 6 - 82 (1978)

6.   Kamoï et coll
      Igaku - no - Ayumi - vol 82 n° u- 208 (1972)

7.   Fossati et coll - société nutrition - Lille, décembre 1977

Health and Sugar Substitutes
Proc. ERGOB Conf., Geneva 1978, pp. 120-122 (Karger, Basel 1978)

MICROBIAL METABOLISM IN THE LOWER GUT

M.J. Hill

Bacterial Metabolism Res. Lab., Central Public Health Lab.,
Colindale, London, NW9, UK.

BACTERIAL METABOLISM OF SUGAR SUBSTITUTES

In the normal healthy person the duodenum, jejunum and upper ileum
contain few organisms, and consequently there is little interaction
between the flora and those sugars readily digested by small intestinal
mucosal enzymes[4]. Any sugar not absorbed from the small intestine,
in contrast, will be metabolised by the flora to a range of fatty acids
and alcohols and gases. In vitro, the fatty acid end-products of
anaerobic bacteria and can be used in their classification[5]. In
addition, a variety of alcohols and aldehydes are produced together
with gases such as CO_2, hydrogen and methane. The results of such
metabolic products are an increase in stool bulk and frequency and
a change in the metabolism of other colonic compounds by the flora.

The mechanism of stool bulking is inknown. About 35g lactulose
is sufficient to induce two soft stools per day (ie. virtually double
the stool frequency and weight per day). One molecule of lactulose
is metabolised to at least 4 molecules of fatty acid or neutral
product and so it has been suggested that the stool bulking is due to
osmotic effects[1]. However, the cathartic effects of lactulose begin
about 2 hours after initial ingestion (ie at about the time that the
lactulose reaches the caecum) indicating an irritant rather than an
osmotic effect. In this respect the fatty acids themselves have
been incriminated as caecal or colonic irritants. The major effect
looked for in the treatment of cirrhosis with lactulose is the
acidification of the large bowel; indeed it has been demonstrated
that, following the ingestion of 35g lactulose the caecal pH falls
well below 6. One result of this is that many compounds excreted in

faeces remain undegraded because so many of the enzymes of faecal bacteria have a pH-optimum greater than 7 and are not produced in acid conditions. We do not know the possible side effects of this failure to degrade colonic components.

There is no doubt that patients are unhappy about the acid and gas produced from lactulose, mannitol etc administered in relatively large amounts therapeutically, and flatulence is a particular problem. However, if we believe (like Burkitt)[2] that stool bulking is important in the treatment and prevention of much gastrointestinal disease (in particular diverticulitis, constipation and haemorrhoids) then the use of sugar alcohols etc as sugar substitutes would be beneficial from this point of view, particularly in view of the fact that so many people find fibre and fibre foods unacceptable.

In addition, we have postulated that large bowel carcinogensis is mediated by the production of bacterial metabolites of bile acids[3]. The enzymes involved have pH optima between 7 and 8 and some are not produced below pH 6; consequently, the use of sugar alcohols etc which give rise to stool bulking and stool acidification might have a further important beneficial side effect - a reduction in the incidence of bowel cancer.

The main questions that I would ask are:-

(1) What is the daily intake of the sugar substitute and what effect will it have on stool bulk and pH ?

(2) What are the main products of metabolism of the sugar substitute by the gut flora and is excessive gas formation and flatulence likely to be a problem ?

(3) Are the sugar substitutes to be used by persons attempting caloric control (in which case the metabolism of absorbed colonic metabolites must be considered), or persons with glucose sensitivity or by other patient groups ?

REFERENCES

1. Neale, G. J. Clin. Path., $\underline{24}$, Suppl. (Roy.Coll.Path.) 5, 22, 1972.

2. Burkitt, D. Cancer, $\underline{28}$, 3, 1971.

3. Hill, M.J. Cancer, $\underline{36}$, 2387, 1975.

4. Drasar, B.S. and Hill, M.J. in Human Intestinal Flora, Academic Press (London) 1974.

5. Holdeman, L.V. and Moore, W.E.C. in Anaerobe Laboratory Manual, 3rd Edition, V.P.I Press (Blacksburg), 1975

III. Practical problems in substituting sugar in various foods

Moderator: D.A.M. Mackay, New York
Co-Moderator: P. M. Vincent, Lestrem

Health and Sugar Substitutes
Proc. ERGOB Conf., Geneva 1978, pp. 124-129 (Karger, Basel 1978)

SORBITOL AS A SUGAR SUBSTITUTE: SOME FACTORS CLOUDING
NEW PRODUCT PROSPECTS

Donald A. M. Mackay, B. A. Ph. D.

Research and Development, Life Savers, Inc., 40 West 57th Street,
New York, N. Y. 10019, U. S. A.

Sorbitol, a hexahydroxyhexane derived from the hydrogenation of glucose
and commonly but loosely called a sugar alcohol, meets the definition of a
sugar substitute very well. It has the bulk and appearance of sugar and it is
fairly sweet; it is colorless, crystalline, and very soluble in water, forming
syrupy solutions. It is safe, being metabolized by the body as if it were
fructose. Since its metabolism does not involve insulin, some doctors think
it valuable in diets for diabetics. Many others, however, who think total
caloric restriction should be the major dietary goal for diabetics, note that
sorbitol is iso-caloric with sugar and frown on unrestricted use. Dentists,
more concerned with events in the mouth than the gut, note that oral bacteria
are unable to utilize sorbitol, since the hydroxyl groups give no ready handle
for attack, and no acid is formed before oral clearance occurs.

The term "sugar substitute" itself is capable of several meanings. It
can mean a substance with (usually intense) sweetness, or one without calories; or one without insulin requirement; or a substance harmless to teeth.
Sorbitol, though only half as sweet as sucrose, has many of the bulk properties of sugar without the diabetic and dental drawbacks. Sorbitol ought to be
the ideal sugar substitute. Yet sorbitol usage in foods is miniscule compared
with sugar usage. Even in confectionery, sorbitol plays a very minor role.
Only in one form of confection, namely "sugarless" gum, is there any significant use at all. In the U. S. an estimated 32 million pounds of sorbitol end
up in sugarless gum for roughly a quarter of the total chewing gum market.
In Europe, excluding France where sorbitol gum is not permitted, sorbitol
may soon account for about one pack of gum out of every three sold. The
anomaly represented by this extremely successful but narrow substitution for
sugar needs to be examined. Why hasn't there been a wider range of success
stories with this "ideal" sugar substitute?

Sorbitol, with a long history of safety, is a permitted additive in most countries, and a large number of food and non-food uses have grown up over the years since sorbitol became a commercial commodity.

Its usage in foods and the regulatory patterns which govern it tend to become intertwined as regulatory pressures, which try to restrain new uses, equilibrate with the counter pressures from sorbitol producers and food manufacturers who have built new markets (or wish to) for their sorbitol-containing products. One consequence is that potential or novel food uses of sorbitol, or of any food additive for that matter, tend to be legislated out of existence on the theory it is easier to regulate and control new dietary inputs than proscribe them after the event. This is certainly not retrograde in public health terms, but, alas, is too frequently tardigrade in regulatory terms in permitting development of new products. The purpose here is not to inveigh against the very desirable control of chemicals added to our food supply, but rather to point out that usage patterns of all kinds are tending to be frozen. For the future, therefore, the food usage of sorbitol (whether considered food or chemical) as a replacement for sugar will almost certainly reflect the current usage pattern.

It should be emphasized that many uses of food grade sorbitol (and also food uses of sorbitol) are not those of a sugar substitute. Sorbitol's humectant properties are useful in a variety of products. Sorbitol consumption, however, as indicated, has risen dramatically in recent years in only one major category of sugar substitution, namely that of a non-cariogenic bulking agent. The other potential major use, as a non-insulin-requiring sweetener, has never been realized as medical opinion, once bitterly divided over sorbitol's safety for diabetics, now seems to stress that sorbitol's use by diabetics should be discouraged for general reasons of caloric restriction, rather than for sorbitol's biochemical specifics in human metabolism.

The word "sugarless" is key to understanding sorbitol's future usage pattern as a sugar substitute. Unlike diet drinks, which are sugarless because they are non-caloric, sugarless confections are based on the traditionally exclusive use of sugar in confectionery, i.e. they are sugarless because they do not contain the sugar historically necessary for confection-

ery. This rationale has been under recent attack in the U.S., particularly
by consumer advocates, on the grounds that "sugarless" means "no
calories" and that dieters, diabetics, etc. will be misled by sorbitol confections which are iso-caloric with sugar. There was vigorous representation by the U.S. dental profession as to the value of the term "sugarless" in its dental context, but soon all sorbitol candy products that claim
a sugarless dental benefit will be required to make it clear they are not
non-caloric, as well as continuing to specify how many calories each confection contributes to the dietary.

Though many foods containing high levels of sugar can be considered
dental threats, these foods, under present regulatory attitudes, are not
(and without meeting rigorous test conditions can not be) candidates for
sorbitol substitution if the intent is to make and identify a dentally
improved product. The trouble lies in the non-sorbitol part of the food,
i.e. starches, proteins, dextrins, etc. Without clinical proof of non-
cariogenicity, which is the technical equivalent of "not promoting tooth
decay", and hence the word "sugarless" in its dental sense, the maker
of such a food has great problems calling the consumer's attention to the
fact that his food now has sorbitol in place of sucrose.

As a result of these factors, it can be seen that only certain types
of sugary foods can be candidates for sorbitol substitution. The food must
be almost 100% sugar, or 100% sugar extractables, to start with, so that
the new product can contribute only sorbitol or similar polyols to the oral
environment. Practically, only confections, and even then only certain
types of these, are candidates. Chewing gum, bubble gum, pressed mints,
hard candy (boiled sweets) and some gelled products can qualify, but for
technical reasons only the chewing gums and pressed tablets (mints) are
capable of even being made with sorbitol under normal processing conditions, and offered to the public as an economic substitute for the sugar-
based product.

There are other products where sorbitol has been substituted for sugar that meet the criteria given, for example, sorbitol chocolate and boiled sweets. But high processing costs, coupled with sorbitol's price differential over sugar, result in a high-priced item for a small market with a compelling, usually medical, reason to buy.

One other important factor determines the likely extent of sorbitol substitution for sucrose in foods. This is the laxation potential of large (50 g) amounts of sorbitol. As a consequence, the emphasis in sugar substitution again moves to confections whose small size (2 g) and consumption pattern effectively preclude the appearance of laxative effects.

For several reasons, therefore, sorbitol's use as a sugar substitute in "foods with dental benefit" is likely to continue in its present highly restricted areas of chewing gum and tabletted confections of the pressed mint type. But this does not explain the present far greater use of sorbitol in gum than in pressed mints. To seek an explanation, at least in the U.S., one must recall the moderate sweetening power of sorbitol and the standard requirement for high sweetness in confectionery. Even when artificial sweeteners were available, mixtures of natural and artificial sweeteners were in general forbidden because of long-standing concepts of pure foods (avoidance of food adulteration), and prevention of deception (economic loss) of customers wishing to buy sugar in food products. For a highly technical reason, U.S. law permitted a special use of saccharin in chewing gum, but in no other confection, on the basis the sweetness of saccharin was needed for the mastic component of the gum and not its nutritive sweetener content.

As a result of marked consumer preference, sorbitol chewing gum has grown rapidly in favor, and perhaps a third of all gums will soon be of the sugarless type. Tabletted confections, until very recently, had a very minor market share, being markedly less sweet than their sugar counterparts.

Sugarless gum with saccharin gradually improved in flavor until consumers either saw no difference between it and sugar gum, or actually began to prefer the "sugarless" taste. The impact of the removal of saccharin from North America upon "sugarless" confections has yet to be seen. Good, safe artificial sweeteners are needed to boost sorbitol's sweetness in order to maintain the conversion rate of between-meal snacks (like sugary confections) to their dentally preferred analogues based on sorbitol.

Xylitol-sweetened sorbitol gums have recently made an appearance, presenting both taste advantages and processing disadvantages, a discussion of which is of interest only to a very narrow audience.

Also outside the scope of this paper, though a general account will be given, is a technical analysis of the various forms and grades of sorbitol available which have very important bearing on ease of manufacture (processing costs) and, in some instances, of consumer acceptance. There have also been related flavor developments which give hope that certain chewing gum products will maintain or improve their consumer acceptance in spite of the loss of artificial sweeteners. Flavor developments such as these may also give impetus to consumer acceptance (on dental grounds) of sorbitol substitution for sugar in products such as jams and jellies where the prerequisites of small portions and absence of dentally compromising food components (such as starch, protein and food acids) can perhaps be met.

To avoid charges of undue pessimism, the prospects of general sorbitol substitution for sugar in the food supply should be re-examined. On the supposition (perhaps not entirely valid) that replacement (even partial) of sugar by sorbitol is a dentally progressive step, the food manufacturer wishing to embrace this dental dogma has four main factors to consider.

1. What additional formulation changes are forced on him by being deprived of sugar's functional properties? How many new food additives will he need? Will public antipathy to these additives affect sales? Will the public pay for the extra cost of sorbitol, additives and reformulation?

2. Is he in a country that permits use of an artificial or non-cariogenic nutritive sweetener in order to compensate for the loss of sweetness consequent to sugar substitution by sorbitol?

3. Will sorbitol used in his product have laxative effects in his customers?

4. Is he willing to make this change silently - except for mandatory ingredient listing - or may he call attention to it? Do regulations in his country permit him to label or advertise his product as sugarless, sugar-free, less sugar, sugar-reduced, less cariogenic, non-cariogenic, less or not harmful to teeth, or even kind, good or better for teeth?

Until the various proponents of less sugar in foods are prepared to use their well-honed powers of advocacy in support of regulatory changes that would give the food manufacturer at least the chance to comply with their wishes, the prospects for further substitution of sugar with sorbitol, or for that matter with other non-cariogenic bulking agents, (or even air or water, were it possible) must appear clouded. Lest it be thought this is an antiregulatory statement (which it is not), one might note that sugarless gum, the one successful example of sorbitol usage, is available in many highly regulated countries, but not all.

As far as sorbitol technology is involved in making dentally improved products, there are only the two major product classes to consider. In pressed mints, standard tabletting technology is used, with various grades of crystal sorbitol from different sorbitol suppliers often having their own peculiarities to be compensated for. In chewing gum, different sorbitol manufacturers produce types of sorbitol which are not readily substitutable one for another. Even minor differences in crystal size and size distribution require great skill and effort by the technologist in reformulation and choice of gum base, and in making apparently minor processing changes which are nevertheless vitally important for economic production and consumer acceptance. There is an art here defying scientific study, and especially obscure when sorbitol is mixed with other polyalcohols. For hard candy, a minor category, the key technology is use of seed crystals to hasten the setting step after the depositing or molding step. This is only the briefest description of processes often so arcane and esoteric the producer himself is hard put to make a product that is consistently acceptable.

SUMMARY

Sorbitol substitution for sugar can be expected to grow in confectionery, with probably increasing emphasis on forms other than sugarless gum, (the presently dominant product) and increasing hopes for dental benefits. In dental terms, hope for progress can be seen for substitution in other foods where requirements for portion control and absence of dentally compromising components can be met, especially where artificial sweeteners or non-cariogenic nutritive sweeteners are available to the food technologist. Hopes for substitution of sorbitol for sugar in the bulk of the food supply may be dentally desirable, but would be wildly impractical, widely implausible, and wisely forgotten.

Health and Sugar Substitutes
Proc. ERGOB Conf., Geneva 1978, pp. 130-137 (Karger, Basel 1978)

XYLITOL: FOOD APPLICATIONS OF A NONCARIOGENIC SUGAR SUBSTITUTE

FELIX VOIROL

Xyrofin Ltd., A Joint Venture of F. Hoffmann-La Roche & Co. Ltd.
and the Finnish Sugar Co., Lättichstrasse 8a, 6340 Baar,
Switzerland.

INTRODUCTION

This presentation is meant to initiate discussion on a hitherto
neglected aspect of xylitol use in foods: Making use of the
characteristic physical, chemical and microbiological properties
of the polyol in formulating new products or procedures.

After a decade of use in parenteral nutrition, industrial
quantities for food use became available in 1974, thus the food
technologist has had only a short interval in which to develop
xylitol products.[1] If, for reasons of compatibility or economics,
the intake of xylitol must be limited, then its most meaningful
use would be to replace sucrose in those foods, which are known
to cause most damage to the teeth. If, however, use on a broader
base would be warranted, specific functional applications should
be considered.

PROPERTIES SUGGESTING NEW APPLICATIONS

A comparison of xylitol with sweeteners normally used in food
processing shows a number of properties, unique for the pentitol.
These properties make xylitol more than a mere sugar substitute.
The sweetener can play new functional roles or simplify
conventional procedures.

Table 1   PROPERTIES OF SOME NATURAL SUGARS AND SUGAR ALCOHOLS

Properties	Sucrose	Dextrose	Sorbitol	Fructose	Xylitol
Molecule	(structure)	(structure)	(structure)	(structure)	(structure)
Molecular Weight	$C_{12}H_{22}O_{11}$ 343.3	$C_6H_{12}O_6$ 180.2	$C_6H_{14}O_6$ 182.2	$C_6H_{12}O_6$ 180.2	$C_5H_{12}O_5$ 152.2
Melting Point	$185^{\circ}C$	$146^{\circ}C$	$110^{\circ}C$	$103^{\circ}C$	$94^{\circ}C$
Stability of Melt	Decomposes	Decomposes	Crystallises	Decomposes	Metastable
Equilibrium Moisture Content at 78% rah + $20^{\circ}C$	0.05%		33%	45%	7%
Solubility in Water at $20^{\circ}C$/100g solution	84g			70g	66g
Viscosity of conc. Solution in Water, $20^{\circ}C$	233cP		150 cP		30 cP
Physical Calories	4cal/g	4cal/g	4cal/g	4cal/g	4cal/g
Non-enzymatic Browning Reactions	after inversion	+	-	+	-
Rel. Sweetness in 10% aqueous solution	1	0.5	0.5	1.25	1
Caloric Density $\frac{(Caloric\ Value)}{(Rel.Sweetness)}$	4	8	8	3.2	4
Cariogenicity	++	++	(-) acidogenic	+	-
Fermentation by Yeasts	+	+	-	+	-
Conditional Suitability for Diabetics	-	-	+	+	+

RELATIVE SWEETNESS

While lending sweetness to food, sucrose will also add to its bulk. Our "standard" everyday sweetener thus fulfils the dual function of sweetening and body-giving. When substituting sucrose in food, the food technologist must attempt to maintain sweetness. All conventional sugar replacers present problems in this area. Fig. 1 exemplifies iso-sweet composite foods.

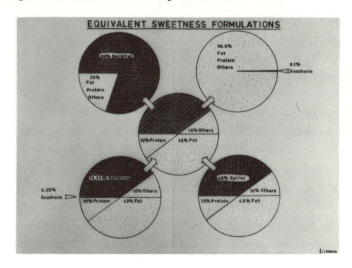

EQUIVALENT SWEETNESS FORMULATIONS

Fig. 1

Sorbitol, being about half as sweet as sucrose, will add twice as much bulk. Artificial sweeteners will bring hardly any bulk at

all. Combinations of both will restore the sweetness/bulk ratio
of sucrose, but they are inferior in taste. Xylitol is the only
sweetener with the same sweetness as sucrose. Although there are
minor deviations caused by low pH or high temperature, the
sweetness of sucrose and xylitol is similar, despite dissimilar
molecules. Besides its demonstrated non-cariogenicity, this is
the most important property of the polyol.[2] Xylitol-sweetened
foods organoleptically approach the quality of standard sucrose-
sweetened foods.

MICROBIOLOGICAL STABILITY

It has been shown, that xylitol is not fermentable by
cariogenic oral microorganisms.[3,4] The main commercial application
at present, based on these findings is chewing gum. Regular
consumption of xylitol chewing gum seems to have an effect on
caries incidence beyond the mere absence of sucrose as evidenced
by the Turku Chewing Gum Study.[5] In part, this may be attributed
to the cumulated effects of a non-cariogenic sweetener combined
with the saliva-stimulating properties of chewing elastomers.

Strains of bacteria, molds and yeasts, known to cause spoilage
in sugar-containing foods have been tested with regard to their
capacity for metabolizing xylitol.[6] Results seem to indicate that
most of the microorganisms tested are unable to utilize low
levels of xylitol as an energy source.

In consequence, xylitol can replace sucrose in applications
involving a syrup phase. Syrups made with sucrose, either in
galenics or in foods must depend on high sucrose concentration to
avoid microbial fermentation. Lowering sugar concentration will
also lower osmotic pressure and the use of preserving agents
becomes necessary. Xylitol solutions being microbiologically
stable, even at low osmotic pressure, allow the formulation of
low-sweetness, thus lower calorie syrups, provided the remaining
ingredients are also non-fermentable.[7]

CHEMICAL STABILITY

The overall chemical stability of xylitol is excellent.
Aqueous solutions are stable at food-processing temperatures.
There is no polymerisation below the boiling point of 216°C.[8]

No esterification, detectable by GC, occurred when heating
xylitol in the presence of citric acid in water at 120°C during
two hours.[9]

In food processing, disaccharides and reducing sugars
sometimes participate in non-enzymatic browning reactions with
amino acids. These so-called Maillard reactions can be either
desirable as in the case of flavour-formation (bread-crust,
roast meat) or unwanted as in the case of discolouration
(caramelisation, off-flavours). Unavoidable they are accelerated
by high processing temperatures and continue during storage.
Aldo- or keto groups, needed in these reactions, are absent in
xylitol, thus substitution of sucrose, lactose, glucose or invert
sugar results in more stable products, i.e. a longer shelf life.

COOLING EFFECT

The heat required to dissolve one gram of xylitol in water,
34.8 cal (145.6 Joules), is the highest known value of sugars or
sugar alcohols.[10]

In food use, the highly endothermic dissolution means that the
consumption of xylitol in solid form results in an actual cooling
of the saliva. This property is considered pleasant by
manufacturers as it is a purely physical phenomenon contrary to
the physiological false "cooling" of menthol.[11] Thus "refreshing"
products become possible with flavours other than peppermint.

Fig.2 shows the temperature drop occurring when variable amounts
of xylitol are dissolved in water. The graph is meant to
illustrate the extent of cooling rather than to advocate the use
of xylitol in self-cooling drink mixes.

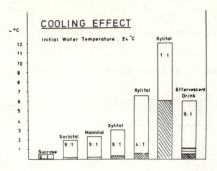

Fig.2

CRYSTALLISATION PROPERTIES

Another outstanding property of xylitol, permitting simplification of conventional techniques in confectionery manufacture, is its crystallisation behaviour. The polyol was first reported to melt at 61°C.[12] Later it was found to exhibit bimorphism: - A monoclinic form, melting at 61°C and a orthorombic form melting at 94°C. The former is metastable and changes into the stable, rhombic form.[13] No melting point depression was shown in a mixture of the two form.[14] Commercially produced xylitol is of the orthorombic form with a melting point of 94°C and a boiling point of 216°. The melt readily recrystallises, yielding 45.3 cal/g (189.2 J/g) in heat of crystallisation.[15] In a closed container, pure xylitol melt or supersaturated solutions are stable, even if contaminated by 1% dust or iron oxide.

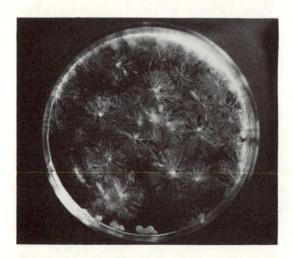

Fig.3

In open containers, dust triggers crystallisation, as does
seeding with xylitol crystals or cavitation with ultrasonics.[16]
Contrary to sucrose or sucrose/glucose systems, recycling of the
crystallisation-melting process is possible without noticeable
change. The fundamental differences in crystallisation properties
between sucrose and xylitol allow the introduction of simplified
procedures in confectionery and pharmaceutical applications.
Hard candies or cough drops can be prepared by the depositing
process using a waterfree mixture of xylitol melt and powdered
xylitol at the melting point. The absence of water makes boiling
unnecessary and the rapid recrystallisation requires less space,
machinery, processing time and energy.[17]

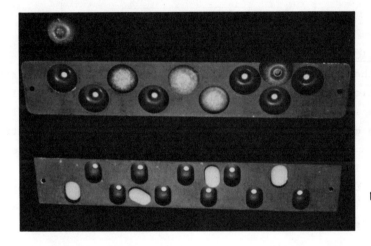

Fig.4

Coated tablets from xylitol or mixtures of xylitol and sorbitol
are possible by sintering the surface of direct compressed tablets
in a hot air stream. Fluidised beds gave best results. The
tablets, suspended in air slightly above the melting point will
melt on the surface, evidenced by their glossy appearance. The
longer the hot air treatment, the deeper the coating layer will
be. After switching to the cold air inlet, the surface
recrystallises leaving a tablet core surrounded by a hard coating.
Ten minutes of fluidisation increased the hardness of one
kilogram pure xylitol tablets from 6.7 to 19.6 strong cobb

units.[18] The procedure may bring substantial savings when used
instead of the conventional pan-coating process, which takes many
hours and requires skilled specialists.

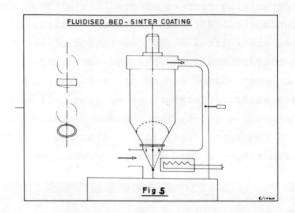

FLUIDISED BED- SINTER COATING

Fig 5

CONCLUSION

At the present time, the main use for xylitol is in caries
prevention. Within the scope of highly cariogenic confectionery,
a replacement of sucrose/glucose is especially indicated in
chewing gum. There are 17 xylitol chewing gums in 11 countries.
For a number of reasons, confectionery will continue to be the
main outlet for some time, but technolgical uses are bound to
follow. One wide-open field of research, both in caries prevention
and application technology, remains in combinations such as
xylitol/sorbitol/Lycasin.

The purpose of this presentation is fulfilled if it can serve
to initiate discussion on new functional applications of xylitol
as a sugar substitute.

REFERENCES

1.   Horecker, B.L. Lang, K. and Takagi, Y. (1969) Pentoses and
      Pentitols, Springer.

2.   Lindley, M.G., Birch, G.G. and Khan, R. (1975) J. Sci. Food
      Agric. 27, 140.

3.   Gehring, F., Mäkinen, K.K., Larmas, M. and Scheinin, A.
      (1975) Acta Odont. Scand. 33, Supplementum 70.

4.   Schneider, P. and Mühlemann, H.R. (1976) Schweiz. Monats-
      schrift für Zahnheilkunde, 86, 150.

5.   Scheinin, A. and Mäkinen, K.K. (1975) Acta Odont. Scand.
      XVIII. 269.

6.   Böhni, E. (1978) F.Hoffmann-La Roche Ltd.Basel. Personal
      Communication.

7.   Nehring, P. (1973) Konserveninstitut, Braunschweig.
      Personal Communication.

8.   Manz, U., Vanninen, E. and Voirol, F. Food R.A., Leather-
      head (1973).

9.   Manz, U. and Meier, H. (1977) F.Hoffmann-La Roche Ltd.Basel.
      Personal Communication.

10.   Mangold, M. (1971) F.Hoffmann-La Roche Ltd.Basel. Personal
      Communication.

11.   Hammond, J.E. and Streckfus, T.K. (1975) U.S. Patent
      3'899'593.

12.   Wolfrom, M.L. and Kohn, E.J. (1942) J.Am. Chem. Soc. 217,251.

13.   Carson, J.F., Waisbrot, S.W. and Jones, F.T. (1943) J. Am.
      Chem. Soc. 65, 1777.

14.   Kim, H.S. and Jeffrey, G.A. (1969) Acta Cryst. 25, 2607.

15.   Guex, W., Kläui,H., Pauling, H. and Voirol, F., German
      (1977) Patent Appl. 2747664.

16.   Voirol, F. International Symposium on Sugar, Science and
      Technology, University of Reading (1978)Appl.Sci.Publishers.

17.   Voirol, F. and Brugger, W. (1976) Swiss Patent Appl. 8633.

18.   Voirol, F. (1978), Swiss Patent Application.

Health and Sugar Substitutes
Proc. ERGOB Conf., Geneva 1978, pp. 138-144 (Karger, Basel 1978)

PALATINIT® - TECHNOLOGICAL PROPERTIES

H. Schiweck

Central-Laboratory of Süddeutsche Zucker-AG, Postfach 1127,
D-6718 Grünstadt 1, Germany

Palatinit®, hydrogenated isomaltulose is the equimolecular mixture of α-D-glucopyranosyl-1,6-sorbitol (isomaltitol, GPS) and α-D-glucopyranosyl-1,6-mannitol (GPM). Both of the substances belong to the group of disaccharide alcohols which have found increasing interest in the field of physiology of nutrition during the last 10 years.

Isomaltitol was first prepared in gramme range by Wolfrom[1] in 1952 by reducing isomaltose with hydrogen in the presence of Raney nickel as catalyst. This method is not suitable for the production of isomaltitol on an industrial scale because of the complicated production of isomaltose - one gramme of isomaltose costs even today over DM 100,--.

A cheaper process is based on isomaltulose which can easily be produced from sucrose with the help of a microbiological process[2] (figure 1).
If the reduction of isomaltulose is carried out in alkaline medium and under definite reaction conditions (pressure, temperature, concentration), one gets isomaltitol over isomaltose which is produced as an intermediate. Reduction of isomaltose in neutral medium and at higher concentrations yields a mixture of isomaltitol and α-D-glucopyranosyl-1,6-mannitol[3]. Because of their different solubility patterns both the components of this mixture can be separated easily through fractional crystallisation from water. Both of the substances, isomaltitol as well as GPM crystallize readily from water and can therefore be prepared with any required purity. Whereas GPM crystallizes with 2 mols of crystal

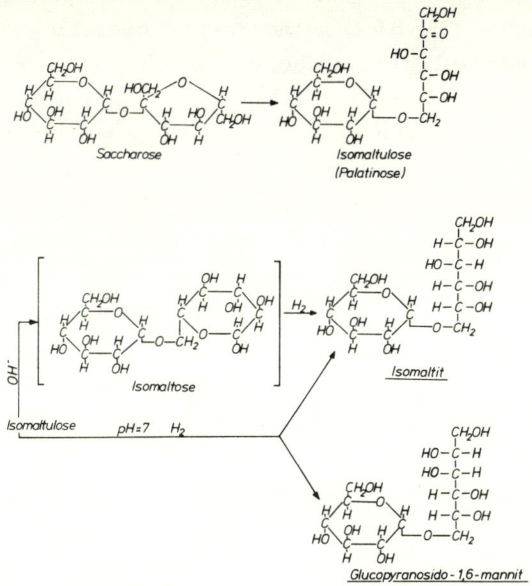

Fig. 1: Preparation of isomaltitol and glucopyranosyl-1,6-
        mannitol from sucrose

water, the crystals of isomaltitol are water free.

Table 1 shows the important chemical and physical properties of
isomaltitol and GPM in comparison with those of other new sugar
substitutes.

Table 1:

	Disaccharide bond	Hydrolysis products	Melting point °C	Specific rotation α	Solubility in water at 20°C g/100 g	Sweetening power sucrose = 1
L-sorbose	-	-	159 - 165	-42,7 → -43,4	44	0,9
maltitol	α-1,4	D-glucose D-sorbitol	?	~ + 90		~ 0,75
maltotriitol	α-1,4; α-1,6		?	~ + 95		~ 0,75
lactitol	β-1,4	D-galactose D-sorbitol	146 (ethanol) ~72 aq.ethanol	+ 14		~ 0,5
isomaltitol	α-1,6	D-glucose D-sorbitol	168	+ 90,5	58	0,45
glucopyranosyl-1,6-mannitol	α-1,6	D-glucose D-mannitol	173,5	+ 90,5	18	0,45

The most important criterion for the enzyme- or acid activated
hydrolysis of disaccharide alcohols is the nature of their di-

saccharide bond. The higher the energy content of a bond between glycosidic hydroxyl groups the easier it is to split (for example sucrose) whereas a bond with the lowest energy content, for example 1,6-bond is the most difficult to split. Thus sucrose can be completely hydrolysed in 0,01 normal hydrochloric acid at 100°C in less than half an hour whereas for the complete hydrolysis of isomaltitol in 1 n hydrochloric acid one needs at least two hours. In 0,1 n hydrochloric acid isomaltitol is split only to an extent of 2/3 even after 10 hours and at 100°C (fig. 2). One needs three hours to completely hydrolyse α-D-glucopyranosyl-1,6-mannitol in 2 n hydrochloric acid at 100°C. In comparison to it the acid activated hydrolysis of lactitol is only negligibly slower than that for lactose[4].

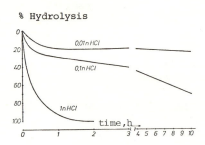

Fig. 2: Hydrolysis of isomaltitol against time at 100°C and different acid concentrations

The extent to which different disaccharide alcohols can be split through enzymatic action, their suitability as substrate for the dextran (plaque) production in the mouth, their cariogenic properties and their importance from the view point of nutritional physiology shall be discussed elsewhere. Besides nutritional and cariogenic properties of sugar substitutes following properties are important for the decision to use these products in food stuffs and beverages:

- their sweetening power and taste-pattern,
- their body giving and
- technological properties like solubility, melting point, stability against heat, acids and alkalis and the property to undergo browning reactions.

Because of their high sweetening power the synthetic sweeteners
constitute only a minor component of formulations and therefore
possess no body giving properties. This is the principal difference between synthetic sweeteners and sweetening hydrocarbons.

As the figures in table 1 show, both GPS and GPM have about the
same sweetening power of 0,45. As the sweetening power of isomaltulose is also about 0,4, these compounds confirm the theory
of Cheang-Kuan Lee and Gordon G. Birch[5] which says that in case of
disaccharides with the same disaccharide bond, only the glucosyl
component is the determining factor for the sweetening power and
that the sweetening power of saccharide alcohols does not differ
much from that of the corresponding reducing sugars[6]. However if
one considers the following figures then the nature of the disaccharide bond does seem to have an influence on the sweetening
power:

sucrose	α-1,2-bond	sweetening power	1,0
maltitol	α-1,4-bond	sweetening power	0,63
isomaltitol	α-1,6-bond	sweetening power	0,45

In case of comparisons of sweetening power in aquous solutions one
must however take into consideration that such comparisons are not
generally valid but that the taste pattern and intensity of
"sweetness" are applicable only to one particular product with
exactly defined composition. Thus it is quite possible that the
sweetening power of one and the same substance is different in a
non-alcoholic beverage from that in chocolate.

In the case of solid foods and sweets which contain the major part
of the sugars in solid or crystalline form, additional taste
feelings can occur as the sugars go into solution. Thus the pronounced cooling effect experienced as the sugar alcohols xylitol
and sorbitol go into solution is a property which may not be
acceptable in all products. Palatinit® does not show this effect,
its taste pattern is pure sweet and very similar to that of sucrose. The melting point is an important technological criterion for
sugars when they are used in foodstuffs like hard or soft drops,
chocolate etc. which contain little or no water. As seen

from table 1 the melting points of isomaltitol and GPM are of the
same order of magnitude as sucrose, the melting point of the mixture, Palatinit® lies between 140° and 145°C.

Further, it is important whether heat treatment causes structural
changes like water elimination which would lead to caramel like
products. This is not the case with α-D-glucopyranosyl-1,6-manni-
tol and α-D-glucopyranosyl-1,6-sorbitol as far as they are pure.
The heat treatment of Palatinit® in solid or liquid form does
neither lead to structural changes nor to reactions with other
components of the formulation. Thus a browning (Maillard reaction)
is also not possible.
Table 1 shows also the solubilities of different sugars in water
at 20°C. The solubilities of crystalline isomaltitol and GPM in
relation to temperature are shown in fig. 3.

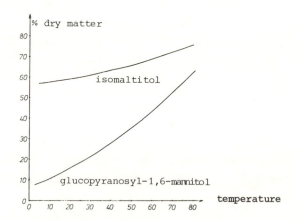

Fig. 3: Solubility of isomaltitol and glucopyranosyl-1,6-
         mannitol in water at different temperatures

The solubility of isomaltitol and glucopyranosyl-1,6-mannitol in
temperature range under 70°C is lower than that of sucrose but it
is still high enough to allow a further processing of these
substances. GPM crystallizes out upon cooling from a saturated
solution of Palatinit® at elevated temperature. This fact must be
taken into consideration if Palatinit® solutions oversaturated
at 20°C as for example in jams with a dry matter content of over

50%, are to be produced. The recrystallization can be prevented through recipe adaptation.

As shown in figure 4 the viscosity of aquous solutions of Palatinit® is of the same order of magnitude as of sucrose solution.

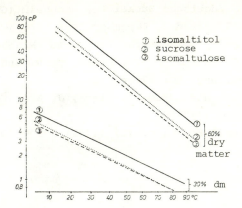

Fig. 4: Viscosities of isomaltitol, sucrose and isomaltulose at differenct concentrations and temperatures

The hygroscopicity of the components used plays an important role in the water retaining power and keeping qualitites of food stuffs. Isomaltitol and glucopyranosyl-1,6-mannitol as well as their equimolecular mixture Palatinit® are not hygroscopic.

At a semi-technical scale Palatinit® has been used to date to produce drops, chocolate slabs, bars, marzipan products, chewing gum, ice cream, jams, pre-mixed doughs and cakes, icings for cookies, puddings and beverages. Moreover crystalline Palatinit® has been used as sweetener for coffee and tea.

REFERENCES

1. Wolfrom, M. L., Thompson, A., O'Neill, A. N.
   and Galkowski, T. T., J. Amer. Chem. Soc. 74: 1062 (1952)
2. DT-PS 2 217 628 dated 12. April 1972
   Patented by Süddeutsche Zucker-AG, Mannheim (Germany)
3. DT-OS 2 520 173 dated 2. December 1976
   Patent applied by Süddeutsche Zucker-AG, Mannheim (Germany)
4. Wolfrom, M. L., Burke, W. J., Brown, K. R. and Rose, R. S.,
   J. Amer. Chem. Soc. 60: 571 (1938)
5. Cheang-Kuan Lee and Gordon G. Birch, J. Sci. Fd. Agric.
   26: 1513 - 1521 (1975)
6. Cheang-Kuan Lee, Fd. Chem. (2) (1977), 95 - 105

Health and Sugar Substitutes
Proc. ERGOB Conf., Geneva 1978, pp. 145-152 (Karger, Basel 1978)

TECHNOLOGICAL PROBLEMS IN THE INCORPORATION OF HYDROGENATED GLUCOSE SYRUPS
AND L-SORBOSE

M. ZIMMERMANN

Food Department - Roquette Frères - 62136 LESTREM (F)

INTRODUCTION

A great number of saccharose nutritive substitutes have been presented
during these ten last years, either in a view to remedy certain metabolic
deficiencies (e. g. sweet diabetes), or to limit dental caries. Fructose and
products obtained by hydrogenation of sugars (Sorbitol, Mannitol, a special
Lycasin 80/55 (hydrogenated Glucose Syrup from Roquette Frères), and Xylitol)
have experienced an impressive development in many fields.

Roquette Frères also found that the L-Sorbose is not or only slightly
fermented by mouth bacterias and that it may have some technological advantages
with regard to other saccharose substitutes, such as polyols.

We shall only discuss the nature, properties and technological applications
of these products. Physiological aspects, regulations and, especially, the
interest in the problems of dental caries are not the subject of our study,
but are mentioned in references.

A/ HYDROGENATED GLUCOSE SYRUP (LYCASIN 80/55)

Lycasin 80/55 is a hydrogenated Glucose Syrup particularly recommended
for production of hard-boiled candy, chewy-toffee, chewing-gum (for the
plastifying phase) and gum candy.

It corresponds to conventional tests proving that it is practically not
fermentable in the mouth by bacterias and enzymes : verified for instance by
statements as "Zahnschonend" according to Swiss legislation.

1. COMPOSITION OF LYCASIN 80/55

The components of LYCASIN 80/55 are the hydrogenated analogues of the
components in the Glucose syrup.

- Dextrose (d-Glucose) $\longrightarrow$ Sorbitol (6 to 8 %)
- Disaccharides $\longrightarrow$ Hydrogenated disaccharides (50 to 55 %)
- Trisaccharides $\longrightarrow$ Hydrogenated trisaccharides (20 to 25 %)
- Polysaccharides $\longrightarrow$ Hydrogenated polysaccharides (10 to 20%)

2. GENERAL PROPERTIES

   2.1. Viscosity : LYCASIN 80/55 is very fluid (see data sheet) and may be
        cold-stored.

   2.2. Crystallization : LYCASIN 80/55 does not crystallize even at high
        concentrations and in dry form. Contrary to other anti-caries powder-
        products such as sorbitol - mannitol - sorbose - xylitol, LYCASIN is
        anticrystallizing.

   2.3. Hygroscopicity : LYCASIN 80/55 gives final products with a lower
        balance moisture content that in sugar candy. LYCASIN 80/55 candy
        are more hygroscopic. In hard-boiled candy for instance, which can
        not recrystallize, the surface will get hygroscopic if moisture is
        present ; therefore it is necessary to use individual and special
        wrapping.

   2.4. Reducing ability - brown colouring : LYCASIN 80/55 has not any redu-
        cing ability. It is therefore very stable and less sensitive to
        reactions of the brown-colouring temperature. At very high temperature,
        it is possible to make a colourless and clear candy.

   2.5. Sweet taste : the sweetness of LYCASIN 80/55 (approx. 75 % of
        Saccharose) is sufficient in most candy types and there is no need
        of any addition of artificial sweeteners. In case of soft drinks, its
        sweet flavour is often insufficient.

   2.6. Flavours : LYCASIN 80/55 has a pleasant taste and goes very well
        together with flavours used in sugar candy. As its sweetness is
        weaker than those of Saccharose, the acidity appears more easily. It
        is possible to substantially reduce the acid quantities generally
        used in classic candy.

3. TECHNOLOGICAL APPLICATIONS

   3.1. Hard-boiled candy (Hart Karamellen - Sucre-cuit)

   The manufacture of hard-boiled candy with LYCASIN 80/55 is very simple
as it is sufficient to dehydrate LYCASIN 80/55 as completely as possible, and
then flavour it.

   Tests have shown that it is necessary to use intense boiling (temperature
and vacuum) to obtain the classical crystal structure of hard candy.

   Rest moisture should be near or inferior to 0.5 % (instead of 2 or 3 %
of classical candy). Over and above that value the structure becomes rapidly
"semi-plastic" (1 % humidity for example).

   Evidently no "inversion" may arise.

   It is, thus, necessary to use flavours without water phase.

If the candy is wrapped immediately (while warm), it is not necessary to have airconditioned packing room, but it should be preferred.

3.2. Chewing-gum / Dental caries

With 25 % gum base for instance.

The powder phase may be composed of Sorbitol, Mannitol, Xylitol or Sorbose (these products are not fermentable by the mouth bacterias). The plastifying phase is LYCASIN 80/55 which should have a concentrated D. S. of 85 % (if boiled to 113-114°C = 235°F at atmospheric pressure). The equilibrium relative humidity (E. R. H.) of chewing-gum should be around 60 %, which determines its good shelf-life stability.

3.3. Chewing-toffees / Dental caries

It is necessary that all ingredients of the recipe do not contain any sugar at all which is fermentable by the mouth bacterias. For example, ordinary milk contains Lactose which is very fermentable and which gives negative result in a dental control.

3.4. Jelly-candy

It is possible to produce jellies with gelatine at 220 blooms - neutral pH. At an acid pH, with Lycasin, the gel of the gelatine is worse. Pectine and arabic gum can also be used. All the recipes and technological details are represented in the manufacturer's brochure (LYCASIN 80/55).

4. CONCLUSION

In the field of "SUGARLESS", LYCASIN 80/55 has the advantages to present all the properties of Glucose Syrup in the traditional products, when other sugar substitutes (Sorbitol, Mannitol, Fructose, Xylitol) are small molecules. Consequently it takes a sole but also a complementary part.

5. REFERENCES

1. Brochure D. 67 "LYCASIN 80/55" - Roquette Frères - 62136 Lestrem (F)

2. British patent N° 1.169.538 (example) - Equivalent in other countries.

3. The Roslagen study - Acta Odont. Scand. 32235 - Frostell. 1974

4. Toxicological study - Ind. Biotest Laboratories (U.S.A.), 1969

5. Study of the clinical and biological tolerance of LYCASIN by Human beings. Prof. A. Tacquet's study in the Calmette Hospital in Lille, 1975, and 1978.

6. "Report on LYCASIN 80/55 candies" - H. R. Mühlemann - Zahnärztliches Institut der Universität Zurich, June 1976.

B/ L-SORBOSE

1. NATURE AND MANUFACTURE OF L-SORBOSE

L-SORBOSE was discovered in 1852 by Pelouze in the spontaneously fermented juice of the sorb berry. It is also found in vinegar[29]. In 1896 Bertrand showed that Sorbose could be produced by fermentation from D-Sorbitol by the "Sorbose bacteria" : this is the principle of the modern production of L-Sorbose. The L-SORBOSE obtained is a reducing sugar belonging to the ceto-hexose family. Most natural sugars belong to the D series, but SORBOSE belongs to the L series and its structural formula is :

```
      CH₂OH
       |
      C = O
       |
HO -  C - H
       |
 H -  C - OH
       |
HO -  C - H
       |
      CH₂OH
```

Basic formula : $C_6H_{12}O_6$

Molecular mass : 180

Other sugars of the L series do exist in the nature : e. g. L-Arabinose, L-Galactose, L-Fructose, L-Rhamnose, etc... SORBOSE is identified and determined in final products by gas chromatography.

2. PHYSICAL PROPERTIES OF L-SORBOSE

SORBOSE, a white odourless powder, is slightly hygroscopic and has a sweet taste near to the one of saccharose (comparative sweetness level app. 90 %). This powder consists of orthorhombic colourless crystals.

2.1. Melting point : 159°-165°C

2.2. Specific rotation power : Solutions of Sorbose are laevorotatory and exhibit only slight mutarotation, i. e. :

at 20°C $\alpha \dfrac{20°}{D}$ =   - 43°4 (concentration of solution : 12 %)

at 30°C $\alpha \dfrac{30°}{D}$ =   - 42°7 (concentration of solution : 5 %)

2.3. Solubility in water

The solubility of SORBOSE is pretty similar to that of dextrose (45 % at 20°C, 65 % at 90°C).

2.4. Stability of SORBOSE in powder form at atmospheric humidity

Tests on Sorbose made at 66 % and 80 % relative humidity in comparison with saccharose, sorbitol, mannitol, xylitol and fructose and dextrose monohydrate indicate the following increasing degrees of hygroscopicity.

- Saccharose - Sorbose and Mannitol show the lowest hygroscopicity.
- After that follows dextrose monohydrate.

- and then xylitol
- and then sorbitol - fructose (levulose) which are the most hygroscopic.

In practice these results are related to the solubility, since the occurence of recrystallisation plays an important part in the stability of finished products stored under humid conditions.

3. CHEMICAL PROPERTIES OF L-SORBOSE

Sorbose exhibits reactions which are typical of cetohexoses. Regarding the use of SORBOSE in food products, it is important to remember that Sorbose is a reducing sugar. Consequently, it develops brown colouration at higher temperatures, viz.

- thermal degradation (caramelisation)
- Maillard's reaction in the presence of amino acids derived from proteins.

These colouring reactions do not, or perhaps rarely, occur with the polyols.

4. L-SORBOSE SWEET FLAVOUR

In non-liquid foods (e.g. confectionery, chocolates) the flavour can be estimated as 0,8 to 1 times that of sucrose.

In liquid foods (soft drinks), it is about 0,8 times that of sucrose in the practical gustative tests.

5. FOOD TECHNOLOGY WITH SORBOSE

5.1. Candy

5.1.1. Hard-boiled candy (sucre-cuit dur - Hart Karamellen)

Like sorbitol and xylitol, SORBOSE slows down the solidification of the hard-boiled candy mass. This means that after the boiling (dehydration) and after cooling down, the hardboiled candy does not vitrify immediately and it is, therefore, impossible to work correctly with standard machinery on an ordinary plastic forming line.

SORBOSE is therefore not recommended for use in hard candy, where LYCASIN is more appropriate.

5.1.2. Bonbons - Toffees - Chewy-toffees

Products of the dairy industry should be free from lactose (which is readily fermentable by mouth-bacteria), when used with Sorbose.

Lycasin is generally used for production of this group of products and is especially recommended for chewy-toffees (Kaubonbons). If caramelisation is necessary, SORBOSE may be added in small quantities.

5.1.3. Compressed candy

SORBOSE G (large-size particles) can be used in the production of compressed candy in presence of usual compression agents (0.5 % of magnesium stearate for example).

5.1.4. Chewing-gum

SORBOSE F (small-size particles), with a particle size of approx. 100 microns can be used as the "powder"-fraction of chewing-gum.

The liquid phase could consist of :

- Either liquid sorbitol of 85 % DS
- Or Lycasin of 85 % DS

The recipe is similar to the standard recipe, i. e. :

- 25 to 30 % gum base
- 50 to 55 % sorbose
- 20 % Lycasin of 85 % DS

NB. To obtain approximately 85 % DS it is sufficient to concentrate by boiling to 113°C. This 85 % DS value is necessary in the final chewing-gum to produce correct equilibrium relative humidity : 60-70 % will give a good shelf-life stability.

SORBOSE F used as a coating mixture on the surface gives a good protection against stickiness.

5.1.5. "Crystallisation" of the surface to cover finished products of a hygroscopic nature (e. g. Jelly-candy)

SORBOSE crystals with pectin, gelatine and arabic gum incorporated in a base of polyols (Sorbitol - Xylitol or Lycasin) on the surface of various jellied candy ensure a good protection of these products.

5.2. Chocolates

It is possible to use SORBOSE in the production of a good tasting chocolate by means of standard chocolate manufacturing procedure without any difficulties. The use of other substitutes in chocolate manufacturing may present some techno-logical problems.

The same process can be applied for milk chocolate recipe. But it is important to use a lactose-free dairy product such as casein or proteins derived from milk or from other proteins.

The Sorbose-chocolate may even be used as an enrobing couverture.

6. OTHER PRODUCTS

The application of Sorbose in various foodstuffs can be suggested as an attempt to overcome the problem of dental caries, which are almost certainly established as directly related to the intake of standard sugars. The proper-ties of SORBOSE already noted would support its use in products such as : Pastries - soft drinks - jams and marmalades - preserved sweet foods - ice-creams, etc...

7. CONCLUSION

SORBOSE is of great interest in particular products which are intended to prevent dental caries, because of the following characteristics :

- It is a "sugar" but it has the "Zahnschonend" characteristics of polyols normally used in this field.
- SORBOSE is a crystallised "sugar" of high purity
- It is non-hygroscopic and some technical applications are very easy to adopt, especially those which need products free from water.

8. REFERENCES

1. Brevet N° 7234 057 (F) - SORBOSE - Société ROQUETTE FRERES.

2. Embden-Griesbach, Z. physiol. Chem. 91 - 251, 1974

3. Verzar, Biochem. Z. 276 - 17, 1935

4. Verzar-Laszt, Biochem. Z. 276 - 28, 1935

5. Grieshaber, Z. Klin. Med. 129 - 412, 1936 - Z. Klin Med. 129 - 422, 1936

6. Judovitz-Verzur, Biochem. Z. 292 - 182, 1937

7. Carr-Forman, J. Biol. Chem. 128 - 425, 1939

8. Thaddea-Sarkady, Schweiz. Med. Wochenschrift 73 - 1331, 1943

9. Thaddea-Sarkady, Schweiz. Med. Wochenschrift 73 - 1400, 1943

10. Thaddea, Schweiz. Med. Wochenschrift 73 - 1578, 1943

11. Thaddea, Klin. Wochschr. 22 - 722 (1943)

12. Leuthardt-Testa, Helv. physiol. Pharmacal. Acta 8 - C 67, 1950

13. Brückner, Helv. physiol. Acta 9 - 259, 1951

14. Crane-Sols, J. Biol. Chem. 210 - 597, 1954

15. Leuthardt-Wolf, Helv.Chim. Acta 37 - 1734, 1954

16. Bean-Hassid, J. Am. Chem. Soc. 77 - 5737, 1955

17. Wolf-Zschocke-Wedemeyer-Hubner, Klin. Wschr.37 - 693, 1959

18. Cadenas-Sols, Biochim. Biophys. Acta 42 - 460 (1960)

19. Woll, Amer. J. Physiol. 198 - 649, 1960

20. Annegers, Amer. J. Physiol. 206 - 1095, 1964

21. Anderson-Kery-Townley, Arch. Dis. Child. 40 - 1, 1965

22. Beyreiss-Willgerodt-Theile, Acta Biol. Med. German 17 - 733, 1966

23. Vaille-Debray-Souchard-Roze, Ann. Pharm. Françaises 25 - N° 78 - 525, 1967

24. Tacquet-Devulder, Faculté Pharm. Lille - Rapports mars 1972 - mars 1974

25. Dupas, Thèse Doct. Pharm. - Lille, 1974

26. Würsch, Symposium "Kalorienarme Stoffe" - Münich - Octobre 1975

27. H. R. Mühlemann / PH Schneider, Helv. Odont. Acta - Vol. 19, Octobre 1975

28. H. R. Mühlemann, Schweiz-Meschr. Zahnheilk. 86 - 1339/23, 1976

29. Elizabeth A. McComb, Carbohydrate Research 42 - pp 200-202, 1975

30. Brochure L-Sorbose - Roquette Frères - 62136 Lestrem.

PERTINENT QUESTIONS REGARDING TECHNOLOGY OF L-SORBOSE IN FOOD-PRODUCTS

- There is a great number of Sucrose nutritive substitutes (Sorbitol, Mannitol, Lycasin 80/55, Fructose, Xylitol). What is the general interest in having additional products ? What does it provide in comparison with other products (for example : chocolate) ?

- Sorbose solubility and hygroscopicity (Table 1).

- Pre-test of fermentescibility by the mouth bacterias : L-SORBOSE - LYCASIN 80/55 (Tables 2 - 3 and 4).

- Technological specificity of Hydrogenated Glucose Syrups (LYCASIN 80/55).

Health and Sugar Substitutes
Proc. ERGOB Conf., Geneva 1978, pp. 153-158 (Karger, Basel 1978)

Practical problems of cyclamate and saccharin
in corporation in foodstuffs.

E. Wolf

1-11 Gereonsmuehlengasse, D5000 Cologne, Germany

Saccharin and cyclamate are artificial sweeteners which
sweeten but at the same time have no calorific value and
contain no carbohydrate. They are very valuable economically
and for enabling a reduction to be made in the amount of sugar
used in foodstuffs. They are ideal for diabetics who cannot
or do not wish to go without sweet foods. They are also suitable
however for slimming diets since the unnecessary wasted calories obtained from sugar can be cut down. For both user groups
the sweeteners cyclamate and saccharin can be presented not
only in the form of sweeteners for table use but also in
sweetened foodstuffs such as soft drinks, desserts, jams, jellies,
biscuits, cakes etc.

Technologically speaking, cyclamate and saccharin must be
defined as substances which are simple to prepare. They are
compatible, almost unreservedly, with all basic food materials.
The sodium or calcium salts of saccharin or cyclamic acid are
very soluble in water so that the sweetening of aqueous, liquid
foods is particularly simple. As the two materials are very
stable over a wide range of temperature, they may be used for
preparing boiled or baked food. They are sufficiently stable
in relation to the pH value to permit of their use in preparing
all sweetened foodstuffs.

Naturally, the specific properties of the sweeteners must be
considered when using them. Weight for weight, both cyclamate
and saccharin are much sweeter than sugar, ie the sodium salts
are about 35 and 400 times as sweet respectively. The amount

of sweetener required to produce a certain sweetness in a foodstuff is considerably less than that for sugar. This dosing
problem however was solved a long time ago by specially developed
forms of presentation. Thus, cold and hot drinks can be sweetened very easily with sweetener tablets, while fruits, desserts,
milk products like yoghurt can be sweetened with sweetener solutions. Sweetener powders are also suitable for purpose. The
sweetening power of these products is normally adjusted such
that 1g of powder corresponds to 10g of sucrose. The sweeteners
are mixed with carriers such as lactose, calcium lactate etc.,
or uniformly distributed by a general spray-drying technique.
Sweetener powders are usually supplied in paper bags containing
1g.

   Recent developments of granular, free-flowing, water-soluble,
low-calorie sweetening compositions having the same general
appearance of sucrose, and (spoon for spoon) the same sweetness,
are of interest. Because of the very low bulk density, the
same volume weighs only one tenth that of sugar. Using these
sugar substitutes, there is a reduction of more than 90% of the
calorie and carbohydrate content compared with sugar. The
products, which appear similar to sugar, are prepared either by
spray-drying [1] or by drum-drying [2]. Certain types of water-
soluble starch hydrolysate are used as support materials for the
sweeteners, sometimes in combination with small amounts of
sodium citrate as taste corrector and for structure-defining
purposes. In addition to calorie reduction, these sweetener
powders also provide psychological advantages because they look
like sugar. Thus, for example, the diabetic need no longer
satisfy his sweetness requirements with small tablets which are
often reminiscent of pills.

   Since sugars are used not only for sweetening in foodstuff
production but also for functional purposes, spezial preparation requirements must often be observed in using sweeteners.
Simple replacement of the sugar by sweetener, particularly in
baked goods, is seldom possible. Thus, sugar also acts here as
a bulking agent and is partly responsible for texture, colour
development etc. Attempts have been made to produce products

which combine both advantages, by simple mixing, spray-drying
and combination of sucrose, lactose, dextrose, sorbitol etc.
with artificial sweeteners. These products have not appeared
on the market to any extent since little baking is done in the
private household and because the sugar-sweetener mixtures do
not provide sufficient cutting down of calories for diabetics
or for slimmers. Moreover, it is simple to make products and
baked goods of acceptable taste by keeping to the recipes specially developed, and made readily available, by the sweetener
industry.

Saccharin has a unique additional property. It suffers the
drawback of having a bitter metallic after-taste especially if
it used in a higher concentration. The sweetening power of
saccharin in aqueous solutions is not directly proportional to
the concentration. Up to a level of sweetness which corresponds
to that of an 8% sugar solution, a doubling of the saccharin
content also doubles the sweetness [3]. Thereafter, the sweetening
increases at a progressively diminishing rate with increasing
amounts of saccharin whereas the bitter taste increases still
further. It is for this reason that only a few persons experience an undesirable taste in coffee sweetened with saccharin
in normal concentrations of 10 to 20 mg compared with coffee
sweetened with 8% of sugar. The position is quite different
where the results of tasting tests of saccharin-sweetened jam
are concerned where up to 70% sugar has to be replaced by the
sweetener.

Many substances have been suggested for eliminating or mini-
mizing the saccharin after-taste. The optimum solution is, in
countries where cyclamate is at present forbidden,
one should say was   to mix 1 part of saccharin
with 10 parts of cyclamate. Sodium cyclamate is approximately
one tenth as sweet as saccharin (sodium compound). 1kg of the
mixture of cyclamate and saccharin in the ratio 10:1 corresponds
to the sweetening power of 100 kg of sugar [4]. This mixture -
even at high concentrations - is practically free from after-
taste.

Suggested combinations of saccharin with pectin, sorbitol, maltose etc. have not solved the problem. HILL found·that the after-taste of saccharin can be masked by adding small quantities of a dipeptide [5]. Those prefered are L-aspartyl dipeptides which have a slightly lingering sweetness which probably masks the bitter saccharin after-taste. The greater the amount of dipeptide used, the less is the after-taste. However, diabetic laws, price and solubility limit the amount of dipeptide.

In addition, mixtures of saccharin with gluco-delta lactone combined with sodium citrate [6], sodium gluconate [7], ribonucleotides [8] etc. were recommended. Since there was little improvement in the taste of these combinations they have not appeared on the market to any extent. The combination of saccharin with lactose [9] suggested by EISENSTADT was more successful. He found that when used in sufficient quantity, lactose reduces the after-taste of saccharin. However, in quantities up to about 1g lactose, it has the undesired effect of changing the taste of the food or beverage in which it is used [10].

A general rule can be derived from our own developments and from studying the existing patent literature. Salts or substances with a salty taste reduce the bitter after-taste of saccharin. Sodiumcitrate or tartrate are the most suitable for this purpose. Even sodium chloride in combination with sodium bicarbonate has a similar effect [11]. On the other hand, it was found that sweetness can mask the bitterness of potassium chloride. Mixtures of potassium chloride with sugars or artificial sweeteners, in amounts sufficiently small that their presence cannot be detected by their taste, do not have the typical bitter metallic after-taste. These types of mixtures can well be used in human food [12].

For diabetics and for those who are placed on a diet, the sweeteners cyclamate and saccharin represent a good and acceptable means for those who like sweet food. They are, in general, a completely suitable alternative for low-sugar food. The sweeteners can be employed for personally preparing drinks and sweet foods. To simplify things for the sugar and calorie conscious but also to meet basic food requirements it would be an advantage if commercially produced sugar-free products having the lowest possible calorie value were also supplied by the industry.

Soft drinks present no problems particularly if the amount of sugar added is only reduced to provide a 50% reduction in the calorie content. It is much more difficult to produce drinks or dry beverage mixtures which are completely free of sugar especially if cyclamate must not be used to make them. Products which taste remarkably well can be made however by suitable choice of additives.

In milk and milk products such as yoghurt, the sugar can usually be replaced by sweeteners without affecting the taste in any way. The lack of volume of the sugar is compensated by an increasedamount of fluid; this is successful for most products which contain a larger amount of water. It is more difficult to prepare sugar-free low-calorie products in which the missing sugar cannot be replaced entirely by water. It ist necessary to use physiologically unobjectionable bulking agents such as cellulose and its derivatives, alginates, gelatin, arabinogalactan [13], pectin, carrageenan etc. which are indigestible or only partially digestible. Bran, in combination with artificial sweetener, is also very suitable for preparing low-calorie baked goods.

Artificially sweetened jams and jellies are desirable food products for those persons who have to limit their normal intake of sugar, and for those who desire a low-calorie diet. Normally, jellies and jams containing sucrose are made with pectin as the gelling agent. Pectin, however, requires sugar and acid to obtain a product having a good appearance and texture. As HORN found, a polysaccharide gum extracted from seaweed is a suitable gelling system for jellies containing artificial sweeteners [14]. Carrageenan extracted from Irish moss is preferred.

Another way of presenting calorie-reduced sugar-free products to the consumer is based on the already mentioned production of spray-dried, low-bulk-density products. Dry beverage mixtures etc. can be produced by this method.

Summarising, it can be stated that with regard to technology and taste, the artificial sweeteners saccharin and cyclamate can be used almost without reservation in place of sugar in human foodstuffs where this is necessary or desired.

REFERENCES

1. Deininger, R. and Wolf, E. CH-Patent 587 023; March 3, 1977.
2. Schmitt, W.H. and Lu Key, R.A. U.S. Patent 3,653,922; April 4, 1972.
3. Fricker, A. et al. Dtsch. Lebensmittel-Rdsch. 71: 138 - 139, 1975.
4. Fricker, A. and Gutschmidt, J. Wiss. Veröff. DGE, Band 20: 60 - 64, 1971. Steinkopf-Verlag Darmstadt, Germany
5. Hill, J.A. and La Via, A.L. U.S.-Patent 3,695,898; October 3, 1972.
6. Kracauer, P. U.S. Patent 3,285,751; November 15, 1966.
7. Liggett, J.J. U.S. Patent 3,684,529; August 15, 1972.
8. Yueh, M.H. U.S. Patent 3,647,482; March 7, 1972.
9. Eisenstadt, B. U.S. Patent 3,259,506; July 5, 1966.
10. Daniels, R. Sugar Substitutes and Enhancers. Noyes Data Corporation, 1973 ISBN: 0-8155-0492-6
11. Yoshida, M. and Yoshikawa, M. U.S. Patent 3,295,993; January 3, 1967.
12. British Patent 1 469 089; June 24, 1975.
13. Stanko, G.L. U.S. Patent 3,294,544; December 27, 1966.
14. Horn, L.J. U.S. Patent 3,563,769; February 16, 1971.

IV. New sweeteners

Moderator: E. Newbrun, San Francisco
Co-Moderator: G.A. Crosby, Palo Alto

ASPARTAME METABOLISM IN HUMAN SUBJECTS

L. D. Stegink, L. J. Filer, Jr., G. L. Baker, M. C. Brummel and T. R. Tephly

Departments of Pediatrics, Biochemistry and Pharmacology, The University of
Iowa College of Medicine, Iowa City, IA 52242, USA

INTRODUCTION

Aspartame (L-aspartyl-L-phenylalanyl-methyl ester) is a dipeptide with a
sweetening power 180 to 200 times that of sucrose. Questions about Aspartame
(APM) safety have arisen (1, 2) because of concern about the potential toxic
effects of its component amino acids (phenylalanine and aspartate) and methanol
which are released from the molecule upon absorption and digestion. Each of
these, like all chemical substances may exert toxic effects at high levels, although species and age susceptibility vary. However, toxic effects of these
components are only noted under conditions when blood aspartate (ASP), phenylalanine (PHE) or methanol (MEOH) levels are grossly elevated. Our studies have
evaluated the effect of Aspartame loads upon blood levels of these components
in normal adults, adults heterozygous for phenylketonuria, and one-year-old
infants. The doses studied include those calculated to be the 99th percentile
of projected daily ingestion, as well as doses in the potential abuse range.

DOSE SELECTION

The Aspartame doses used were selected on the following basis. A 70 kg
man may be considered to have a caloric requirement of about 2500 kcal per day.
Approximately 17% of these calories are ingested as sucrose. Thus, daily sucrose ingestion is about 1.5 gm/kg body weight. This is equivalent to 7.5 to
8.5 mg/kg Aspartame, considering its range of sweetening power is about 180 to
200 times that of sucrose. If we assume the subject's total carbohydrate intake to be 50% of total calories, about 313 gm of carbohydrate are ingested.
If all this carbohydrate is ingested as sucrose, the subject would ingest 4.47
gm/kg. If the sweetening equivalent of this amount of sucrose were ingested as
Aspartame, the subject would ingest between 22 to 25 mg/kg over the course of
an entire day. Thus, the 99.9th percentile of total daily ingestion would be
about 34 mg/kg.

ADULTS GIVEN 34 MG/KG IN JUICE

We evaluated the effect of Aspartame administration upon plasma amino acid levels in 12 normal adult subjects (6 male, 6 female) given 34 mg Aspartame per kg body weight as a single dose dissolved in 250 ml cold orange juice (3). As shown in Table 1 below, mean ($\pm$ S.D.) plasma aspartate levels were unchanged from fasting levels, while phenylalanine levels peaked 45 to 90 minutes after Aspartame ingestion.

Table 1: PLASMA ASP AND PHE LEVELS (μmoles/dl) AFTER APM INGESTION (34 MG/KG)

	0 hr	½ hr	1 hr	1½ hr	2 hr	3 hr	4 hr
ASP	0.3 $\pm$ 0.1	0.3 $\pm$ 0.1	0.3 $\pm$ 0.2	0.3 $\pm$ 0.1	0.3 $\pm$ 0.1	0.3 $\pm$ 0.2	0.3 $\pm$ 0.1
PHE	5.7 $\pm$ 1.2	11 $\pm$ 2.5	11 $\pm$ 1.7	9.5 $\pm$ 1.8	8.8 $\pm$ 1.4	7.7 $\pm$ 1.6	7.1 $\pm$ 2.4

The plasma phenylalanine levels observed were similar to those noted post-prandially in normal infants (4), and were far below those associated with toxic effects. These results clearly demonstrate that plasma aspartate and phenylalanine levels are not elevated above normal postprandial levels after the administration of large doses of Aspartame.

ADULTS GIVEN 34 MG/KG WITH MEALS AND MONOSODIUM GLUTAMATE

It has been suggested that the addition of monosodium glutamate (MSG) and Aspartame (APM) to a meal might result in a decreased metabolism of these two food additives when ingested together as part of a high protein meal (1,2). Such conditions were postulated to result in elevated plasma glutamate and aspartate levels, and the potential for neurotoxicity. Six normal adult subjects were studied after ingestion of test meals providing 1 gm protein/kg body weight. The subjects ingested the meal alone, and the identical meal to which MSG and APM were added at a level of 34 mg/kg body weight. The meals were fed in a randomized cross-over design. Mean ($\pm$ S.D.) plasma glutamate (GLU) and aspartate levels in these subjects are shown in Table 2. Plasma glutamate and aspartate levels did not differ significantly between groups.

Table 2

PLASMA GLU AND ASP (μmoles/dl) AFTER INGESTION OF MEAL ALONE

	0 hr	½ hr	1 hr	1½ hr	2 hr	4 hr	6 hr
ASP	0.3 $\pm$ 0.2	0.4 $\pm$ 0.2	0.4 $\pm$ 0.3	0.4 $\pm$ 0.3	0.6 $\pm$ 0.4	0.7 $\pm$ 0.4	0.5 $\pm$ 0.4
GLU	4.0 $\pm$ 1.8	5.7 $\pm$ 3.3	6.9 $\pm$ 4.5	6.2 $\pm$ 2.6	8.2 $\pm$ 3.0	7.8 $\pm$ 3.2	7.2 $\pm$ 3.4

PLASMA GLU AND ASP (μmoles/dl) AFTER INGESTION OF MEAL + APM AND MSG

	0 hr	½ hr	1 hr	1½ hr	2 hr	4 hr	6 hr
ASP	0.3 $\pm$ 0.1	0.3 $\pm$ 0.3	0.4 $\pm$ 0.3	0.5 $\pm$ 0.4	0.7 $\pm$ 0.5	1.1 $\pm$ 0.7	0.6 $\pm$ 0.3
GLU	4.7 $\pm$ 3.0	7.3 $\pm$ 4.4	7.0 $\pm$ 2.9	8.8 $\pm$ 3.4	11 $\pm$ 3.1	11 $\pm$ 2.9	8.6 $\pm$ 4.4

PHENYLKETONURIC HETEROZYGOTES

Individuals affected with the disease phenylketonuria (PKU), fail to
metabolize phenylalanine effectively, resulting in abnormally elevated plasma
phenylalanine levels. Since the incidence rate for the heterozygous state of
PKU is estimated at 1:50, such individuals will ingest Aspartame when it enters
the market. Plasma amino acid levels were measured in four female subjects,
known to be heterozygous for phenylketonuria, after ingestion of Aspartame
(34 mg/kg body weight) dissolved in orange juice. As shown in Table 3, plasma
aspartate levels were not affected in these heterozygous subjects. However,
plasma phenylalanine levels in PKU heterozygous subjects (Table 3) showed a
somewhat higher and broader absorption curve than that noted in normal subjects
(Table 1). This was expected in view of the decreased levels of the phenylalanine hydroxylase system. Despite this, maximal phenylalanine levels noted
were only at the upper edge of the normal postprandial range noted in infants
(4), and were below 18 μmoles/dl (3 mg%). The data indicate that the PKU
heterozygote rapidly metabolizes large doses of Aspartame, and suggest no
hazard from the phenylalanine content of Aspartame at the level tested.

Table 3

PLASMA ASPARTATE AND PHENYLALANINE LEVELS (μmole/dl) IN PKU HETEROZYGOTES

	0 hr	½ hr	1 hr	1½ hr	2 hr	3 hr	4 hr
ASP	0.3 $\pm$ 2.2	0.2 $\pm$ 0.1	0.2 $\pm$ 0.1	0.2 $\pm$ 0.1	0.1 $\pm$ 0.1	0.1 $\pm$ 0.1	0.1 $\pm$ 0.1
PHE	6.6 $\pm$ 1.7	15 $\pm$ 3.5	16 $\pm$ 1.5	13 $\pm$ 0.9	13 $\pm$ 0.8	10 $\pm$ 1.6	9.3 $\pm$ 1.3

ASPARTAME INGESTION BY LACTATING WOMEN

We also studied whether Aspartame ingestion by the lactating female would
affect blood or milk amino acid levels. Six healthy women with well established lactation were studied after administration of either Aspartame or lactose at 50 mg/kg body weight dissolved in orange juice. As shown in Table 4,
neither Aspartame or lactose administration had a significant effect upon
plasma aspartate levels. As expected, plasma phenylalanine levels increased
after Aspartame loading to a mean ($\pm$ S.D.) peak value of 16 $\pm$ 6 μmoles/dl, but
were not affected by lactose.

Table 4

PLASMA ASPARTATE AND PHENYLALANINE LEVELS (μmoles/dl) AFTER LACTOSE INGESTION

	0 hr	½ hr	1 hr	1½ hr	2 hr	3 hr	4 hr
ASP	0.3 + 0.2	0.2 + 0.1	0.4 + 0.4	0.2 + 0.1	0.2 + 0.1	0.2 + 0.2	0.2 + 0.1
PHE	5.0 + 1.1	4.5 + 0.8	4.5 + 0.9	4.3 + 0.8	4.3 + 0.8	4.4 + 0.9	5.0 + 1.2

PLASMA ASPARTATE AND PHENYLALANINE LEVELS (μmoles/dl) AFTER ASPARTAME

	0 hr	½ hr	1 hr	1½ hr	2 hr	3 hr	4 hr
ASP	0.4 + 0.3	0.5 + 0.5	0.3 + 0.2	0.3 + 0.2	0.3 + 0.2	0.2 + 0.1	0.2 + 0.2
PHE	4.6 + 1.8	15 + 4.5	14 + 4.1	16 + 6.2	13 + 3.8	8.1 + 2.3	6.4 + 2.0

Breast milk phenylalanine and aspartate levels (Table 5) showed a small increase after Aspartame administration, when compared to lactose loading. However, levels of these amino acids after Aspartame loading were no higher than levels noted in these subjects after ingestion of meals (8 & 12 hours).

Table 5

MILK ASPARTATE AND PHENYLALANINE LEVELS (μmoles/dl) AFTER LACTOSE

	0 hr	1 hr	2 hr	3 hr	4 hr	8 hr	12 hr
ASP	2.6 + 0.8	3.1 + 0.5	3.6 + 0.9	3.9 + 1.5	3.8 + 1.8	3.8 + 1.5	4.1 + 2.5
PHE	0.8 + 0.4	0.9 + 0.4	0.9 + 0.3	1.4 + 1.9	0.9 + 0.5	0.8 + 0.3	0.9 + 0.6

MILK ASPARTATE AND PHENYLALANINE LEVELS (μmoles/dl) AFTER ASPARTAME

	0 hr	1 hr	2 hr	3 hr	4 hr	8 hr	12 hr
ASP	2.3 + 1.1	2.8 + 0.9	4.5 + 1.5	4.5 + 2.2	4.8 + 1.7	5.6 + 2.4	5.6 + 3.2
PHE	0.5 + 0.3	2.0 + 1.1	2.3 + 1.1	2.0 + 0.9	2.0 + 0.9	2.2 + 1.7	1.2 + 0.5

DOSES OF ASPARTAME IN THE POTENTIAL ABUSE RANGE

The effects of potential abuse doses of Aspartame on blood amino acid levels were also studied. Three separate groups of 6 normal adult subjects each, were administered graded doses of Aspartame (100, 150 and 200 mg/kg) dissolved in orange juice. Peak plasma aspartate and phenylalanine levels in these subjects are shown in Table 6. Small changes in plasma aspartate levels were noted after Aspartame ingestion at 150 and 200 mg/kg, with no significant changes noted at the 100 mg/kg body weight dose. Peak plasma phenylalanine levels showed a dose-related response to increasing doses of Aspartame (Table 6). At the highest dose, plasma phenylalanine levels reached a mean value (+ S.D.) of 49 umoles/dl at 45 to 90 minutes after Aspartame ingestion, and then declined rapidly. The phenylalanine levels observed are below those which would be expected to cause any toxic effects upon such short term elevation of plasma phenylalanine. No ill effects have been reported in normal subjects and phenylketonuric heterozygotes showing similar plasma phenylalanine levels resulting from phenylalanine loading while testing for the heterozygous condition (5). These data indicate rapid metabolism of Aspartame doses in the potential abuse range.

Table 6

PEAK PLASMA ASPARTATE AND PHENYLALANINE LEVELS (μmoles/dl)

Dose	0	34 MPK	50 MPK	100 MPK	150 MPK	200 MPK
ASP	0.3 + 0.2	0.3 + 0.2	0.5 + 0.5	0.4 + 0.2	1.0 + 0.7	0.8 + 0.6
PHE	5.6 + 1.2	11 + 2.5	16 + 6.2	20 + 6.8	29 + 8.8	49 + 15

INFANTS VS ADULTS

It has been suggested that infants metabolize Aspartame less well than adults (1, 2). We examined the effects of Aspartame ingestion upon blood amino acids and methanol levels in normal adults and one-year-old infants given 34, 50 or 100 mg Aspartame/kg body weight. Plasma concentrations of aspartate were unchanged from fasting levels in both infants and adults at all ingestion levels, indicative of rapid aspartate metabolism. Phenylalanine levels in plasma peaked 45 to 90 minutes after Aspartame ingestion. The increase was dose, but not age, related. The phenylalanine absorption curves were similar in both groups, as were peak levels (mean + S.D.) as shown in Table 7.

Table 7

PEAK PLASMA PHENYLALANINE LEVELS (μmoles/dl)

Subjects	Dose	0	34 MPK	50 MPK	100 MPK
Infants		6.1 + 1.2	9.7 + 2.7	11.5 + 3.1	22.5 + 11.6
Adults		5.7 + 1.2	11.1 + 2.5	16.2 + 4.6	20.2 + 6.8

METHANOL

Methylated compounds present in food are hydrolyzed in the gut, releasing methanol. However, little data are available on methanol clearance. Our data show blood methanol levels peak 60 - 120 minutes after Aspartame ingestion. Methanol absorption curves were similar for both infants and adults. Peak methanol levels (mean + S.E.M.) are shown in Table 8.

Table 8

PEAK BLOOD METHANOL LEVELS (mg%)

Subjects

Dose	34 MPK	50 MPK	100 MPK	150 MPK	200 MPK
Infants	0.18 + 0.14	0.31 + 0.15	1.0 + 0.	----	----
Adults	0.24 + 0.22	----	1.2 + 0.	2.1 + 0.4	2.6 + 0.8

The data indicate that one-year-old infants absorb and metabolize Aspartame as well as adults.

The data in Table 8 also show peak methanol levels in normal adults given potential abuse doses of Aspartame (150 and 200 mg/kg). It now appears that toxic effects of methanol ingestion result from formate accumulation. We assayed for the presence of formate in the blood and urine of subjects receiving Aspartame at 200 mg/kg. No formate was detected, with the limits of detection being 1 mg%.

SUMMARY

The data presented indicate rapid metabolism of Aspartame by normal adults, one-year-old infants and individuals who are heterozygote for phenylketonuria. In view of the rapid metabolism, there appears little chance for significant accumulation of aspartate, phenylalanine or methanol in these subjects under normal use conditions of the product.

REFERENCES

1. Olney, J. W., Fd. Cosmet. Toxicol. 13, 595-596 (1975).

2. Olney, J. W. In: Sweeteners, Issues and Uncertainties, Academy Forum National Academy of Sciences, U.S.A, Washington, D. C., 1975, 189-195.

3. Stegink, L. D., Filer, L. J., Jr. and Baker, G. L., J. Nutr. 107, 1837-1846 (1977).

4. Stegink, L. D., Schmitt, J. L., Meyer, P. D. and Kain, P. H., J. Pediat. 79, 648-654 (1971).

5. Tocci, P. M. and Beber, B., Pediatr. 52, 109-113 (1973).

ACKNOWLEDGEMENTS:

Supported in part by G. D. Searle and General Foods.

Health and Sugar Substitutes
Proc. ERGOB Conf., Geneva 1978. pp. 166-171 (Karger, Basel 1978)

DIHYDROCHALCONE SWEETENERS

R. M. Horowitz and Bruno Gentili

U.S. Department of Agriculture, Science and Education Administration,
Fruit and Vegetable Chemistry Laboratory, 263 South Chester Avenue,
Pasadena, California 91106

INTRODUCTION

The flavonoid constituents of Citrus have remarkable taste properties, yield valuable byproducts and are available in large quantity. Among the large array of flavonoids are eight flavanone glycosides, four of which are bitter and all of which can be reduced to dihydrochalcones. In work done in the early 60's it was found that some of these dihydrochalcones are intensely sweet.[1] It now appears likely that certain of these compounds will eventually be used in various applications of sweeteners.

Three sweeteners that are of particular interest are neohesperidin dihydrochalcone, naringin dihydrochalcone and hesperetin dihydrochalcone 4'-β-D-glucoside (HDG). These were among the first compounds prepared in this series and a large body of information about their taste and toxicology is now available. Many variants of the substances have been synthesized, including both glycosidic and non-glycosidic derivatives. Although some of the newer derivatives are of interest, none of them appears to offer any major improvement in properties over those of the earlier compounds. Since, of all the sweeteners in the series, neohesperidin dihydrochalcone would probably be the first to gain acceptance, we will deal mainly with it and the closely related substances naringin dihydrochalcone and HDG.

SOURCE, PREPARATION AND PROPERTIES

The starting compounds, plant sources and products are shown in Table 1.

Table 1. Sources of Dihydrochalcone Glycosides

Starting compound	Plant source	Product
Neohesperidin (bitter)	Seville orange (*c. aurantium*)	Neohesperidin dihydrochalcone (sweet)
Naringin (bitter)	Grapefruit (*c. paradisi*)	Naringin dihydrochalcone (sweet)
Hesperidin (tasteless)	Sweet orange (*c.sinensis*) Lemon (*c. limon*)	Hesperetin dihydrochalcone 4'-β-D-glucoside (sweet)

Two of the starting compounds, neohesperidin and naringin, contain as their sugar component the disaccharide β-neohesperidose (2-$\underline{O}$-α-L-rhamnopyranosyl-β-D-glucopyranose);[2] the third compound, hesperidin, contains the disaccharide β-rutinose (6-$\underline{O}$-α-L-rhamnopyranosyl-β-D-glucopyranose). Experience has shown that many (but not all) phenolic or flavonoid glycosides are taste-eliciting (bitter, sweet or bitter-sweet) if their sugar component is β-neohesperidose or β-glucose.[3] On the other hand, analogous compounds in which the sugar component is β-rutinose have thus far been found to be tasteless. When hesperidin is used as starting material it is essential to alter the taste-abolishing β-rutinosyl group if one wishes to obtain a taste-eliciting substance. One way to do this is by hydrolysis to remove rhamnose.

The conversion of neohesperidin and naringin to their respective dihydrochalcones can be done simply by dissolving them in dilute alkali, which yields the chalcone, and hydrogenating the chalcone solution with the aid of a standard hydrogenation catalyst. The products are formed rapidly in almost quantitative yield and crystallize easily. The reduction of hesperidin in dilute alkali yields hesperidin dihydrochalcone, a tasteless compound. Partial hydrolysis of this dihydrochalcone, either by acid or by dissolved or immobilized enzymes, gives rise to the sweet hesperetin dihydrochalcone 4'-β-D-glucoside (HDG) in an overall yield of 40-50%.[4]

Because hesperidin could be produced in abundance as a byproduct of the orange- or lemon-processing industry, hesperidin-based sweeteners, such as HDG, are attractive candidates for further study. On the other hand, the large-scale preparation of neohesperidin dihydrochalcone is hampered by the fact that neohesperidin is not available on a commercial scale from its best natural source, the Seville orange. To get around this impasse it is neces- sary to convert the readily available naringin to neohesperidin and thence to the dihydrochalcone by the following reactions: naringin + NaOH → phloracetophenone 4'-β-neohesperidoside (PN); PN + isovanillin + NaOH → → neohesperidin; neohesperidin + H_2 (Pd/C) + NaOH → neohesperidin dihydro- chalcone. The overall yield in this process averages about 20-30% but could doubtlessly be improved through further study.[5]

The dihydrochalcones are crystalline solids that are colorless and odorless when pure. Neohesperidin dihydrochalcone is soluble to the extent of about 1.2 grams per liter of distilled water. Stability would probably not be a major problem in most applications of dihydrochalcones. Dilute aqueous solu- tions have been kept for periods of years with little change in appearance or sweetness. It has been reported that the compounds are resistant to hydro- lysis by acids at pH's > 2 at normal room temperature.[6] At high temperature (75-100°C) free sugars arising from hydrolysis can be detected in a matter of minutes or hours in the pH range 1.5-3.6.

TASTE

In general, dihydrochalcones have a pleasant sweetness, somewhat slow in its onset and of varying (usually long) duration. The sweet aftertaste is usually not marred by bitterness, but is often described as having a slight cooling or licorice-like quality. It has been reported that the delay in on- set of sweetness can be reduced by combining the dihydrochalcone with gluconic acid or δ-gluconolactone.[7] No way has yet been found to reduce the lingering

of the sweetness. Most tasters agree, however, that monosaccharyl derivatives, such as HDG, have less of the sweet aftertaste than disaccharyl derivatives.

Quantitative studies of dihydrochalcone sweetness have been reported by
Guadagni, et al.[8] At threshold neohesperidin dihydrochalcone is almost 1900
times sweeter than sucrose, while naringin dihydrochalcone and HDG are almost
300 times sweeter. As concentration increases, the relative sweetness of the
dihydrochalcones decreases. Thus, the relative sweetness at the 2.5% sucrose
level is only 20-35% of the values at threshold.

An unexpected property of these sweeteners is their ability to mask or
interfere with the perception of bitterness.[8] Sucrose, even at relatively
high concentration, is not very effective in raising the threshold of the
bitter flavanone, naringin, and it has almost no effect at all on the bitter
triterpenoid, limonin. On the other hand, neohesperidin dihydrochalcone and
particularly HDG give, at relatively low concentrations, striking increases
in the threshold values of these bitter principles.

OTHER COMPOUNDS

It was mentioned above that many dihydrochalcone variants have been synthesized. Hesperetin dihydrochalcone 4'-β-D-galactoside and hesperetin
dihydrochalcone 4'-β-D-xyloside are both sweeter (1.5 - 2x) than the 4'-β-D-
glucoside (HDG) and, in addition, have quite good taste characteristics.[9]
Both are difficult to synthesize. A number of other hesperetin dihydrochalcone 4'-monosaccharides and 4'-disaccharides have been reported;[10] all
are difficult to make and there is no evidence that any of them are superior
to the older compounds. It was recognized early that the sugar moiety is
neither necessary nor sufficient to confer sweetness on a dihydrochalcone
aglycone.[3] For example, the aglycone hesperetin dihydrochalcone was found to
be sweet, if essentially insoluble. A large number of 4'-O-carboxyalkyl and

4'-O-sulfoalkyl derivatives of hesperetin dihydrochalcone have been synthesized recently.[11] Many of these compounds have excellent solubility and several are good sweeteners but, again, they seem to provide no significant improvement in taste over that of the older compounds. Moreover, because alkyl
substituents of this type are not found in naturally occurring flavonoids,
their introduction does away with one of the chief attractions of the citrus-
based dihydrochalcones, i.e., that they are only a short step removed from
natural products usually regarded as inoccuous.

APPLICATIONS

Dihydrochalcone sweeteners obviously work best where long-lasting sweetness
is advantageous. These applications would include products such as chewing
gums, confections of various sorts, toothpastes, mouthwashes and similar preparations. It is likely that in these applications dihydrochalcones could be
substituted for existing synthetic sweeteners without drastic reformulation of
the product. It also appears that, with proper formulation, dihydrochalcones
could be used successfully to provide some of the sweetness in soft drinks.

Other applications of the dihydrochalcones would be in products where it is
desirable or necessary to reduce bitterness. These include a very large number of pharmaceuticals and a few fruit juices, such as grapefruit juice. Recent work has shown that the addition of as little as 12 ppm of neohesperidin
dihydrochalcone to moderately bitter grapefruit juice leads to a dramatic
increase in its acceptability to taste panels (D. Guadagni, unpublished data).

TOXICOLOGY AND METABOLISM

Long-term (2-year) feeding studies of neohesperidin dihydrochalcone in rats
and dogs have been carried out by M. R. Gumbmann and coworkers. A summary of
the results has been published.[12] In general, the data indicate that this
dihydrochalcone has a very low order of toxicity. The compound has also been
studied for mutagenicity in the Ames bacterial mutant test; the results were
negative.[13] When neohesperidin dihydrochalcone labeled with ^{14}C in the car-

bon atom adjacent to the B-ring was fed to rats, over 90% of the radioactivity was excreted in the urine within 24 hours and only one major metabolite was detected.

REFERENCES

1.   Horowitz, R. M. and Gentili, B. U. S. Patent 3,087,821 (1963); J. Agr.
      Food Chem. 17: 696, 1969; in Symposium: Sweeteners, edited by Inglett,
      G. E. pp. 182-193, Avi Publishing Company, Westport, Connecticut, 1974.

2.   Horowitz, R. M. and Gentili, B. Tetrahedron 19: 773, 1963.

3.   Horowitz, R. M. in Biochemistry of Phenolic Compounds, edited by
      Harborne, J. B. pp. 543-571, Academic Press, New York, 1964.

4.   Horowitz, R. M. and Gentili, B. U. S. Patent 3,429,873 (1969); U. S.
      Patent 3,583,894 (1971); Krasnobajew, V. Ger. Offen. 2,402,221 (1974).

5.   Horowitz, R. M. and Gentili, B. U. S. Patent 3,375,242 (1968);
      Krbechek, L., Inglett, G. E. et al. J. Agr. Food Chem., 16: 108, 1968;
      Robertson, G. H., Clark, J. P. and Lundin, R. E. Ind. Eng. Chem., Prod.
      Res. Develop. 13: 125, 1974.

6.   Inglett, G. E., Krbechek, L. et al. J. Food Sci. 34: 101, 1969.

7.   Huber, U., Kossiakoff, N. and Vaterlaus, B. Ger. Offen. 2,445,385
      (1975).

8.   Guadagni, D. G., Maier, V. P. and Turnbaugh, J. H. J. Sci. Food Agric.
      25: 1199, 1974.

9.   Horowitz, R. M. and Gentili, B. U. S. Patent 3,890,296 (1975); U. S.
      Patent 3,890,298 (1975).

10.   Kamiya, S., Esaki, S. and Konishi, F. Agr. Biol. Chem. (Japan) 40: 1731,
      1976.

11.   DuBois, G. E., Crosby, G. A. and Saffron, P. Science 195: 397, 1977;
      DuBois, G. E., Crosby, G. A., Stephenson, R. A. and Wingard, R. E.
      J. Agr. Food Chem., 25: 763, 1977; Rajky-Medveczky, G. et al. Nahrung
      21: 131, 1977.

12.   Gumbmann, M. R., Gould, D. H., Robbins, D. J. and Booth, A. N. in
      Sweeteners and Dental Caries, edited by Shaw, J. H. and Roussos, G. G.,
      pp. 301-308, Information Retrieval Inc., Washington, 1978.

13.   Batzinger, R. P., Ou, S. L. and Bueding, E. Science, 198: 944-946, 1977;
      Brown, J. P., Dietrich, P. S. and Brown, R. J. Biochem. Soc. Trans. 5:
      1489-1492, 1977.

Health and Sugar Substitutes
Proc. ERGOB Conf., Geneva 1978, pp. 172-177 (Karger, Basel 1978)

TALIN - A NOVEL SWEET PROTEIN FROM T. DANIELLII

J.D. Higginbotham

Tate & Lyle, Limited, Group Research & Development,

Philip Lyle Memorial Research Laboratory, P.O. Box 68, Reading RG6 2BX, Berks. UK

INTRODUCTION

With the ever increasing world demand for sucrose, there is a parallel increase in demand for complementary low calorie sweeteners. All the existing sweeteners have either undesirable organoleptic qualities or suspected or proven toxicity, and the search for alternative sweeteners is becoming increasingly urgent. Tate & Lyle are proposing the use of a sweet extract of the West African plant - Thaumatococcus daniellii (T.d.), the fruit of which contains an extremely intense sweet protein.

HISTORY AND BOTANY

In the Pharmaceutical Journal of 1855[1], W.F. Daniell, a British Surgeon, described a 'number of red triangular-shaped pods' observed in trading canoes while travelling in Nigeria in 1839. He originally mistook them for kola nuts, but two years later he tasted them for himself and experienced 'an indescribable but intense degree of dulcidity'. He reported the name of the fruit as Katemfe, the Yoruba name, or 'the Miraculous fruit of Soudan'.

The fruit is not used commercially in West Africa today, but Daniell mentions that the plant was cultivated in colonists' gardens in Sierra Leone in 1853 using seeds imported from Nigeria, and the fruit was offered for sale in colonial markets. at one halfpenny each.

In modern West Africa, the plant is quite extensively used - its leaves for thatching, wrapping and boiling food, its petioles (stalks) for weaving mats and baskets and the pith from inside the petioles is compressed into a paper-like material. The fruit is occasionally eaten or used for improving the palatability of acidulated palm wine or sour fruit.

Botanically, <u>Thaumatococcus daniellii</u> (Benth) belongs to the Marantaceae family [2], a monoecious perennial, and is common throughout the West African rain forest zone from Sierra Leone to Zaire.

The plant has broad, oval, papery leaves on petioles up to 3 metres tall in dense thickets, growing only inches apart. The fruit is fleshy, trigonal, maturing from a dark green, through brown and orange, to bright red when fully ripe. Each fruit contains 1 to 3 hard, black seeds each capped with a membranous sac, called an aril, which contains the sweet substance.

STRUCTURE OF TALIN

Talin is a mixture of naturally-occurring closely related sweet proteins; predominantly, these occur as Thaumatin I and II [3], with traces of other sweet proteins (T_o). They all have very similar amino acid constitutions (Table 1) and molecular weights <u>circa</u> 21,000 and only differ significantly in their ionic charge, caused by a differing degree of amide substitution on the glutamic and aspartic acid residues. Separation into the constituent sweet proteins can be achieved by exploiting their charge differences by elution through a cation exchange resin. However, the separated sweet proteins are individually less sweet than their mixture and are less stable to denaturants.

Interestingly, it is found that Td fruit collected from the east of the Volta river in Ghana only contain TI and traces of To whereas western Ghanaian fruit always contain several sweet proteins.

Antibodies raised to the thaumatins are being used in structural studies in combination with protein sequencing to learn more about the features important in conferring the sweet taste. Other studies relate to the development of the proteins in the ripening aril and the underlying protein synthesis mechanism which is responsible for generating such a high sweet protein concentration (<u>circa</u> 200 mg/ml) in the aril tissue.

Table 1. Amino Acid Composition (residues per mole) of the Thaumatins

AMINO ACID	Thaumatin I TI	Thaumatin II TII	Thaumatin To To
Alanine	15	14	15
Arginine	11	12	11
Aspartic Acid	21	19	21
Half-cystine	14	14	14
Glutamic Acid	10	10	10
Glycine	23	22	24
Histidine	0	0	0
Iso-leucine	7	7	7
Leucine	9	9	9
Lysine	10	11	10
Methionine	1	1	1
Phenylalanine	10	10	10
Proline	12	12	12
Serine	12	10	10
Threonine	19	17	17
Tryptophan	3	3	3
Tyrosine	7	8	7
Valine	9	8	9
TOTALS	193	187	190

SWEETNESS OF TALIN

Talin is one of the sweetest substances known, either natural or synthetic, hence only small quantities are required in food and drink formulations.

The sweet taste of Talin is characterised by delay in perception of the sweet taste. The time that elapses between application of Talin to the tongue and response, is much longer than that of sucrose.

The period of developing sweetness, that is, the interval between the start of the sweet response and the point of maximum sweetness, is also longer than that of sucrose. Talin has a lingering sweet after taste. At high concentrations, this can last for up to an hour.

The delay in sweetness perception of Talin can be overcome by combining it with another sweetener such as sucrose, glucose, fructose or saccharin, and the lingering sweet taste can be reduced, or completely eliminated by taste modifiers.

Talin solutions have a threshold level of sweetness approximately 5500 times that of sucrose on a weight basis and the sweetness intensity decreases when compared with sucrose concentrations down to circa 1000 times at the 17% sucrose level.

For convenience, the sweetness of Talin for most of the proposed applications may be taken to be approximately 3000 times as sweet as sucrose on a weight basis.

Increasing temperature to 45°C enhances Talin sweetness intensity. At higher temperatures than 45°C Talin begins to lose sweetness, if not specially treated.

NOTES ON THE USE OF TALIN IN FOOD PRODUCTS

On a weight for weight basis Talin has approximately the same calorific value as the carbohydrate sweeteners. But since the levels of use are so very much smaller the effective calorific value is negligible. Hence Talin may be used in all kinds of reduced calorie, non calorie, diet or diabetic foods as well as sugar-reduced and sugar-free products.

Talin may be used as a sweetener in its own right in many food or pharmaceutical compositions where a novel sweet sensation and a lingering sweetness is desirable.

For many potential uses it is however desirable to provide a sweet sensation as similar as possible to that of sucrose.

The delay in sweetness perception is related to the high molecular weight (app. 20,000) of Talin, and if an immediate sweetness impact is required, Talin must be used in combination with another sweetener such as sugar and/or saccharin.

When two or more sweeteners are combined, the effective sweetness of each is different to that found when they are tasted separately. For example, sucrose and saccharin act synergistically together, to produce more sweetening power in combination than would be expected from the sum of their individual sweetness levels.

A similar effect is noted when Talin is used with various other sweeteners. The most effective combinations have approximately half the total sweetness from Talin. The addition of Talin to saccharin is particularly advantageous, as the bitter after-taste of saccharin is minimised by the developing sweetness of Talin.

It is possible to modify the flavour of Talin by the use of specific 'taste modifiers'. The effect of the taste modifiers is to minimise the sweetness duration and the after-taste and to give a more 'rounded' sweetness profile to combinations of Talin with alternative sweeteners. These modifiers include glucuronic acid and arabinogalactan.

STABILITY

Freeze dried Talin is stable indefinitely; existing as a stable free-flowing powder, which may be readily formed into tablets or agglomerates. Aqueous solutions are susceptible to bacterial attack, but this may be prevented by the addition of permitted preservatives.

The effect of pH and temperature on the sweetness of Talin is complex and is also dependent on the other solutes (e.g. salts, polysaccharides) present.

At room temperature, there is no appreciable sweetness change between pH 2.0 and 10.0 but between pH 1.8 and 2.0, and pH 10.0 and 11.0 there is a 20% loss of sweetness. Sweetness is rapidly lost below pH 1.8 and above 11.0, reaching zero by pH 1.5 and 11.7 respectively.

APPLICATIONS

Talin is a low calorie, protein sweetener and, as such, may be used in many products suitable for diabetics and slimmers. It may be used either as the sole sweetener, for a novel taste profile, or in combination with other low calorie or carbohydrate sweeteners.

Several types of drink have been formulated using Talin. A wide range of flavours was possible in powder or syrup-based instant drinks, squashes, carbonated and whole fruit beverages. It was found that the presence of Talin in low calorie drinks, particularly carbonated ones, produced a well-rounded, full flavour effect, known as 'body' which is normally lacking from low calorie drinks.

Talin has been incorporated into sweetening tablets for tea and coffee, in combination with a carbohydrate, or low calorie sweetener for best results.

Talin is suitable for many desserts, including gelled, whipped, frozen, instant and dairy products.

Several compressed, confectionery products have been formulated, which contain Talin and a tablettable base material with various flavouring agents.

In addition to its intense sweetness, Talin has a distinct flavour, characterised by a long-lasting sweet after-taste. It is this property which is utilised in many food and pharmaceutical applications. It is desirable to prolong the flavour of products such as toothpaste, mouthwash and chewing gum. It has been found that Talin lends itself well to such applications - not only is the taste of Talin itself prolonged, but it also perpetuates the flavours of other components, particularly mint and spices.

The distinct and long-lasting flavour of Talin can also be employed in therapeutic drug products, where low levels of the sweetener are able to mask the unpleasant tastes of some chemicals.

SAFETY EVALUATION

Talin has shown no adverse effects when tested for acute oral toxicity (LD_{50} in excess of 20g/kg) and in 13 week dietary administration to rats; also no allergenic, mutagenic or teratogenic effects were noted.

REFERENCES

1.   Daniell, W.F. Pharm. J. 14 : 158-159, 1855.
2.   Dalziel, J.M. in The Useful Plants of West Tropical Africa, Crown Agents, London, 1937.
3.   Van der Wel, H. and Loeve, K. Eur. J. Biochem. 31 : 221-225, 1972.

Health and Sugar Substitutes
Proc. ERGOB Conf., Geneva 1978, pp. 178-183 (Karger, Basel 1978)

ACESULFAME-K, A NEW NONCALORIC SWEETENER

H.-J. Arpe

Hoechst AG, Postfach 800320, 6230 Frankfurt (M) 80,
Federal Republic of Germany

INTRODUCTION

When reactions were carried out with the reactive intermediate
fluorosulfonyl isocyanate ($F-SO_2-N=C=O$) in the Hauptlabor of
Farbwerke Hoechst (now Hoechst AG) in 1967, it was noted for the
first time that substances incorporating the newly discovered
ring system of dihydro-oxathiazinone dioxide[1] have a sweet taste.
This chance observation made in the laboratory soon became the
starting point for an extensive research programme, the objective
of which was the development of a new sweetener.

CHEMICAL STRUCTURE AND SWEETNESS

The first problem to be dealt with was an investigation of the
connection between the substituents on the heterocycle and the
resulting sweetness. It was found that substituents in the 5 and
6 position on 3.4-dihydro-1.2.3-oxathiazine-4-one-2.2-dioxide
can change the organoleptic properties from barely sweet and
metallic via sweet and more or less bitter to a pure, sweet
taste.

R^1, R^2 =H, CH_3, C_2H_5, C_6H_5

Additional control of the organoleptic properties is possible
by way of the cation which is present in a salt-like bond with
the hetero nitrogen of the strongly acidic sweetener acid. The
purity of the sweet taste increases markedly if sodium is
replaced by potassium or calcium.

In consequence, 3.4-dihydro-6-methyl-1.2.3-oxathiazine-4-one-
2.2.-dioxide potassium salt was selected, on the basis of the
criteria discussed above, for further development:

This sweetener has been registered under the generic name
'acesulfame potassium salt' by the WHO in Geneva.

SYNTHESIS AND PROPERTIES

Acesulfame can be seen as a derivative of acetoacetic acid and
can thus be produced inexpensively from tert-butylacetoacetate
which is first reacted with fluorosulfonyl isocyanate to form
the addition product α-(N-fluorosulfonylcarbamoyl)-acetoacetic
acid tert-butyl ester. When heated slightly this ester gives off
CO_2 and isobutene, and is converted in high yield to N-
fluorosulfonyl acetoacetic acid amide which can be cyclized in
the presence of potassium hydroxide to the oxathiazinone dioxide
derivative, by elimination of hydrogen fluoride:

Both starting products required are readily accessible; tert-
butylacetoacetate by reacting ketene with tert-butanol, and
fluorosulfonyl isocyanate from SO_3 and chlorocyan via the

subsequent exchange of chlorine for fluorine in the intermediate
product chlorosulfonyl isocyanate.

The solubility temperature gradient of the potassium salt in
water (27 g/100 ml at 20 $^{\circ}$C; approx. 130 g/100 ml at 100 $^{\circ}$C) is
particularly steep. In consequence, the potassium salt can be
readily obtained by recrystallization in a purity exceeding 99 %.
In this form the heavy metal content is far less than 10 ppm and
the fluorine content considerably lower than the limit permitted
for food additives. Further suitable solvents for the sweetener
are aqueous solutions of ethanol or glycerol.

The stability of a sweetener is of special importance, as the
sweetness of products sweetened with it should not decrease to
any great extent over a long period of time. In aqueous solutions
decomposition due to hydrolysis at the sulfonic ester group is
possible; this is dependent not only on the temperature but also
on the pH of the medium. The stability to hydrolysis of
Acesulfame-K was tested with buffered aqueous solutions at
different pH values at temperatures up to 120 $^{\circ}$C. Acesulfame-K
can be considered largely stable in the temperature range, pH
range and time range applicable in respect of foods (up to
40 $^{\circ}$C; pH 3-8; for several months). Hydrolysis, producing mainly
acetone, CO_2, as well as ammonium and sulfate ions, takes place
preferably under extreme conditions, in other words only below
pH 2.5 and in the strongly alkaline range. Moreover, the aqueous
solutions can be sterilized; up to pH 4 and 120 $^{\circ}$C there is no
detectable decomposition. Nor does subsequent storage of the
sterilized solution for a period of one month at 40 $^{\circ}$C result
in any detectable hydrolysis, so that there is no decrease in
sweetness.

Since Acesulfame-K, on account of the nitrogen atom contained
in its heterocycle, can in principle form a nitrosamide, trials
were conducted to introduce the N-nitroso group into the molecule
under various experimental conditions. Any nitrosamide that might
have formed was tried to analyze photometrically. It was found
that the risk of a N-nitroso group being introduced into the
Acesulfame-K under the conditions prevailing in the organism is
very small compared to other nitrogen-containing compounds.

SWEETNESS AND USE

The relative sweetness of Acesulfame-K is about 200 times that
of a 3 % saccharose solution. The sweetness is perceptible very
quickly and falls off gradually without being unpleasant. As a
rule no unpleasant taste is noticeable in the normal
concentrations applied. Thus Acesulfame-K can be used in a large
number of different foods[2]. Additions in hot and cold drinks
and juices, in bakery products, milk products, fish salads, etc.
have been very favourably assessed from the organoleptic aspect.
Acesulfame-K is also very suitable for imparting a sweet taste
to toothpastes, mouthsprays, mouthwashes, as well as chewing
gums used for cleaning the teeth, and also for pharmaceutical
preparations.

A further field is animal nutrition, where a physiological
adaption to the sweet taste of the mother animal's milk is
achieved by improving the taste of rearing feed. This renders
less problematical the acceptance of food when changing from the
mother animal's milk to dry feed.

PHARMACOLOGICAL AND TOXICOLOGICAL PROPERTIES

Acesulfame-K has been subjected to many pharmacological trials,
including tests for an analgesic, antiphlogistic, psychotropic,
diuretic and broncholytic action. Special tests were carried out
in the dog, viz. analyses of the cardiovascular system and
antiarrhythmic examinations. In addition, the influence of the
coagulation parameters and a possible influence on the lipid
metabolism were investigated.

All tests have shown that Acesulfame-K is an 'inert substance'
in pharmacological respect.

The extensive investigations of the toxicological properties of
Acesulfame-K were carried out by the toxicological department at
Hoechst and university institutes in the Federal Republic of
Germany and the USA, as well as in testing establishments, for
example, in the Netherlands. The results are summarized in the
following.

Determination of the acute oral toxicity shows that Acesulfame-K
is a virtually nontoxic substance (LD_{50} = 6.9 - 8.0 g/kg body

weight). The <u>acute intraperitoneal toxicity</u> resulted in an LD_{50}
of 2.2 g/kg body weight.
The <u>subchronic toxicity</u> (90-day test) was examined in albino
rats in the feed in the following doses: 0/1.0/3.0/10.0 %.
The no-effect level in the feed is 3 %. At 10 % there is slight
diarrhoea and slightly reduced growth. The latter effect was
noted in several long-term trials too. It can be interpreted as
an osmotic effect due to the high potassium ion concentration;
this activity can be simulated by means of an equivalent
potassium chloride dose in parallel examinations with a
similar effect.
The doses 0.3/1 and 3 % in the feed were derived from the
subchronic toxicity test for virtually all long-term trials.
The <u>chronic toxicity</u> was tested in two animal species (dogs and
rats) over a period of 2 years. The test in dogs has been
completed; neither mortalities nor any toxic effects were noted.
The two-year trial in rats was designed as a combined test for
determining the chronic toxicity and <u>carcinogenicity.</u> For this
purpose rats of the F_1^a generation were used whose dams had been
subjected to intra-uterine exposure with Acesulfame-K according
to the dosage level in the two-year trial.
The histological examination of this trial will not be completed
until mid-1979. At the present time no findings at variance with
the control group have been made. The <u>carcinogenicity</u> was
investigated in addition in mice in an 80-day trial. Acesulfame-
K did not exhibit any carcinogenic effect in this trial. A
possible <u>mutagenic</u> activity of the sweetener was determined in
vivo by the following methods:
1.   Dominant lethal assey in rats.
2.   Micronucleus test in mice.
3.   Bone marrow examinations in hamsters.
Trials 1 and 2 have been completed. There are no indications of
a mutagenic activity of Acesulfame-K. In addition to the afore-
mentioned trials, in order to obtain further confirmation of the
absence of <u>mutagenicity,</u> the Ames test was carried out using
several salmonella strains; the results were negative. Cell
transformation tests on cell cultures from Chinese hamsters
and mice were also conducted. According to these tests

Acesulfame-K is neither cytotoxic nor mutagenic.
Reproduction tests with rats to the 3rd filial generation
showed that the fertility, number of young per litter, the
birth weight, growth rate and mortality are not affected when
Acesulfame-K is administered in the feed.
In a similar way it was demonstrated that there is no
teratogenic influence of Acesulfame-K during the pregnancy of
rats on skeleton and internal organs of the foetuses.

^{14}C-labelled Acesulfame-K was used for investigating the
metabolism. It was found that the sweetener is not metabolized
in man, dog, pig and rat. It is excreted unchanged in the form
of the original substance, even after several doses; this was
established in rats after 10 consecutive doses. No other
radioactive substance is detectable alongside that administered.

Pharmacokinetic tests were carried out in man, dog, pig and rat.
Absorption is very rapid and nearly complete. Excretion takes
place preponderantly in the urine. After multiple application
there is no cumulation or accumulation in tissues or organs.

Thus, if the final results of the two-year rat trials are
favourable, a new sweetener will be available which it is
hoped will meet all requirements of the licensing authorities.

REFERENCES
1.   Clauss, K. and Jensen, H., Angew. Chemie 85, 965-973 (1973)
     and Angew. Chemie Internat. Edit. 12, 869-876 (1973)
2.   von Rymon-Lipinski, G.-W., Lück, E. and Dany, F.-J.,
     Kosmetik und Aerosole 49, 243 - 244 (1976)

Health and Sugar Substitutes
Proc. ERGOB Conf., Geneva 1978, pp. 184-190 (Karger, Basel 1978)

POTENTIAL INTENSE SWEETENERS OF NATURAL ORIGIN

G. E. Inglett

Northern Regional Research Center, Federal Research, Science and Education
Administration, U.S. Department of Agriculture, 1815 N. University
Street, Peoria, Illinois 61604, USA

INTRODUCTION

Many people around the world use intensely sweet materials of natural
origin. Plant parts containing intensely sweet principles are used for
sweetening foods or they are used for medicinal purposes as a part of
some societies daily lives. Intense sweetness of natural origin is
tasted in these societies today as it has been done throughout the
ages[1].

PHYLLODULCIN

A sweet tea, Amacha, is served at Hanamatsuri, the flower festival
celebrating the birth of Buddha. Amacha is the dried leaves of Hydranga
macrophylla Seringe var. Thunbergii Makino. The sweet principle, phyllodulcin,
was isolated, and its absolute configuration was shown to be the 3R
configuration at the asymmetric center at C(3) by identification of a
malic acid from ozonized phyllodulcin[2]. Recently, an analog of phyllodulcin,
2-(3-hydroxy-4-methoxyphenyl)-1,3-benzodioxan, was found to be intensely
sweet[3].

STEVIOSIDE

The sweet herb of Paraguay (Yerba dulce), has long been the source
of an intense sweetener. Natives use the leaves of this small shrub,
Stevia rebaudiana (Bert.) Hemsl, to sweeten their bitter drinks. The
sweet, crystalline glycoside that has been extracted from the leaves of
S. rebaudiana, is named stevioside.

Pomaret and Lavieille[4] reported that stevioside readily passes
through human elimination channels in its original form. It did not
appear to be toxic to guinea pigs, rabbits or chickens. Furthermore,
there are no recorded reports of ill effects in Paraguayan users of the
leaves of S. rebaudiana.

Also from the leaves of Stevia rebaudiana, two new sweet glucosides,
rebaudiosides A and B, were isolated besides the known glucosides,
stevioside and steviolbioside. On the basis of IR, MS, IH and ^{13}C NMR,
as well as chemical evidences, the structure of rebaudioside B was
assigned as 13-O-[β-glucosyl(1-2)-β-glucosyl(1-3)]-β-glucosyl-steviol
and rebaudioside A was formulated as its β-glucosyl ester[5].

GLYCYRRHIZIN

Licorice, well-known for centuries and widely used, is obtained
from the roots of Glycyrrhiza glabra, a small shrub, grown and hand-
harvested in Europe and Central Asia. The roots contain from 6 to 14%
glycyrrhizin.

Glycyrrhizic acid exists in licorice root as the calcium-potassium
salt in association with other constituents[6]. Glycyrrhizic acid is a
glycoside of the triterpene, glycyrrhetic acid, which is condensed with
O-β-D-glucuronosyl-(1'→2)-β-D-glucuronic acid. The absolute configuration
of the aglycone, glycyrrhetic acid, is determined as the result of
investigations too numerous to cite completely. Important contributions
were made by Ruzicka et al.[7-11], Voss et al.[12,13] and Beaton and Spring[14].
Although two isomers (18-α and 18-β) have been isolated, Beaton and
Spring have indicated that only the 18-β-glycyrrhetic acid is the natural
isomer that occurs in glycyrrhizin.

The extracts are universally employed in the flavoring and sweetening
of pipe, cigarette and chewing tobaccos, and they are regularly used in
confectionery manufacture. Some segments of the flavor industry have
long utilized these extracts in root beer, chocolate, vanilla, liqueur
and other flavors. Ammonium glycyrrhizin (AG), the fully ammoniated salt
of glycyrrhizic acid, is commercially available. Further treatment and
repeated crystallizations yield the more costly, colorless salt, monoammonium
glycyrrhizinate (MAG). Both derivatives have the same degree of sweetness
but they differ markedly from each other in solubility properties and
sensitivity to pH. AG is the sweetest substance on the FDA list of
natural GRAS flavors and is 50 times sweeter than sucrose.

LO HAN FRUIT (MOMORDICA GROSVENORI) SWINGLE

Lo Han Kuo (Lo Han fruit), from Momordica grosvenori Swingle, is a dried fruit from Southern China. The brownish-gray pulp dries to a light fibrous mass. Swingle[15] also reported that 1000 tons of the green fruits were delivered every year to the drying sheds at Kweilin (Kwangsi Province). The dried fruit is a valued folk medicine used for colds, sore throats, and minor stomach and intestinal troubles. Lee[16] found that the sweet principle could be extracted by water from either the fibrous pulps or from the thin rinds of Lo Han Kuo; 50% ethanol was also found to be a good extractant. Rinds afforded a more easily purified extract. Sweetness of Lo Han sweetener was accompanied by a lingering taste described as licorice-like, somewhat similar to that of stevioside, glycyrrhizin and the dihydrochalcones. Structural studies indicate the sweetener to be a triterpenoid glycoside with 5 or 6 glucose units[17]. The purified sweetener has a more pleasant sweet taste than the impure material. The purest sample is about 400 times sweeter than sucrose.

OSLADIN

The sweet taste of rhizomes of the widely distributed fern, Polypodium vulgare L., has attracted the interest of many chemists and pharmacists. Osladin comprised only 0.03% of the dry weight of the rhizomes; its chemical structure was revealed as a bis-glycoside of a new type of steriodal saponin[18]. The glycoside that results by replacement of the monosaccharide radical with hydrogen was isolated separately and named polypodosaponin. Its absolute configuration was determined by Jizba et al.[19]. The disaccharide of osladin was shown to be neohesperidose, 2-O-α-L-rhamnopyranosyl-β-D-glucopyranose.

MIRACLE FRUIT (SYNSEPALUM DULCIFICUM)

An important approach to sweet taste perception is the study of the strange properties of the miracle fruit (Synsepalum dulcificum). Although the miracle fruit's capacity to cause sour foods to taste sweet has been known in the literature since 1852, scientific investigations of the fruit were not made until Inglett and his associates found some experimental evidence that the active principle was macromolecular[20]. This berry posseses a taste-modifying substance that causes sour foods such as lemons, limes, grapefruit, rhubarb and strawberries to taste delightfully sweet. The berries are chewed by West Africans for their sweetening effect of some sour foods. The taste-modifying principle was independently isolated by two different research groups[21,22]. Kurihara and Beidler[21] separated the active principle from the fruit's pulp with a carbonate buffer (pH 10.5). Destroying the active principle by trypsin and pronase suggested its proteinaceous character. The taste-modifying protein was also separated from the fruit's pulp with highly basic compounds, salmine and spermine[22].

The basic glycoprotein has a molecular weight between 42,000 and 44,000. The purified glycoprotein has no inherent taste. Sweetening of acid taste was observed at 5×10^{-8}M concentration of the glycoprotein solution and reached a maximum at 4×10^{-7}M and slowly declines over a period up to 2 hr.

SERENDIPITY BERRIES (DIOSCOREOPHYLLUM CUMMINSII DIELS)

While studying various natural sweeteners previously mentioned, the author discovered the intense sweetness of some red berries indigenous to tropical West Africa. The fruit was called the serendipity berry, and its botanical name, Dioscoreophyllum cumminsii, was established many months later[23-26].

Researchers at the Monell Senses Center and the Unilever Research Laboratorium, working independently, confirmed the protein nature of the serendipity sweetener[27,28]. Amino acid composition of monellin was determined by van der Wel and Loeve[29] and Morris et al.[30]. The most outstanding observation is the complete absence of histidine. Monellin is composed of two dissimilar polypeptide chains with known amino acid sequences that are noncovalently associated[31,32]. The sweetness of monellin is approximately 2500 times sweeter than sucrose on a weight basis. The molecular weight of the sweetener is 11,000.

KATEMFE (THAUMATOCOCCUS DANIELLI)

Besides studies on miracle fruit and the serendipity berry, a large variety of plant materials were examined systematically by Inglett and May[24] for intensity and quality of sweetness. Another African fruit containing an intense sweetener was katemfe, or the miraculous fruit of the Sudan. Botanically the plant is Thaumatococcus danielli of the family Marantaceae. The mucilaginous material around the seeds is intensely sweet and causes other foods to taste sweet. Katemfe yields two sweet-tasting proteins which are called thaumatin I and II[33,34].

The purified sweetener is 1600 times sweeter than sucrose on a weight basis. Thaumatin I contains 193 amino acids[33,34]. Polyacrylamide gel electrophoresis in the presence of sodium dodecyl sulfate indicated that the protein is a single polypeptide chain with alanine as the N-terminal amino acid. Thaumatin I was crystallized and physical characteristics and diffraction data of the crystals were obtained[35]. A process for extraction of the thaumatins from the fruit was reported[36] and commercial interest in this sweetener is developing.

REFERENCES

1. Inglett, G. E.   J. Toxicol. Environ. Health. 2: 207-214, 1976.
2. Arakawa, H. and Nakazaki, M.   Chem. Ind. (London) 671, 1959.
3. Dick, W. E., Jr. and Hodge, J. E.   J. Agric. Food Chem. (in press).
4. Pomaret, M. and Lavieille, R.   Bull. Soc. Chim. Biol. 13: 1248-1252, 1931.
5. Kohda, H., et al.   Phytochemistry 15: 981-983, 1976.
6. Nieman, C.   in Advances in Food Research, Vol. 7, Academic Press, New York, 1957.
7. Ruzicka, L., Furter, M. and Leuenberger, H.   Helv. Chim. Acta 20: 312-325, 1937A.
8. Ruzicka, L., Jeger, O. and Ingold, W.   Helv. Chim. Acta 26: 2278-2282, 1943.
9. Ruzicka, L. and Leuenberger, H.   Helv. Chim. Acta 19: 1402-1406, 1936.
10. Ruzicka, L., Leuenberger, H. and Schellenberg, H.   Helv. Chim. Acta 20: 1271-1282, 1937.
11. Ruzicka, L. and Marxer, A.   Helv. Chim. Acta 22: 195-201, 1939.
12. Voss, W., Klein, P. and Sauer, H.   Ber. 70B: 1212-1218, 1937A.
13. Voss, W. and Butter, G.   Ber. 70B: 1212-1218, 1937C.
14. Beaton, J. M. and Spring, F. S.   J. Chem. Soc. 3126-3129, 1955.
15. Swingle, W. T.   J. Arnold Arbor. Harv. Univ. 22: 198, 1941.
16. Lee, C. H.   Experientia 31(5): 533-534, 1975.
17. Lee, C. H.   Personal communication.   General Foods Corporation, Tarrytown, N.Y., 1977.
18. Jizba, J., Dolejs, L., Herout, V. and Sorm, F.   Tetrahedron Lett. 18: 1329-1332, 1971.
19. Jizba, J., et al.   Chem. Ber. 104: 837-846, 1971.
20. Inglett, G. E., Dowling, B., Albrecht, J. J. and Hoglan, F. A.   J. Agric. Food Chem. 13: 284-287, 1965.
21. Kurihara, K. and Beidler, L. M.   Science 161: 1241-1243, 1968.
22. Brouwer, J. N., van der Wel, H., Francke, A. and Henning, G. J. Nature (London) 220: 373-374, 1968.

23. Inglett, G. E. and Findlay, J. C. Abstr. Pap. 75A presented to the Division of Agriculture and Food Chemistry, 154th Am. Chem. Soc. Meeting, Chicago, Ill., 1967.

24. Inglett, G. E. and May, J. F. Econ. Bot. 22: 326-331, 1968.

25. Inglett, G. E. and May, J. F. J. Food Res. 34: 408-411, 1969.

26. Inglett, G. E. in Symposium: Sweeteners, edited by G. E. Inglett, Avi Publishing, Westport, Conn. 1974.

27. Morris, J. A. and Cagan, R. H. Biochim. Biophys. Acta 261: 114-122, 1972.

28. van der Wel, H. FEBS Lett. 21: 88-90, 1972.

29. van der Wel, H. and Loeve, K. FEBS Lett. 29: 181-184, 1973.

30. Morris, J. A., Martenson, R., Deibler, G. and Cagan, R. H. J. Biol. Chem. 248: 534-539, 1973.

31. Bohak, Z. and Li, S-L. Biochim. Biophys. Acta 427: 153-170 1976.

32. Hudson, G. and Biemann, K. Biochim. Biophys. Res. Commun. 71: 212-220, 1976.

33. van der Wel, H. and Loeve, K. Eur. J. Biochem. 31: 221-225, 1972.

34. van der Wel, H. in Symposium: Sweeteners, edited by G. E. Inglett, Avi Publishing Co., Westport, Conn., 1974.

35. van der Wel, H., Soest, Van T. C. and Royers, E. C. FEBS Lett. 56(2): 316-317, 1975.

36. Higginbotham, J. D. U.S. Pat. 4,011,206. March 8, 1977.

V. Sugar substitutes in oral health Metabolic criteria indicative for cariogenicity

Moderator: H.R. Mühlemann, Zurich
Co-Moderator: B. Guggenheim, Zurich

Health and Sugar Substitutes
Proc. ERGOB Conf., Geneva 1978, pp. 192-198 (Karger, Basel 1978)

SOME BACTERIOLOGICAL ASPECTS OF SUGAR SUBSTITUTES.

R. Havenaar, J.H.J. Huis in 't Veld, O. Backer Dirks and J.D. de Stoppelaar.

Departments of Preventive Dentistry and Oral Microbiology, University of Utrecht
School of Dentistry, Sorbonnelaan 16, Utrecht, The Netherlands.

INTRODUCTION

Dental caries is initiated by decalcification of the dental enamel by organic acids. These acids are produced through fermentation of dietary carbohydrates by micro-orgamisms accumulated in dental plaque adhering to the surface of the teeth. Many in vivo experiments have shown that consumption of sugars, e.g. sucrose, glucose or other mono- and disaccharides, results in a pH-drop in plaque to values far below the critical pH (5.5) at which enamel starts to dissolve. In addition various plaque-bacteria have the ability to synthesize intracellular polysaccharides (IPS) from different sugars. These glycogen-like glucans will be broken down when exogenous carbohydrates have been exhausted, resulting in prolonged acid production.

Sucrose has received special attention because of the production of extracellular polysaccharides (EPS) by certain oral streptococci (S. mutans). These glucans are believed to play a role in adhesion and accumulation of bacteria on the tooth surface, thus contributing to plaque formation and caries.

Our most common dietary sweetener is sucrose and one area of research in caries prevention is the (partial) replacement of sucrose in the diet by non-cariogenic sweeteners. In this respect the main criterium to be met by such sugar substitutes is that they will not - or only slowly - be fermented to acid by plaque bacteria and do not exhance plaque formation.

The following substances have received considerable attention: sorbitol, xylitol, lactitol, maltitol, L-sorbose and lycasin. Various animal experiments as well as some clinical studies have demonstrated that these substances are less cariogenic than sucrose. Even a partial substitution of sucrose by xylitol has been shown to cause less carious lesions in rats than sucrose alone.

Why do these sugar substitutes have such low cariogenic potential? Which bacteriological aspects are involved? In the present study these sugar substitutes were tested in a series of experiments:

1) acid formation in growing cultures by predominant oral bacteria;

2) influence of addition of xylitol to glucose in growing cultures of S. mutans;

3) acid production and adaptation in resing cell suspensions of S. mutans and
   Lactobacillus casei;

4) IPS and EPS production from the sugar substitutes.

MATERIALS AND METHODS

Bacterial reference strains were obtained from the department of Oral Microbiology. Fresh isolates of Streptococci and Actinomyces strains were obtained
from caries-free and caries active subjects at the department of Preventive Dentistry.

The following sugar substitutes were used in this study: sorbitol (Difco),
xylitol (Hoffmann-La Roche), lactitol (Amsterdam Chemie Combinatie, A.C.C.),
maltitol (A.C.C.), L-sorbose (Roquette Frères) and Lycasin types 05.60, 80.33
and 80.55 (Roquette Frères). Lycasin is an hydrogenated starch hydrolysate, containing sorbitol, maltitol and higher polyols.

The ability to produce acid from glucose and the sugar substitutes in growing
cultures was tested using micro-titer plates (Dynatech). The cups were filled
with 0.2ml Phenol Red Broth (PRB; Difco) with addition of 1% glucose or sugar
substitute and 0.15% agar and inoculated with 25 µl of a bacterial suspension in
PRB without carbohydrates. After incubation for 72 hours at $37^{o}C$, a colour change indicated acid formation. In this way it was possible to test many strains in
a relatively short time. Of each species at least twenty strains were tested in
duplicate.

For fermentation experiments of non-growing cells of S. mutans and L. casei
standardized resting cell suspensions were used. Overnight cultures of S. mutans
C67-1 and L. casei in trypticase yeast-extract medium supplemented with 0.1%
glucose were centrifuged, washed twice with a phosphate-citric acid buffer (pH
7.0) and suspended in the same buffer to an optical density of 6.0 at 565 nm.

Growth of S. mutans serotype c and e in glucose broth with or without added
xylitol was recorded automatically. At regular intervals, samples for pH measurements were taken.

Adaptation of the strains tested was obtained by subculturing twenty times in
a medium containing 1% of the sugar substitutes, while the stability of the
adaptation was tested by re-culturing the adapted strain once in 0.1% glucose
medium.

IPS formation by S. mutans was determined by measuring the optical density of
the IPS-Iodine complex (1) in the resting cell suspensions after the addition of
2% glucose or sugar substitute for 2 hours at $37^{o}C$.

Adherence of S. mutans cells to glass surfaces in the presence of sucrose and
sugar substitutes was tested using the method of Mukasa and Slade (2). That
method is based on measuring the optical density of the dislodged adhered cells.

RESULTS

FERMENTATION OF DIFFERENT SUGAR SUBSTITUTES BY PREDOMINANT ORAL BACTERIA.

The results of the fermentation in growing cultures are shown the table below.

	Glucose	Sorbitol	Xylitol	Lactitol	Maltitol	Lycasin	L-sorbose
S. mutans	+	+	−	+	+	+	−
S. sanguis	+	−/(+)	−	−/+	−	−	−
S. mitior	+	−/(+)	−	−	−	−	−
S. milleri	+	−	−	+/(−)	−	−	−
A. viscosus	+	+	−	−/+	−/(+)	+/−	−
A. naeslundii	+	+	−	+/(−)	−	−/(+)	−
A. odontoliticus	+	−	−	−/(+)	−	+	−
Lactobacillus	+	+	−	+	+	+/(−)	+/−

(+/− 50-90% +; −/+ 50-90% −; +/(−) 90-100% +; −/(+) 90-100% −)

As expected glucose was fermented by all strains tested. No acid production from xylitol by any of the bacterial strains was observed. In addition to reference strains of L. casei, several freshly isolated oral lactobacilli could ferment L-sorbose. S. mutans produced acid from: sorbitol, lactitol and lycasin, while maltitol was slowly fermented. Actinomyces species were also able to ferment sorbitol, lactitol and lycasin.

In other series of experiments, a variety of predominant oral bacteria (not shown in the table) were found to be incapable of fermenting any of the sugar substitutes tested.

Figure 1 shows that addition of small amounts of xylitol to glucose medium inhibited the initial growth of S. mutans (dotted lines), but had little influence on the final pH (solid lines).

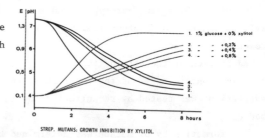

STREP. MUTANS: GROWTH INHIBITION BY XYLITOL.

figure 1

FERMENTATION BY STANDARDIZED RESTING
CELL SUSPENSIONS OF S. MUTANS.

Figure 2 shows that resting cell
suspensions of S. mutans very slightly
fermented the sugar substitutes, except
xylitol and L-sorbose. The fast fermentation of glucose was not inhibited by
the addition of varying amounts of xylitol (0-4%).

Adaptation of S. mutans by frequent
subculturing in lycasin, sorbitol,
lactitol and maltitol resulted in a
marked increase in fermentation, as
shown in figure 3.

However, when the adapted strain
subsequently was subcultured once in
glucose, most of this adaptation was
lost (figure 4), indicating that the
adaptation was rather unstable. No
adaptation to xylitol and L-sorbose
was observed.

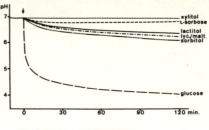

STREP. MUTANS C67-1:   NON-ADAPTED STRAIN.

figure 2

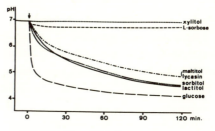

STREP. MUTANS C67-1 :   ADAPTED STRAINS.

figure 3

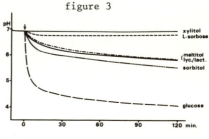

STREP. MUTANS C67-1:   DIS-ADAPTED STRAINS.

figure 4

INTRACELLULAR AND EXTRACELLULAR POLYSACCHARIDE SYNTHESIS BY S. MUTANS C67-1.

Resting cell suspensions of the non-adapted strain of S. mutans were not
able to produce detectable levels of IPS from the sugar substitutes within two
hours.

However, after adaptation to sorbitol and lactitol some IPS formation occurred; the extinction value of the iodine/polysaccharide complex was only about
25% of the value obtained with glucose. This capacity disappeared after one subsequent cultivation of the adapted strain in glucose.

Since iodine also forms a coloured complex with lycasin, IPS synthesis from
lycasin could not be determined with this method.

Addition of xylitol (0-4%) to a medium containing glucose (1-2%), inoculated

with S. mutans and incubated for 18 hours had no influence on the IPS synthesis
by S. mutans from glucose.

Adherence can be used as a parameter for the synthesis of different kinds of
EPS (2). Addition of different percentages of sugar substitutes to cell suspensions of S. mutans in sucrose buffer, did not influence the initial adherence
of S. mutans to glass surfaces caused by sucrose alone.

No adherence of S. mutans by the individual sugar substitutes was observed.

FERMENTATION BY STANDARDIZED RESTING CELL SUSPENSIONS OF L. CASEI.

Resting cell suspensions of L. casei
were tested for fermentation of and adaptation to L-sorbose and lycasin. Figure
5 shows that acid production from L-sorbose by the non-adapted strain is poor.
Only one subculturing in L-sorbose resulted in a remarkable adaptation:
a drop to pH 4 within 60 minutes.

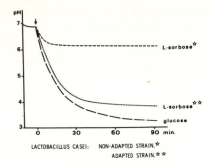

figure 5

Similarly, adaptation to (2%) lycasin
could be demonstrated (figure 6). In contrast to the other sugar substitutes and
to S. mutans figure 6 also shows two
other phenomena concerning the initial
fermentation of lycasin by L. casei:
a) 1 or 2% lycasin was still not an excess;
the addition of 4% lycasin resulted in a
faster and lower pH-drop than 2% lycasin; b) the pH curve shows an irregular
pH-drop, probably indicating different
enzymes involved in the fermentation of
the various components of lycasin.

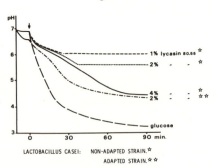

figure 6

DISCUSSION.

In the present study no predominant oral micro-organisms were found capable
of fermenting xylitol and L-sorbose, while sorbitol, lactitol, maltitol and lycasin were (slowly) fermented in growing cultures by some streptococci, actinomyces and lactobacilli. In resting cell suspensions, S. mutans could slowly ferment sorbitol, lactitol, maltitol and lycasin and L. casei L-sorbose. The above
in vitro results are essentially in agreement with the findings of various other
investigators (3; 4).

In vivo plaque pH measurements in numerous studies have shown little or no
pH-drop after rinsing with solutions of sugar substitutes or after eating candies containing them (e.g. 5; 6; 7). Only lycasin has been reported in some studies to cause a significant pH-drop in plaque (8; 9). The chemical composition
of lycasin, which varies from one type to another, may be responsible for
slightly conflicting results.

The non-fermentation of xylitol by oral bacteria agrees with in vivo plaque
pH measurements (10).

The fermentation of L-sorbose and lycasin by some strains of lactobacilli
seems to be of little concern because lactobacilli in general constitute only
a small fraction of the plaque flora.

Our experiments demonstrate that S. mutans is able to adapt (acid production,
some IPS formation) to the sugar substitutes tested except xylitol and L-sorbose. It is likely that this is caused by the induction of enzymes, necessary for
the fermentation of these sugar-alcohols. The adaptation is partly lost after
one subculturing in glucose. Since sugar substitutes are virtually always consumed in combination with other sugars, it seems unlikely that gross adaptation
will occur in vivo. This was also suggested in a recent clinical study with sorbitol by Birkhed and Edwardsson (11).

Addition of xylitol to cultures of S. mutans in media containing glucose or
sucrose had little influence on the final pH but slowed the growth of the organisms. Similar observations were reported by Knuuttila and Mäkinen (12), although they used larger amounts of xylitol. From these bacteriological findings
per se a possible caries preventive effect of xylitol/sucrose combinations cannot be expected. Nevertheless, recent results from animal experiments in our
laboratory (Havenaar and Huis in 't Veld, unpublished results) showed a caries
inhibition when xylitol was added to a sucrose diet. Other than bacteriological
effects, such as changes in the composition of saliva, may play a role.

In conclusion, bacteriological laboratory studies with sugar substitutes
provide valuable information concerning their possible effect on caries and are
a good basis for further biochemical, clinical and animal experiments.

REFERENCES.

1. Van Houte, J. and Jansen, H.M. Caries Res. 2 : 47-56, 1968.

2. Mukasa, H. and Slade, H.D. Infect. Immun. 8 : 555-562, 1973.

3. Gehring, F.   Dtsch. zahnärztl. Z. 26 : 1162-1171, 1971.

4. Edwardsson, S., Birkhed, D. and Mejàre, B.
   Acta Odont. Scand. 35 : 257-263, 1977.

5. Neff, D.   Caries Res. 1 : 78-87, 1967.

6. Schneider, Ph. and Mühlemann, H.R.   Schweiz. Mschr.
   Zahnheilk. 86 : 150-166, 1976.

7. MacFadyen, E.E.   et al. Caries Res. 11 : 114, 1977.

8. Mühlemann, H.R.   Schweiz. Mschr. Zahnheilk. 79 : 117-145, 1969.

9. Frostell, G. Odont. Revy 24 : 217-226, 1973.

10. Mühlemann, H.R. et al. Caries Res. 11 : 263-276, 1977.

11. Birkhed, D. and Edwardsson, S.   25th ORCA-congress, abstract no. 75, 1978.

12. Knuuttila, M.L.E. and Mäkinen, K.K.   Caries Res. 9 : 177-189, 1975.

CARBOHYDRATES, SUGAR SUBSTITUTES AND ORAL BACTERIAL COLONIZATION

J. van Houte

Department of Microbiology, Forsyth Dental Center
140 Fenway, Boston, MA 02115

INTRODUCTION

Carbohydrates serve as substrates for a variety of bacterial metabolic
activities. The magnitude and frequency of their consumption are known to
influence the mass, composition, and metabolism of the bacterial flora present
on different oral surfaces. Topics that will be briefly discussed are: 1)
bacterial metabolism related to the presence of carbohydrates in the mouth, 2)
the influence of dietary carbohydrates on the composition of the oral flora,
and 3) the effect of sugar substitutes on the colonization of oral bacteria.

METABOLIC PROCESSES ASSOCIATED WITH CARBOHYDRATE UTILIZATION

The colonization of the mouth by bacteria involves two distinct processes.[1]
First, bacteria must adhere to an oral surface with sufficient strength to prevent their removal by the existing cleansing forces. Second, once attached,
bacteria must initiate growth and multiplication. On certain surfaces such as
the teeth, large bacterial masses, termed dental plaque, can accumulate. Such
bacterial accumulation requires besides initial cell attachment and growth,
interbacterial adhesion that allows the formation of different bacterial layers.[1]

Fermentation of carbohydrates by bacteria, leading to the formation of
organic acids, provides energy for their growth, multiplication and maintenance. Carbohydrates are a major, if not sole, source of energy for many
numerically-important oral bacteria. Carbohydrate fermentation by bacteria
concentrated in dense masses such as dental plaques may lead to the accumulation of high concentrations of acids and a low pH which is generally considered a prerequisite for caries development.

Carbohydrates also serve as substrates for the synthesis of glycogen-like
polymers[2] and extracellular polymers[3]. Many oral bacteria store intracellularly glycogen-like polymers that are synthesized from common dietary carbohydrates. Carbohydrate consumption leads to rapid bacterial fermentation and
acid production in plaque as well as bacterial glycogen accumulation. Bacterial degradation of intracellular glycogen to acid after oral depletion of the

carbohydrate consumed may contribute to prolonged acid production in plaque. Glycogen accumulation by certain streptococci also increases their rate of acid production[2] presumably because this process requires energy that must be generated via carbohydrate fermentation. Glycogen accumulation can possibly also promote the survival of bacteria by acting as a reserve of energy.[4] Glycogen synthesis by plaque bacteria has been implicated in the etiology of dental caries based on the prolonged and increased acid production associated with this metabolic process, but conclusive evidence for its significance in caries development is still lacking.

The synthesis of extracellular homo- and heteropolysaccharides from various carbohydrates is common among oral bacteria.[3,5] Streptococci such as S. mutans and S. sanguis or certain lactobacillus sp. can synthesize glucans, e.g. dextran or mutan, especially from sucrose. Sucrose may also be converted to fructan, e.g. levan, by streptococci such as S. salivarius and by Actinomyces sp.[6] or to inulin-like fructan by S. mutans.[7] Extracellular polysaccharides may promote bacterial attachment to and accumulation on teeth and may serve as an energy reserve. Glucans clearly enhance the accumulation of S. mutans on teeth by promoting intercellular binding; it is not clear whether they also promote initial attachment of S. mutans cells to teeth.[8] At present, glucans do not appear to play a role in the attachment of other glucan or non-glucan-synthesizing oral bacteria.[1,8] Glucans may also play a minor role as energy reserves since they can be slowly degraded by various oral bacteria.[1] Levans are rapidly degraded by oral bacteria and may serve, similar to glycogen, as energy reserves; they have not been associated with bacterial adherence.[1] Lactobacillus casei can synthesize a glucose-rhamnose capsule from sucrose, lactose, maltose and fructose and especially from glucose which can serve as an energy reserve.[9] Actinomyces sp. form a different heteropolysaccharide from various common carbohydrates but its role in the organisms' colonization has not yet been clarified.[10]

INFLUENCE OF DIETARY CARBOHYDRATE ON THE ORAL FLORA

Studies with tube-fed rodents,[11] dogs,[12] monkeys[13,14] and humans[15] or with subjects fed a diet with negligible carbohydrate content[16,17] indicate that plaque development per se can occur when little or no dietary carbohydrate enters the mouth. However, the amount of plaque formed under these conditions is generally lower than that in subjects consuming a "normal" diet. This difference may not always, or entirely, reflect the absence of dietary carbohydrate in the mouth because of other concomitant changes, f.e. in the consistency of the diet,[18] that are known to influence plaque formation. In some studies with humans, sucrose has been found to specifically promote plaque formation[19,20,21] whereas in others with humans[22] or dogs[23] no difference has been noted. This variation may be partly due to differences in the basal sucrose level of the diets consumed, or in the plaque flora between humans or between humans and dogs with respect to organisms such as S. mutans that can benefit in their colonization from the presence of sucrose.

Information about the role of different dietary carbohydrates in the colonization of individual oral bacteria is very incomplete. Only a few of the bacteria such as S. mutans and lactobacilli, mainly due to their suspected involvement in dental caries, have been studied in this respect. Studies with rodents, monkeys and humans have clearly demonstrated the favorable effect of sucrose on the colonization of teeth by S. mutans.[1,24,25] Replacement of sucrose in the diet by glucose, fructose, maltose, starch, or other carbohydrates or its deletion from the diet leads to a rapid decrease of the S. mutans numbers on the teeth whereas an increase in sucrose consumption leads to higher numbers. As mentioned earlier, sucrose influences the colonization of S.mutans mainly via adherence mechanisms. To date, sucrose does not appear to specifically influence the colonization of other plaque bacteria such as S. sanguis, S. salivarius, lactobacilli, or A. viscosus;[1] data for other plaque bacteria are unavailable.

Changes in total carbohydrate intake affect various plaque organisms. Restriction of carbohydrate consumption in normal individuals or subject suffering from hereditary fructose intolerance or tube feeding of humans or monkeys, leads to a decrease in S. mutans, streptococci (undifferentiated), lactobacilli, yeasts and S. salivarius whereas a high carbohydrate consumption is associated with relatively high oral levels of these organisms.[13,14,15,17,26,27] The fluctuation of the populations of these organisms according to the carbohydrate supply may be partly due to the fact that carbohydrate serves as their main source of energy for growth and/or is a required substrate for the synthesis of polymers involved in their adhesion to oral surfaces. Also, lactobacilli, yeasts, and S. mutans are relatively acid-tolerant organisms. Thus, a low plaque pH associated with a high carbohydrate intake provides these organisms with a selective growth advantage over less acid-tolerant plaque organisms. Shifts in the populations of these organisms in plaque may therefore also be due to changes in plaque pH. This is also suggested by studies with subjects suffering from xerostomia (=dry mouth). Such individuals have a negligible salivary flow, have generally a high carbohydrate intake, may develop rampant caries unless treated adequately, and exhibit increased plaque proportions of lactobacilli, yeasts, S. mutans and catalase-positive diphtheroids.

SUGAR SUBSTITUTES AND COLONIZATION OF ORAL BACTERIA

Data on the influence of sugar substitutes on plaque development or the colonization of different oral bacterial species are limited and nearly exclusively concern sorbitol and xylitol. Studies with monkeys[25] and humans[29,30] suggest that consumption of sorbitol does not decrease the amount of plaque in comparison to the consumption of sucrose. Partial replacement of dietary sucrose by xylitol appears to lead to somewhat less plaque in humans[31,34] whereas almost complete replacement of dietary sucrose by fructose or xylitol for 2 years has been found to reduce the plaque quantity in subjects on the diet with xylitol to 50% of that of subjects consuming the other diets.[35] Rinsing with xylitol solution does not appear to interfere with early plaque formation in humans.[36] Consumption of candy with Lycasin, a mixture of sorbitol, maltitol and hydrogenated saccharides and dextrins, has also been reported to decrease plaque formation as compared to candy with sucrose.[37]

Nearly complete replacement of dietary sucrose by sorbitol in studies with monkeys, by xylitol in studies with rats and humans, or by Lycasin in rats and hamsters, causes a marked decrease in plaque populations of S.mutans or impairs its implantation on the teeth but other streptococci remain unaffected.[25,38,39,40,41] Nearly complete long-term replacement of sucrose by xylitol also lowers the salivary numbers of lactobacilli and Candida sp. in humans.[42] In vitro, xylitol does not interfere with the colonization of S. mutans on rat teeth in presence of sucrose[36] or with the growth of oral Candida albicans strains.[43] Aspartame has been reported to interfere with plaque formation by S. mutans in presence of sucrose in vitro whereas saccharine enhanced this process and cyclamate was without effect.[44]

The influence of sugar substitutes on the oral flora appears to be similar to that of restriction of dietary carbohydrates. This is not unexpected since sugar substitutes are selected because they are poorly metabolized by oral bacteria and their consumption does not cause dangerous plaque pH drops.[36,45] Sorbitol and Lycasin are only slowly metabolized by a variety of oral bacteria whereas only L. salivarius has been found so far to ferment xylitol.[36,46-51] It may be anticipated therefore that other potential, poorly fermentable, sugar substitutes such as sorbose[51] or maltitol[45,50] will exert a similar influence on the oral flora as the other sugar substitutes.

Aspects of sugar substitution in relation to the composition of the oral flora that deserve attention include: 1) its effect on potentially cariogenic bacteria other than S. mutans and lactobacilli, e.g. Actinomyces sp., that have not been studied, and 2) its effect on the balance of the oral flora in relation to disease. With respect to the latter, restriction of dietary carbohydrate

has not been found to lead to obvious ecological imbalances of the oral flora
or to disease. However, substantial dietary changes may have more subtle
effects. For example, the higher plaque pH resulting from such a regimen may
favor the establishment and growth of certain groups of Gram-negative bacteria
that are implicated in periodontal disease.

REFERENCES

1. Gibbons, R.J. and van Houte, J. Ann. Rev. of Micro. 29: 19-44, 1975.

2. Gibbons, R.J. and van Houte, J. Ann. Rev. of Med. 26: 121-136, 1975.

3. Newbrun, E. in Microbial aspects of dental caries, edited by Stiles,
   H.M., Loesche, W.J. and O'Brien, T.C. pp. 649-664, Information Retrieval
   Inc., Washington, D.C., 1976.

4. van Houte, J. and Jansen, H.M. J. Bacteriol. 101-1083-1085, 1970.

5. Guggenheim, B. Int. dent. J. 20: 657-678, 1970.

6. Howell, A. and Jordan, H.V. Archs. Oral Biol. 12: 571-573, 1967.

7. Rosell, K. and Birkhed, D. Acta Chem. Scand. B28: 589, 1974.

8. van Houte, J. in Microbial aspects of dental caries, edited by Stiles,
   H.M., Loesche, W.J. and O'Brien, T.C. pp. 3-32, Information Retrieval
   Inc., Washington, D.C., 1976.

9. Hammond, B.F. Archs. Oral Biol. 11: 1199-1202, 1966.

10. Vander Hoeven, J.S. Caries Res. 8:193-210, 1974.

11. Kite, O.W., Shaw, J.H. and Sognnaes, R.F. J. Nutr. 42: 89-105, 1950.

12. Egelberg, J. Odont. Revy. 16: 50-60, 1965.

13. Bowen, W.H. and Cornick, D.E. Int. dent. J. 20: 382-395, 1970.

14. Bowen, W.H. Archs. Oral Biol. 19: 231-239, 1974.

15. Littleton, N.W., McCabe, R.M. and Carter, C.H. Archs.Oral Biol. 12:601-609,
    1967.

16. van Houte, J. Archs. Oral Biol. 9:91-93, 1964.

17. deStoppelaar, J.D., van Houte, J. and Backer-Dirks, O. Caries Res. 4: 114-123,
    1970.

18. Egelberg, J. Odont. Revy. 16: 31-41, 1965.

19. Carlsson, J. and Egelberg, J. Odont. Revy. 16: 112, 1965.

20. Kinoshita, S., Schait, A., Brebou, M. and Mühlemann, H.R. Helv. odont.
    Acta 10: 134-137, 1966.

21. Fry, A.J. and Grenby, T.H. Archs. Oral Biol. 17:873-882, 1972.

22. Staat, R.H., Gawronski, T.H., Cressey, D.E. Harris, R.S. and Folke, L.E.A.
    J. dent. Res. 54: 872-880, 1975.

23. Carlsson, J. and Egelberg, J. Odont. Revy. 16: 42-49, 1965.

24. van Houte, J. Upeslacis, V.N., Jordan, H.V., Skobe, Z. and Green, D.B.
    J. dent. Res. 55: 202-215, 1976.

25. Cornick, D.E. and Bowen, W.H. Archs. Oral Biol. 17: 1637-1648, 1972.

26. Hoover, C.I. and Newbrun, E. Int. Assoc.Dent.Res. 57, Abstr.#555, 1978.

27. Jay, P. Am. J. Orth and Oral Surg. 33: 162-184, 1947.

28. Dreisen, S. and Brown, L.R. in Microbial aspects of dental caries,
    edited by Stiles, H.M., Loesche, W.J. and O'Brien, T.C. pp. 263-273,
    Information Retrieval Inc., Washington, D.C.,1976.

29. Scheinin, A. and Mäkinen, K.K. Acta odont. Scand. 30: 235-257, 1972.

30. Ainamo, J., Asikainen, S., Ainamo, A., Lahtinen, A. and Sjoblom, M.
    Int. Assoc. Dent. Res. 57, Abstr. #993, 1978.

31. Scheinin, A. and Mäkinen, K.K. Int. dent J. 21: 302-321, 1971.

32. Mouton, C., Scheinin, A. and Mäkinen, K.K. Acta odont.Scand. 33: 33-40, 1975.

33. Mouton, C., Scheinin, A. and Mäkinen, K.K. Acta odont.Scand. 33: 27-31,1975.

34. Larmas, M., Scheinin, A., Gehring, F. and Mäkinen, K.K. Acta odont. Scand.
    33, Suppl. 70: 321-336, 1975.

35. Mäkinen, K.K. and Scheinin, A. Acta odont. Scand. 33,Suppl.70:129-171, 1975.

36. Mühlemann, H.R., Schmid, R., Noguchi,T., Imfeld, T. and Hirsch,R.S. Caries
    Res. 11: 263-276, 1977.

37. Frostell, G., Blomlöf, L., Blomquist, T., Dahl, G.M., Edwards, S.,
    Fjellström, A., Henrikson, C.O., Larje, O., Nord, C.E. and Nordenvall,K.J.
    Acta odont. Scand. 32: 235-254, 1974.

38. Karle, E. und Gehring, F. Dtsch. Zahnärztl. Z. 30: 356-363, 1975.

39. Gehring, F., Mäkinen, K.K. Larmas, M. and Scheinin, A. Acta odont. Scand.
    33, Suppl. 70: 223-237, 1975.

40. Frostell, G., Keyes, P.H. and Larson, R.H. J. Nutr. 93: 65-76, 1967.

41. Larje, O. and Larson, R.H. Archs. Oral Biol. 15: 805-816, 1970.

42. Larmas, M., Mäkinen, K.K. and Scheinin, A. Acta odont. Scand. 33,
    Suppl. 70: 173-216, 1975.

43. Makinen, K.K., Ojanotko,A.and Vidgren,H.J. dent. Res. 54: 1239, 1975.

44. Olson, B.L. J. dent. Res. 56: 1426, 1977.

45. Fosdick, L.S., Englander, H.R., Hoerman,K.C. and Kesel, R.G.,
    J. Amer. Dent. Ass. 55: 191-195, 1957.

46. Edwardsson, S., Birkhed, D. and Mejare, B. Acta odont. Scand. 35: 257-263,
    1977.

47. Frostell, G. Dtsch. Zahnärztl. Z. 26: 1181-1187, 1971.

48. Gehring, F. und Patz, J. Dtsch. Zahnärztl. Z. 29: 1026-1029, 1974.

49. Gehring, F. Dtsch. Zahnärztl. Z. 26:1162-1171, 1971.

50. Trautner, K. Dtsch. Zahnärztl. Z. 26: 1172-1180, 1971.

51. Havenaar, R. Huis in 't Veld, J.H.J., Backer-Dirks, O. and deStoppelaar,
    J. D. Caries Res. 12: 118, 1978.

52. Mühlemann, H.R. and Schneider, Ph. Helv. odont.Acta 19: 76-80, 1975.

Health and Sugar Substitutes
Proc. ERGOB Conf., Geneva 1978, pp. 205-210 (Karger, Basel 1978)

POTENTIALS OF THE ORAL MICROFLORA TO UTILIZE SUGAR SUBSTITUTES AS ENERGY SOURCE

J. Carlsson

Department of Oral microbiology, University of Umeå,
S-901 87 Umeå, Sweden

INTRODUCTION

The microbial flora of the oral cavity is proverbially rich and varied. The nutritional environment of this flora is subjected to constant fluctuations and there could also be gradual profound nutritional shifts. The ability of the flora to adapt to a changing environment is dependent not only on its range of phenotypic adaptability but also on the flexibility of the genetic apparatus of the organisms of the flora[1,2].

CATABOLIC PATHWAYS OF SUGAR AND SUGAR SUBSTITUTES

Before discussing the potentials of the oral microflora to utilize various sugar substitutes, we have to examine the catabolic pathways of sugars and sugar substitutes. The first step of these pathways is the transport of the compound into the cytoplasm of the organism. The compound could be transported by a carrier-mediated (permease) system or by a phosphotransferase system. In the carrier-mediated system the compound is delivered unaltered into the cytoplasm and in the phosphotransferase system it is delivered phosphorylated. Both these transport systems usually require proteins that are specific for the sugar or the sugar substitute. When the compound has entered the cytoplasm it has to be converted by specific enzymes to a metabolic intermediate that can be introduced into the common sugar-degradative pathway of the organism *i.e.* in most organisms into the EMP pathway. This means that a compound is not utilized, *if* it is unable to enter the cell, *if* there are no enzymes that convert it to suitable metabolic intermediates or *if* the compound is an inhibitor of an essential cellular activity[3]. In addition, the catabolic pathway usually has to be integrated into the cellular processes by control mechanisms that regulate the enzymes and transport systems by modulating the synthesis or the activity of the proteins. Thus the evolution of a physiologically effective catabolic pathway requires the acquisition of a full set of structural and regulatory genes[4].

VARIOUS WAYS OF ADAPTATION OF THE MICROFLORA

Very little is known about the mechanisms of sugar utilization in oral microorganisms. So when we have to consider the potentials of the oral microflora to utilize sugar substitutes as energy source we have to extrapolate from results gained in studies of other microorganisms. An adaptation of the oral microflora for growth on a specific sugar substitute could be accomplished in the following ways. The ability to utilize the compound may already exist in some members of the flora and the synthesis of the specific proteins for its utilization only has to be induced or derepressed in these organisms. The utilization may be more effective if other members of the flora gain this ability by genetic transfer of genomes from the previous organisms. A third possibility is that a new function arises in some members of the flora by mutational events. However, very often mutations are attended by impairment or by loss of function. But recent works, in which xylitol has been used in search of models for studying acquisitive biochemical evolution, indicate that new functions could develop in an organism as a result of sequential mutational steps [2,5].

MODEL STUDIES OF ACQUISITIVE BIOCHEMICAL EVOLUTION

An example of such a study is when *Klebsiella aerogenes* 1033 became able to utilize xylitol as new source of carbon and energy. First one mutant (X1) was isolated which grew on xylitol with a doubling time of four hours. From strain X1 a secondary mutant (X2) was selected with a doubling time of two hours, and from X2 a mutant (X3) was obtained which was very effective in utilizing xylitol as substrate[5]. The superiority of X2 over X1 in its ability to use xylitol was demonstrated in a xylitol-limited continuous culture of strain X1[6]. When 20 cells of strain X2 was inoculated into a steadily growing culture of 5×10^{11} cells of strain X1, strain X2 displaced strain X1 in the culture within a few days.

What had happened in these strains? In strain X1 a mutation derepressed a ribitol dehydrogenase and this dehydrogenase also could

use xylitol as substrate. Strain X2 constitutively produced a
structurally altered ribitol dehydrogenase with increased affini-
ty for xylitol. At least two amino acid substitutions had taken
place in that enzyme[7]. Strains X3 had acquired a constitutive a-
bility to transport xylitol into the cell. This strain had a constitutive expression of the D-arabitol pathway and xylitol was
transported by a derepressed D-arabitol permease. The ability to
use xylitol thus developed in strains X1, X2 and X3 by a successive
recruitment of pre-existing gene-enzyme systems belonging to different pathways. The relationship of these pathways is illustrated
in the figure.

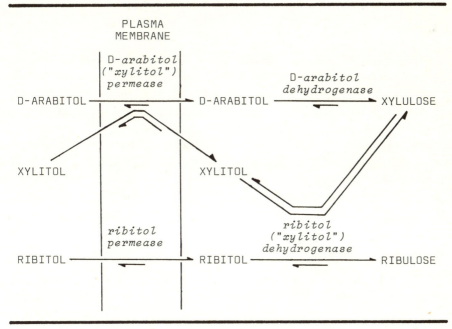

Figure. Relationships among the pathways for the dissimilation
of D-arabitol, xylitol and ribitol.[2]

A new catabolic pathway for xylitol has also been constructed in
Escherichia coli K-12 by derepressing other existing enzymes which
fortuitously act on xylitol[8]. *E. coli* K-12 has no pathways for the
natural pentitols ribitol and D-arabitol, but xylitol can be transported by a D-xylose permease and converted to D-xylose by a pro-
pandiol dehydrogenase. However, xylitol is not able to induce
these enzymes. By sequential selection of mutants a strain was obtained with a derepressed D-xylose permease and a derepressed pro-

pandiol dehydrogenase and this strain was able to grow on xylitol
as sole carbon and energy source[8]

   This type of adaptation by sequential mutations can only be expected to occur if strong selective pressures are applied to large
bacterial populations with short generation times.

REQUISITES FOR THE ADAPTATION OF THE ORAL MICROFLORA

   When the oral microflora is provided with a sugar substitute,
there may thus be some members of the flora which have the potential of utilizing the compound. However, before the compound can
be utilized, specific proteins for the transport and dissimilation
of the compound have to be synthesized. To be able to synthesize
new proteins the bacteria must be in an environment where they are
growing. This is a very important point. If the bacteria are exposed to the compound when they are not growing, they are not able
to utilize the compound. Another important point is that even
growing bacteria may not be able to synthesize these proteins, if
glucose is present. An example of such a condition we find in
Escherichia coli. In *E. coli* glucose is transported by a constitutive phosphotransferase system and sorbitol by an inducible system.
If glucose and sorbitol are present at the same time only glucose
can be utilized. Synthesis of the proteins of the sorbitol phosphotransferase system is inhibited[9,10]. This phenomenon has been
called catabolite repression.

   The proteins of the transport system and the enzymes that convert the transported compound to a suitable metabolic intermediate
are usually induced at the same time. This is very important in
cases where the compound is transported via the phosphotransferase
system. The phosphorylated compound could be toxic and had to be
converted immediately in a suitable metabolic form. Recently xylitol and D-arabitol were reported to be toxic in *E. coli* K-12[11].
Although the phosphotransferases are induced only by specific sugars, they sometimes are able to transport and phosphorylate also
a number of related sugars. In *E. coli* K-12 xylitol was transported and phosphorylated by a derepressed fructose phosphotransferase
and D-arabitol by derepressed galactitol phosphotransferase and
sorbitol phosphotransferase. The phosphorylated intermediates of
the pentitols had no route of further catabolism and poisoned the
organism.

Various members of the oral microflora are able to use sugar substitutes like sorbitol, maltitol and xylitol[12]. Normally these members of the flora make up a minor part of the flora. So far there are no reports of a significant increase in that part of the flora when these substitutes have been eaten regularly. This lack of adaptation may have the following explanation. The growth of the oral microflora is limited by the restricted availability of nutrients. An important fact is that the source of carbon does not seem to limit the growth of the bacteria in the oral cavity. Free glucose has been demonstrated in dental plaque[13] and addition of sugar to the mouth does not increase the bacterial yield[14]. Thus eating sugar substitutes in snacks between meals is not probable to induce growth of those bacteria that have the potential to use these sugar substitutes because their growth is limited by other nutrients than the carbon source. When they are not growing, they will not be able to syntesize the enzymes required for utilizing the sugar substitutes. In addition, the presence of free glucose may cause catabolite repression. The synthesis of inducible enzymes is inhibited also when the bacteria are actually growing.

The probability of aquisition of new functions by sequential mutations has also to be considered, but this probability will be very low, because sugar substitutes are only intermittently supplied to the oral cavity and the generation time of the bacteria of the oral cavity is probably very long with only a few doublings each day.

CONCLUSIONS

Bacteria have the potential to adapt to new carbon and energy sources. The successful competition by an organism in a complex microbiota depends not only on the range of phenotypic adaptability of the organism but also on the flexibility of its genetic apparatus.

Sugar substitutes are catabolized by inducible pathways. To be able to use these pathways the bacteria have to grow when they are confronted with the sugar substitute in order to be able to synthesize the proteins of the pathway and the glucose concentration in the environment of the bacteria has to be low in order to avoid catabolite repression effects. Neither of these conditions seems to be prevailing in the oral cavity. The bacteria are growing very

slowly or not at all and the carbon and energy source is not limiting the growth.

The slow growth rate of organisms of the oral cavity also seems
to exclude an adaptation to sugar substitute by sequential mutational events.

From clinical experiences on the use of sugar substitutes and
from microbial physiological considerations one has to conclude
that there is a low risk of adaptation of the oral microflora to
sugar substitutes as main carbon and energy source.

REFERENCES

1. Lerner, S.A., Wu, T.T. and Lin, E.C.C. Science 146:1313-1315,
    1964.
2. Lin, E.C.C., Hacking, A.J. and Aguilar, J. BioScience 26:
    548-555, 1976.
3. Clarke, P.H. in Evolution in the Microbial World, edited by
    Carlile, M.J. and Skehel, J.J. pp. 183-217, Cambridge Univer-
    sity Press, Cambridge, 1974.
4. Ornston, L.N. and Parke, D. Biochem. Soc. Trans. 4:468-472,
    1976.
5. Wu, T.T., Lin, E.C.C. and Tanaka, S. J. Bacteriol. 96:447-
    456, 1968.
6. Hartley, B.S. in Evolution in the Microbial World, edited by
    Carlile, M.J. and Skehel, J.J. pp. 151-182, Cambridge Univer-
    sity Press, Cambridge, 1974.
7. Burleigh, Jr. B.D., Rigby, R.W.J. and Hartley, B.S. Biochem.
    J. 143:341-352, 1974.
8. Wu, T.T. Biochim. Biophys. Acta 428:656-663, 1976.
9. Lengeler, J. and Lin, E.C.C. J. Bacteriol. 112:840-848, 1972.
10. Lengeler, J. J. Bacteriol. 124:39-47, 1975.
11. Reiner, A.M. J. Bacteriol. 132:166-173, 1975.
12. Edwardsson, S., Birkhed, D. and Mejàre, B. Acta Odont. Scand.
    35:257-263, 1977.
13. Hotz, P., Guggenheim, B. and Schmid, R. Caries Res. 6:103-121,
    1972.
14. Carlsson, J. and Johansson, T. Caries Res. 7:273-282, 1973.

Health and Sugar Substitutes
Proc. ERGOB Conf., Geneva 1978, pp. 211-217 (Karger, Basel 1978)

ACID PRODUCTION FROM SUCROSE SUBSTITUTES IN HUMAN DENTAL PLAQUE

D. Birkhed and S. Edwardsson

Departments of Oral Microbiology and Cariology, University of Lund,
School of Dentistry, S-214 21 Malmö, Sweden

INTRODUCTION

Owing to the fact that the bacterial formation of organic acids in the dental plaques plays a central role in the etiology of dental caries we have evaluated the effects of various sucrose substitutes on the acid production in individual plaque samples from many subjects using two different methods: (1)
measurement of acid production rate in plaque suspensions (in vitro)[1], and (2)
measurement of pH-changes of pooled plaque samples after mouth rinses[2,3]. This
paper will briefly review these methods and the data we have obtained with them.

MEASUREMENT OF ACID PRODUCTION RATE IN PLAQUE SUSPENSIONS (IN VITRO)

Subjects are instructed not to clean their teeth for 2 days before the experiment and not to eat or drink anything the morning of the examination. No
professional cleaning of the teeth is performed before this 2-day period. In
the forenoon the third day the subject rinses his mouth with distilled water
for 10 sec to remove loose debris. As completely as possible plaque material
is scraped from the buccal, lingual, and approximal surfaces of the teeth with
an amalgam carver, and is transferred to a plastic spoon kept in a moist chamber. The wet weight is determined to the nearest 0.1 mg. The material is homogenized at 4-6°C in 0.01 M sodium potassium phosphate buffer, pH 6.8, in a
glass mortar. There are 5-10 mg wet weight of plaque/ml. Aliquots (1.0 ml) of
the suspension are immediately distributed to micro-titration glass vessels
and kept cold (4-6°C) until tested. The storage time of the suspension is always kept as short as possible, usually not exceeding 2 h.

The titration vessel is then placed in a thermostat jacket of a micro-titration assembly maintained at 37°C. An automatic burette delivering approximately 0.01 ml of 0.002 N NaOH at each impulse is fitted to the titration vessel. The autoburette is connected with an automatic titrator and a recorder.
The titrator is set to maintain pH constant at 6.8. One ml of an aqueous solu-

tion (37°C) of 0.2 M glucose is added to the titration vessel and acid production is followed for approximately 10 min. The acid production rate is expressed as E x 10^{-9} (E = equivalent weight) of acid/mg plaque (wet weight)/min.

Repeated acid production experiments are performed with 1.0 ml-aliquots of
the same plaque suspension and with 1.0 ml of the substrates to be tested. In
order to check the acid production stability of the plaque suspension and to
determine the error of the method another experiment with glucose is performed.
The acid production rate from the test substances is expressed as described
above and as per cent of the acid production rate from glucose. With this
automatic titration method[1] (ATM) it is possible to investigate the fermentability of up to 10-15 substances with plaque material from one subject. The
equipment for the titration experiment is manufactured by Radiometer A/S,
Copenhagen, Denmark.

MEASUREMENT OF pH-CHANGES OF POOLED PLAQUE SAMPLES AFTER MOUTH RINSES

Subjects are instructed not to clean their teeth for 2 days, not to eat or
drink anything on the morning of the third day, and then to rinse their mouth
with distilled water, as described above. An amalgam carver is used to remove
small amounts of dental plaque from at least 20 different tooth areas. The material is immediately pooled in a drop of distilled water in a one drop glass
electrode connected to a pH-meter, and the pH of the material is determined
(0-min value) at room temperature. The subject is then instructed to rinse his
mouth for 30 sec with 10 ml of a concentrated solution of glucose (or sucrose).
Pooled plaque samples for pH-determination are then taken at 2, 5, 10, 20 and
30 min after the mouth rinse. The pH-meter should be read at a fixed interval
after sampling. The error of a single pH-measurement is determined when the
pH-meter is calibrated against standard buffers at pH 5.00 and 6.00.

Mouth rinse experiments are repeated at one week intervals with the substances to be tested. Usually another test with glucose (or sucrose) is used
as control. This method[3] is subsequently called the pH-method (pH-M).

RESULTS

The error of the ATM has been calculated to be 10-15 % in duplicate experiments with glucose. The acid production rate from various sucrose substitutes has been determined and the results are presented in Table 1. Fructose,
glucose syrups (DE 40 and 60, Reppe Glykos AB, Växjö, Sweden), invert sugar,
and sucrose are fermented with comparable high rates. Swedish Lycasin (candy
quality, no longer available, Lyckeby Stärkelseförädling AB, Lyckeby, Sweden)

Table 1. Acid production rate in dental plaque suspensions from sucrose and sucrose substitutes expressed as per cent of the rate from glucose. Mean values of experiment with 5-20 subjects. Part of the result has been published[1]

Substrate	Acid production rate
Mannitol, xylitol	0
Maltitol, sorbitol	10-30
French Lycasin (80/55)	20-40
Lactose	40-60
Swedish Lycasin (candy quality)	50-70
Fructose	80-100
Glucose syrups (DE 40 and 60), invert sugar, sucrose	100

contains more high molecular weight hydrogenated polysaccharides than French Lycasin (80/55, Roquette Frères, Lille, France) and is therefore rather fermentable, approximately comparable to boiled soluble starch (not shown). The acid production rate from French Lycasin (80/55), maltitol, mannitol, sorbitol, and xylitol is either low or not detectable.

The error of the single observation of the pH of the pooled dental plaque samples (pH-M) judged from measurements at pH 5.00 and at pH 6.00 has been calculated to be approximately ± 0.06 and ± 0.05, respectively, when the pH-meter was calibrated against the standard buffers. The results obtained with the pH-M are presented in Fig. 1. French Lycasin (80/55), mannitol[4] (not shown), maltitol, and xylitol increase or in some cases only slightly decrease the plaque pH. Lactose[5] (not shown) and Swedish Lycasin (candy quality) decrease the plaque pH but not to the same extent as fructose, glucose[5] (not shown), and sucrose.

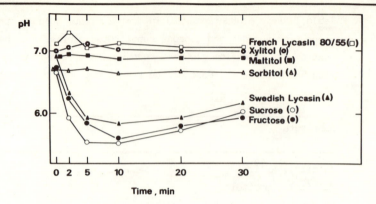

<u>Figure 1</u>. Changes in pH of dental plaques after a mouth rinse for 30 sec with 50 % (w/v) solutions of sucrose and sucrose substitutes. Mean values from experiments with various groups of 18-20 subjects. Part of the results has been published[5].

DISCUSSION

The characteristic of the ATM and pH-M is that they are simple to perform, require only standard laboratory equipment, and many subjects can easily be studied in a short time. It is also possible to screen many substances or products and to evaluate the results statistically (see below). The methods can be used to investigate various specific groups of individuals, e.g. subjects with high caries activity, with low saliva flow rate, buffering capacity etc. For both methods it is preferable to include only subjects with at least 20 natural teeth and moderate to marked predisposition to dental plaque formation.

We have recently applied the ATM and pH-M for studying the risk of "adaptation" of the plaque flora to sorbitol[6] and to lactose (unpublished observations) in two separate studies. The results indicate that the methods are sensitive, since relatively small differences in the fermentability of these substrates in the plaques could be detected.

The advantage with the ATM compared to the pH-M is that many substances can be tested with plaque material from one subject. However, ATM cannot reproduce completely the conditions in the oral cavity. First, dental plaque is pooled from several tooth surfaces and thus, the acid production rate constitute overall averages. Second, the plaque material is diluted about 100 times so that unidentified extracellular enzymes, inhibitors, and activators are diluted. Third, in the homogenized plaque suspension the microorganisms are in close contact with the substrate and the result is not influenced by such factors as the solubility of the substrate and the diffusion rate of the substrate into plaque.

The pH-M provides information of pH-changes in superficial dental plaque (mainly collected from buccal and lingual tooth surfaces) following exposure to different test products in vivo. Lower pH-values are obtained if the pH of interdental plaques is measured[7]. Moreover, the pH-M does not give information of the pH of a certain site of a tooth but overall averages.

A factor of importance for both ATM and pH-M is the substrate concentration. In vivo experiments (pH-M) with different concentrations of sucrose (0.05-50%) have shown that the pH-drop in the plaques increases with increasing sucrose concentration[8]. It can be expected that this is valid also for other fermentable substrates than sucrose. Hence, by comparing the pH-curve obtained with a test product with the corresponding results from various sucrose (or glucose) concentrations it is possible to state that the fermentability of the test product corresponds to a certain sucrose (or glucose) concentration range, e.g. 0.5-5 %. In studies on the possible "adaptation" of the plaque flora to various sucrose substitutes (with low fermentability) a high substrate concentration (usually 50 %, w/v) has been used to secure a high sensitivity of the pH-M[9]. In other experiments[6] when testing sucrose substitutes, however, we have used a concentration which can be expected in the saliva immediately after consumption of a foodstuff containing the substitute in question.

When using the ATM an optimal final substrate concentration of about 3 % (w/v) has been used[10], which for many mono- and disaccharides corresponds to 0.1-0.2 M. The ATM should only be used to determine the fermentability of well caracterized substrates and not of e.g. foodstuffs with unknown concentration of carbohydrates and other substances which may influence the microbial metabolism.

Regarding cariogenicity it is of interest to know if a "critical" acid production rate (ATM) or a "critical" pH-value (pH-M) can be advocated. It is here suggested that an acid production rate of not more than 30 % of that from glucose (or sucrose) can be considered as acceptable. A "critical" pH-value of 5.7 has been accepted by the Swiss Office of Health for telemetric recordings of interdental plaque in vivo[7]. This corresponds to approximately pH 6.5 with the pH-M[7]. However, since the initial (0-min) pH-values found with the pH-M may vary between different subjects and to some extent may influence on the subsequent pH-values it is also important to consider the maximum mean pH-decrease (usually at 5-10 min). It is here suggested that a maximum mean pH-decrease of at most 0.4 can be accepted using the pH-M on indication of "safety for teeth", providing that this pH-value does not drop below 6.5. If these "critical" values for the ATM and pH-M are considered, French Lycasin (80/55), maltitol, sorbitol, and xylitol and foodstuffs containing high concentrations of these sucrose substitutes will pass the tests. On the other hand, carbohydrates such as fructose, glucose syrups and invert sugar and foodstuffs containing high concentrations of these carbohydrates will not pass the tests.

It is important to consider that the measurements with both methods should be based on experiments with a group of subjects and not on a single observation since the amount of plaque[11], saliva flow rate and buffering capacity of the saliva and of the plaque[12] strongly affect the results.

Both ATM and pH-M give information about the fermentability and to some extent also of the acidogenicity[14] of the products tested. They do not give complete information about the cariogenicity of a certain product, because cariogenicity is influenced also by other factors. However, when the cariogenicity of a certain sucrose substitute or foodstuff is assessed, its fermentability by the dental plaques is probably one of the most important factors to take into consideration.

STATISTICAL EVALUATION

When comparing the fermentability of various substrates with the ATM, Student's t-test for paired observations has been applied on both the percentage and the absolute values[1]. With the pH-M the same statistical method has been used on the: (1) pH-values[3], and (2) differences between 0-min value and pH at a certain time point[3]. On: (3) pH-minimum[13], and (4) sum of all pH-depressions below the fasting basline level a ranking test has been used[13].

In a study on the effects of frequent consumption of pastilles containing various sucrose substitutes on the possible "adaptation" of the plaque, analysis of variance applied on the results obtained with the ATM and the pH-M was also included[9]. Differences observed with the Student's t-test on a 5 % level disappeared when the same data was analyzed with analysis of variance. The discrepancy between the results of the two statistical methods may depend on the possibility that the application of a great number of paired t-tests imply a risk of obtaining a few significant differences by chance only.

SUMMARY

Two methods are here described - measurement of acid production rate in plaque suspensions (in vitro) and measurement of pH-changes of pooled plaque samples after mouth rinses. These methods have been used to compare the fermentability of sucrose substitutes by plaque material from many subjects. The "critical" acid production rate and the "critical" plaque pH-value for evaluation of cariogenicity is discussed.

REFERENCES

1.   Birkhed, D.   Caries Res. 12: 128-136, 1978.

2.   Englander, H.R., Carter, W.J. and Fosdick, L.S.   J. Dent. Res. 35: 792-799 (1956).

3.   Frostell, G.   Acta Odontol. Scand. 28: 599-608, 1970.

4.   Ahldén, M.-L. and Frostell, G.   Odontol. Revy 26: 1-6, 1975.

5.   Frostell, G.   Odontol. Revy 24: 217-226, 1973.

6.   Birkhed, D., Edwardsson, S., Svensson, B., Moskowitz, F. and Frostell, G. Archs Oral Biol., 1978 (accepted for publication).

7.   Imfeld, T.   Helv. Odontol. Acta. 21: 1-28, 1977.

8.   Frostell, G.   Acta Odontol. Scand. 27: 3-29, 1969.

9.   Birkhed, D., Edwardsson, S., Ahldén, M.-L. and Frostell, G.   Acta Odontol. Scand., 1978 (accepted for publication).

10. Frostell, G.   Acta Odontol. Scand. 20: 335-347, 1962.

11. Strålfors, A.   Odontol. Tidskr. 58: 155-341, 1950.

12. Edgar, W.M.   Caries Res. 10: 241-254, 1976.

13. Edgar, W.M., Bibby, B.G., Mundorff, S. and Rowley, J.   J. Amer. Dent. Ass. 90: 418-425, 1975.

14. Frostell, G.   Acta Odontol. Scand. 28: 609-622, 1970.

Health and Sugar Substitutes
Proc. ERGOB Conf., Geneva 1978, pp. 218-223 (Karger, Basel 1978)

IN VIVO ASSESSMENT OF PLAQUE ACID PRODUCTION. A LONG-TERM
RETROSPECTIVE STUDY

Th. Imfeld

Department of Cariology, Periodontology and Preventive Dentistry,
Dental Institute, University of Zurich, Plattenstrasse 11,
8028 Zurich, Switzerland

INTRODUCTION

Intra-oral plaque-pH telemetry is an in vivo method to measure
the hydronium ion concentration under an undisturbed layer of
plaque at the level of the enamel surface of the tooth. At
present it is the quickest and most accurate way to assess the
acidogenicity of diets and it is the only method to do so in
vivo. In contrast to in vitro sampling techniques pH-telemetry
allows for and does not disturb any of the factors influencing
plaque-pH, such as carbohydrate permeation and fermentation rate,
buffer capacity of saliva and plaque, dietary acids, etc. pH-
telemetry continuously records plaque-pH, it thus reflects oral
clearance times of fermentable dietary carbohydrates and/or
dietary acids.

Intra-oral radio-telemetry was first described in 1965 [1] and
1966 [2] and reviewed in 1971 [3]. Intra-oral wire-telemetry,
currently used for testing in this laboratory, was described
in detail in 1977 [4].

Plaque-pH telemetry has proved to be an excellent instrument
with which to evaluate the potential cariogenicity of foods,
beverages and drugs. The Swiss Office of Health allows
manufacturers to label and advertise a carbohydrate containing
product as "safe for teeth" ("zahnschonend") only if they submit
plaque-pH telemetric tests showing that the pH of interdental
plaque is not depressed below 5.7 by glycolysis during, and for
30 minutes after, normal consumption of the product. Typical

test results from commercially available confectionary products
have been published previously [4-9] as well as tests of the
cariogenic potential of several cough-mixtures [10]. All telemetric
test participants are volunteers. Several have been in the
program for over 5 years and the data from standard control
procedures for these volunteers were available for retrospective
examination.

The purpose of the present study was to examine this data to
determine if there was inter- and intraindividual consistancy
in the rate and amount of intraplaque acid production.

EXPERIMENTAL

The pH of interdental plaque telemetrically recorded during
and for 15 minutes following 2-minute rinses with 15 ml of 10%
sucrose solutions was used as a measure of plaque glycolytic
activity.

The lowest pH value recorded and the time in minutes after
expectorating the sucrose solution it occurred were noted for
plaques 3 to 7 days old.

This information was available for 8 volunteers. For two
volunteers (J.S. and E.B.) data were accessible over a 5-year
period and two readings per year, at least 6 months apart, for
each plaque age were examined. For 6 volunteers data were
available for a 2-year period and six readings per year, one
every second month, for each plaque age were examined.

RESULTS AND DISCUSSION

The average pH values, times and standard deviations are
given in Table I and illustrated in Figures 1-8.

TABLE I

		\overline{\text{3 d}}		4 d		5 d		6 d		7 d		$\overline{\overline{x}}$
		pH	min	pH	min	pH	min	pH	min	pH	min	pH
E.B.	$\overline{x}$	4.35	8.3	4.08	9.1	4.13	10.3	4.02	10.4	4.10	9.1	4.14
	SD	0.42	3.4	0.27	3.3	0.26	2.1	0.21	3.1	0.20	3.2	
J.S.	$\overline{x}$	4.29	10.6	4.03	10.0	4.02	10.3	4.00	9.2	3.92	10.4	4.05
	SD	0.55	2.7	0.22	3.3	0.24	3.1	0.31	2.9	0.21	4.0	
H.W.	$\overline{x}$	4.21	11.4	4.24	9.1	4.22	9.0	4.22	8.5	4.17	8.3	4.21
	SD	0.24	3.6	0.36	3.5	0.28	2.6	0.34	2.7	0.24	2.0	
E.C.	$\overline{x}$	4.24	10.9	4.33	9.8	4.25	9.8	4.25	11.0	4.10	9.9	4.23
	SD	0.40	3.0	0.25	2.6	0.31	2.1	0.22	2.7	0.37	3.5	
G.J.	$\overline{x}$	4.13	12.0	4.29	8.0	4.13	10.1	3.98	8.3	4.19	8.5	4.14
	SD	0.24	2.5	0.31	3.7	0.35	2.8	0.16	3.1	0.36	2.3	
J.T.	$\overline{x}$	4.21	9.9	4.30	8.7	4.16	7.7	4.31	7.2	4.27	8.9	4.25
	SD	0.37	2.7	0.41	3.5	0.39	2.2	0.29	2.3	0.22	2.8	
M.L.	$\overline{x}$	4.36	10.4	4.16	10.9	4.15	11.0	4.06	9.6	4.13	12.0	4.17
	SD	0.25	3.2	0.38	2.8	0.28	4.0	0.34	3.6	0.19	1.8	
H.H.	$\overline{x}$	4.60	10.2	4.36	10.8	4.29	11.9	4.43	10.5	4.36	13.1	4.41
	SD	0.42	3.0	0.31	3.8	0.36	2.4	0.22	3.0	0.46	0.9	
	$\overline{\overline{x}}$	4.30	10.5	4.22	9.5	4.17	10.0	4.16	9.3	4.16	10.0	

d = age of plaque

Fig.1

Average values and SD of lowest interdental pH reached and
time taken after 2min rinses with 15ml 10% sucrose solution.
Values are from one proband (E.B.) over a 5 year period,
2 readings per year and plaque age.   N = 10

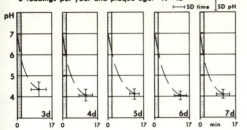

Fig.2

Average values and SD of lowest interdental pH reached and
time taken after 2min rinses with 15ml 10% sucrose solution.
Values are from one proband (J.S.) over a 5 year period,
2 readings per year and plaque age.   N = 10

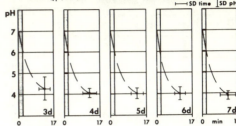

Fig.3

Average values and SD of lowest interdental pH reached and
time taken after 2min rinses with 15ml 10% sucrose solution.
Values are from one proband (H.W.) over a 2 year period,
6 readings per year and plaque age.   N = 12

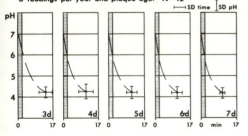

Fig.4

Average values and SD of lowest interdental pH reached and
time taken after 2min rinses with 15ml 10% sucrose solution.
Values are from one proband (E.C.) over a 2 year period,
6 readings per year and plaque age.   N = 12

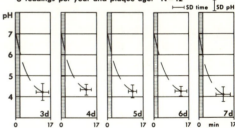

Fig.5

Average values and SD of lowest interdental pH reached and
time taken after 2min rinses with 15ml 10% sucrose solution.
Values are from one proband (G.J.) over a 2 year period,
6 readings per year and plaque age.   N = 12

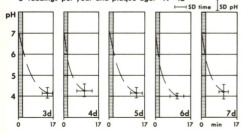

Fig.6

Average values and SD of lowest interdental pH reached and
time taken after 2min rinses with 15ml 10% sucrose solution.
Values are from one proband (J.T.) over a 2 year period,
6 readings per year and plaque age.   N = 12

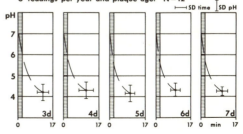

Fig.7   Fig.8

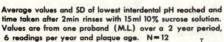

Average values and SD of lowest interdental pH reached and
time taken after 2min rinses with 15ml 10% sucrose solution.
Values are from one proband (M.L.) over a 2 year period,
6 readings per year and plaque age. N=12

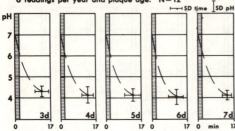

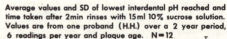

Average values and SD of lowest interdental pH reached and
time taken after 2min rinses with 15ml 10% sucrose solution.
Values are from one proband (H.H.) over a 2 year period,
6 readings per year and plaque age. N=12

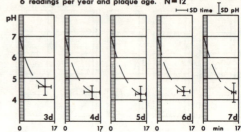

During the period reviewed, the average pH minima reached
were 4.30 in 3-day old plaque, 4.22 in 4-day old plaque and 4.17
or 4.16 in 5-, 6- and 7-day old plaque, respectively. In an
analysis of variance the slight decrease from 4.30 to 4.16 was
significant ($p < 0.05$). The difference between the lowest pH
values of the 8 volunteers was highly significant ($p < 0.001$).
Volunteer H.H. showed the highest average of pH values (4.41),
while J.S. showed the lowest (4.05).

Regarding the time (min) required to reach the lowest pH
values, which was close to 10 minutes (average 9.88), there was
a small, but significant variation between the different
volunteers ($p < 0.001$), but not between different ages of plaque.

The consistency of the results is noteworthy when one
considers that at no time during the period covered in this
study were the volunteers under any special dietary instructions.
In addition, the results of this study emphasize the
reproducibility of telemetric in vivo plaque-pH measurements.

REFERENCES

1. Graf, H. and Mühlemann, H.R.   J.dent.Res. (Abstract) 44:
    1139, 1965

2. Graf, H. and Mühlemann, H.R.   Helv.odont.Acta 10: 94-101,
    1966

3. Mühlemann, H.R.   Int.dent.J. 21: 456-465, 1971

4. Imfeld, Th.   Helv.odont.Acta 21: 1-28.In Schweiz.Mschr.
    Zahnheilk. 87: 437-464, 1977

5. Mühlemann, H.R.   Schweiz.Mschr.Zahnheilk. 79: 117-145, 1969

6. Schneider, Ph. and Mühlemann, H.R.   Schweiz.Mschr.Zahnheilk.
    86: 150-166, 1976

7. Imfeld, Th. and Mühlemann, H.R.   J.Prev.Dent. 4: 8-14, 1977

8. Mühlemann, H.R. and Imfeld, Th.   Quintessenz 2: 97-108,
    1978

9. Mühlemann, H.R. and Imfeld, Th.   Proceedings "Methods of
    Caries Prediction". Sp. Supp. Microbiology Abstracts.
    pp. 241-244, 1978

10. Imfeld, Th.   Schweiz.Mschr.Zahnheilk. 87: 773-777, 1977

Health and Sugar Substitutes
Proc. ERGOB Conf., Geneva 1978, pp. 224-228 (Karger, Basel 1978)

TESTING OF SUGAR SUBSTITUTES IN ANIMALS WITH SPECIAL
REFERENCE TO NON-SPECIFIC EFFECTS

K.G. König

Institute of Preventive and Community Dentistry,
University of Nijmegen, The Netherlands

INTRODUCTION

The taste of food does not only influence the pattern of
intake in man. Analogous to consumer acceptance of a certain
foodstuff in a human population, experimental animals may
definitely prefer one food component above another. In case of
administration as a homogenous experimental dietary mix, one
component may determine either acceptance or rejection[1].

THE TASTE OF TEST DIETS DETERMINES THE EATING PATTERN

When two groups of rats are offered a control and a test
diet respectively, chances are high that there will be a
difference in taste which results in differences between the
groups as to amount of food consumed, frequency of intake of
food and sometimes of liquid as well. Since the differences
in eating and drinking pattern are not always accompanied by a
conspicuous difference in weight gain between the groups, the
whole phenomenon may escape the laboratory technician's and
herewith the experimenter's attention.

ORGANOLEPTIC JUDGEMENTS ARE SPECIES SPECIFIC

For instance, replacing tap water by a sweetened beverage
may easily more than double the intake of liquid (Fig. 1),
whereas addition of 5 per cent calcium gluconate to an experimental diet will significantly reduce eating time and amount
of food consumed[1,2]. The rat seems to dislike the diet with
the supplement although the human taste organ cannot detect a
difference from the control diet. Usually human subjects in
organoleptic testing report an unpleasant aftertaste of

saccharine whereas sodium cyclamate is not objectionable at comparable concentrations[3]. Nobody knows the sensations of rats, but they seem to have taste sensations different from those of man: rats accept a saccharine-sweetened test diet without changes of their pattern of food intake, whereas they decrease their eating frequency and food intake when cyclamate is added.

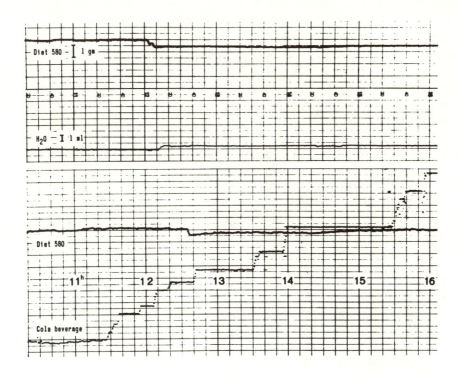

Fig. 1   Recordings of intake of diet and water by the same rat (age 45 days, weight 140 gm) on two successive days during the resting phase between 10:20 AM 16:00 PM. On the first day (top), normal behavior with a meal consisting of one eating-drinking cycle; on the second day (bottom), water was replaced by a cola beverage, which stimulated abnormally frequent and excessively high intake[2].

POSITIVE CORRELATION BETWEEN EATING FREQUENCY AND CARIES ACTIVITY

Caries activity tends to increase with higher frequency of intake and more frequent/longer availability of readily fermentable sugars in the oral cavity and the microbial plaque on teeth. The Vipeholm experiment[4] and observations on children[5] (Fig. 2) as well as controlled-feeding studies on rats[1,6] (Fig.3) have convincingly shown the positive correlation between frequency of sugar intake and caries activity. Because of this correlation, any influence of taste on eating frequency automatically implies unspecific effects on caries activity.

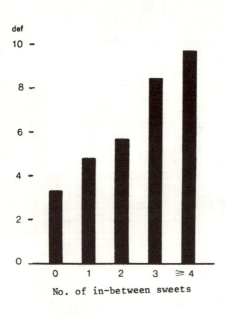

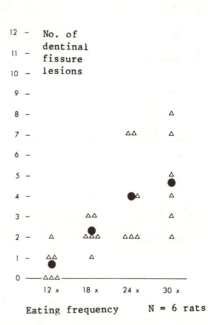

Fig. 2 Correlation between admitted number of in-between sugar-containing snacks and drinks and caries (def) in deciduous teeth[5]

Fig. 3 Caries incidence of individual rats (triangles) and group averages (circles) on programmed feeding, 12 to 30 times per day[1]

SUGAR ALCOHOLS DECREASE FOOD INTAKE AND MAY THEREFORE LOWER CARIOGENIC CHALLENGE UNSPECIFICALLY

Whenever the nature of dietary components like sugar alcohols results in a change of the normal eating pattern of rats (Table I), the obvious solution of the problem is to change the experimental conditions from ad-libitum feeding to controlled feeding[6]. This requirement should always be fulfilled in animal experiments in order to exclude the possibility that the caries reduction observed was due to an unspecific effect, viz. low eating frequency and not to the failure of oral microorganisms to break down the sugar alcohol in question to acid. Controlled-feeding experiments with sugar alcohols have shown, however, that rats have an aversion to these carbohydrates to such an extent that they rather die from starvation than accept high percentages of

Diet 2000 f with	Food intake(g)	Water intake(ml)	Weight gain(g)	Av.No. of lesions
0% xylitol	11.7	23.3	122	2.7
10% xylitol	10.3	24.7	97	1.2
20% xylitol	10.7	50.6	68	2.2
30% xylitol	9.4	58.0	44	2.8
0% sorbitol	10.0	19.0	103	1.7
10% sorbitol	10.1	25.7	100	4.3
20% sorbitol	10.6	43.9	77	4.1
30% sorbitol	11.6	79.3	51	4.3

Table I Average daily intake of food and water, weight gain and number of dentinal carious lesions in rats 33 days on free-fed xylitol or sorbitol diets in which the 64-per-cent flour component was in part substituted. The differences in intake and weight gains reflect the presence of unspecific effects[9].

e.g. sorbitol in their diet[7]. When used in low concentrations,
and when the animals get gradually accustomed to substances
like sorbitol and xylitol, it could be shown that they are
consumed and that their cariogenicity is very low in comparison
to sucrose[8]. Nevertheless the rat caries model which in general
gives reliable information relevant to the understanding of
mechanisms of cariogenicity or caries inhibition in man,
cannot be used in such studies without precautions and
restrictions.

REFERENCES

1. König, K.G. J. dent. Res. 49: 1327-1332, 1970.
2. König, K.G., Savdir, S., Marthaler, T.M., Schmid, R. and
   Mühlemann, H.R. Helv. Odont. Acta 8 (Suppl): 82-96, 1964.
3. Unpublished results.
4. Gustafsson, B.E., Quensel, C.E., Swenander Lanke, L.,
   Lundqvist, C., Grahnen, H., Bonow, B.E. and Krasse, B.
   Acta Odont. Scand. 11: 232-364, 1954.
5. Weiss, R.L. and Trithart, A.H. Amer. J. Pub. Health 50:
   1097-1104, 1960.
6. König, K.G., Schmid, P. and Schmid, R. Arch. Oral Biol. 13:
   13-26, 1968.
7. Unpublished results.
8. Karle, E.J. Dtsch. zahnärztl. Z. 32 (Suppl)S82-S95, 1977.
9. Mühlemann, H.R., Regolati, B. and Marthaler, T.M.
   Helv. odont. Acta 14: 48-51, 1970.

Health and Sugar Substitutes
Proc. ERGOB Conf., Geneva 1978, pp. 229-234 (Karger, Basel 1978)

CARIOGENIC PROPERTIES OF SUGAR SUBSTITUTES EXAMINED IN GNOTOBIOTIC RAT EXPERIMENTS

F. Gehring

Department for Experimental Dentistry,
Dental School, University of Würzburg,
Pleicherwall 2, D 8700 Würzburg

INTRODUCTION

Beside conventional laboratory animals the advantage of gnotobiotic experimental animals, above all rats, has been recognised and is used to test the cariogenic properties of sugar substitutes or microorganisms of dental plaque[1,2,3]. These gnotobiotic animals are kept in plastic isolators under sterile conditions; they are mono-, di-, tri-, or polyassociated with certain bacterial strains; and are fed diets containing the sugar
substitute to be tested. In the rule the animals are sacrificed
after an experimental period of 6 weeks and caries is determined
as in conventional animals. The caries rate represents a measure
for the cariogenicity of the tested substances, respectively the
inoculated microbial species. We should, however, consider that
gnotobiotic conditions vary considerably from conventional animal experiments, on account of which results obtained by gnotobiotic experimental technics should be interpreted with great
care, as they merely demonstrate the potential cariogenic properties of a substance or a certain microorganism.

SORBITOL

Sorbitol is a sugar substitute which has been known for some
time. Probably due to osmotic properties and the poor absorption
of sorbitol by the intestinal tract conventional rats already
show considerable dilatation of the caecum with laxative effect
when fed a sorbitol diet. Thus gnotobiotic rats, whose caecum is
enlarged anyway, presumably experience such decisive changes in
the mucosae of the caecum and the colon by feeding on a sorbitol
diet, that the animals would not be able to survive.

XYLITOL

Little is known on the microbial degradation of xylitol and its acidic metabolic endproducts[4],[5]. During the course of the "Turku sugar studies"[6] several streptococci strains with the ability to catabolise xylitol and slowly produce small amounts of acids were isolated from human dental plaque[7]. These streptococci could not yet be classified, but 80% of the characteristics can be associated with the serogroup Q. The descriptions of this serogroup all name xylitol utilization as a positive property [8],[9]. Further reference to xylitol degradation can be found in Bergey's Manual[8] on page 580, which mentions that Lactobacillus salivarius subsp. salivarius is able to ferment xylitol. However, a recent renewed description of this species does not mention xylitol utilization[10].

The cariogenic properties of xylitol utilising, serogroup Q analog streptococci mentioned above were tested in gnotobiotic experimental arrangements. The monoassociations of rats and microorganisms received xylitol, fructose, or sucrose chocolate diets for a period of 12 weeks[11],[12]. The total caries incidence of the

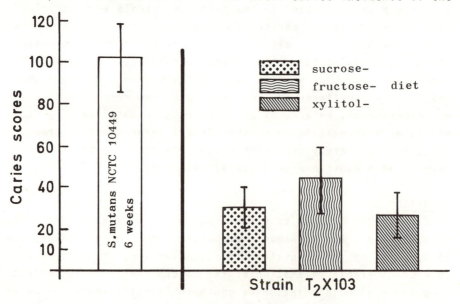

Fig. 1: Caries incidence on the lower jaws of gnotobiotic rats. Mean values and standard deviations (Wistar, 6 animals/litter, 12 weeks).

gnotobiotic rats is shown in Fig. 1. Compared to the caries produced by the monoassociation of a Streptococcus mutans reference strain with gnotobiotic rats that were fed a cariogenic sucrose diet for <u>six weeks</u>, a considerably shorter experimental
period, the cariogenic effect of the xylitol degradating test
strains can practically be neglected. This very low cariogenic
potential of xylitol degradating microorganisms could also be
demonstrated in the clinical tests of the "Turku sugar studies".
After two years of xylitol diet no increase in caries could be
observed in the test persons under consideration[6].
A further gnotobiotic rat experiment showed that the reference
strain of the serological streptococci group Q, which readily
metabolises xylitol, also does not produce noteworthy caries
scores under similar conditions and results mentioned above and
in comparison to S.mutans monoassociations with the sucrose diet.

L-SORBOSE

Like xylitol, l-sorbose[13,14] is not fermented by the more important and frequently occurring oral streptococci species such

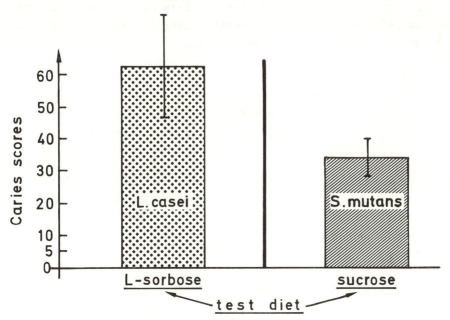

Fig. 2: Caries incidence on the lower jaws of gnotobiotic rats.
Mean values and standard deviations. n=7.

as S.mutans, S.sanguis, S.salivarius, S.mitis, S.milleri. But
l-sorbose is definitely utilised to acids (lactic acid) by
strains of the serological streptococci group Q (e.g. Streptococcus avium), furthermore by the hitherto not classified, but
serogroup Q similar, xylitol degradating strains, and eventually
by Lactobacilli, especially Lactobacillus casei, a species which
is more or less frequently present in human dental plaque. As
the high cariogenicity of L.casei with sucrose as substrate is
a well established finding[15], it was interesting to know what
cariogenic potential l-sorbose would have in gnotobiotic rat experiments. Fig. 2 shows the results of an experiment with L.ca-
sei strains isolated from human dental plaque and monoassociated
with gnotobiotic rats that were fed a l-sorbose diet[16]. The results are again compared to monoassociations with S.mutans
strains and the cariogenic sucrose diet.

The caries incidence of the L.casei monoassociations and l-sorbose diet was surprisingly high, significantly higher than the
monoassociation with S.mutans and the sucrose diet. A possible
explanation for the high caries scores seems to be the particular ability of all Lactobacilli to remain metabolically active
at low pH-values and thus to further produce acids; especially
in the case of gnotobiotic experiments, i.e. without other com-
peting microorganisms. This result clearly shows the limits of
gnotobiotic arrangements. Beginning and progress of the caries
process in vivo, depending on the synergistic and antagonistic
effects of the entire plaque flora, are completely different
and much more complicated than under gnotobiotic conditions.

PALATINIT

A novel sugar substitute is palatinit[17]. Rats do not seem
to particularly like it and it has thus to be fed alternatively with basic diet in gnotobiotic S.mutans monoassociation experiments. Caries incidence after a 5 week period is illustrated by fig. 3. The caries scores of the sucrose diet are again
very high, whereas caries by palatinit diet is to be neglected.
The negative effects of the palatinit diet on the intestinal
tract of the gnotobiotic rats can possibly either be reduced
or eliminated completely by polyassociation with microorganisms
from the normal intestinal flora of the rat.

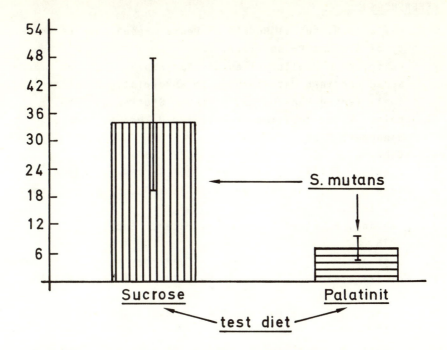

Fig.3: Caries incidence on the lower jaws of gnotobiotic rats. Mean values and standard deviations.

THE MOST PERTINENT QUESTIONS

1.   General validity and significance of gnotobiotic animal experiments for investigations of the cariogenic properties of microorganisms and sugar substitutes?

2.   Compatibility of sugar substitutes with gnotobiotic animals?

3.   Feeding behaviour/habits of gnotobiotic animals compared to conventional animals?

4.   Side effects of sugar substitutes in gnotobiotic rats? Unspecific effects?

5.   Suitable selection of microorganisms for inoculation of gnotobiotic rats in cariogenicity tests (mono-, di-, tri-, or polyassociations)?

REFERENCES

1. Navia, J.M. Animal Models in Dental Research, The University of Alabama Press, 1977.

2. König, K.G. Möglichkeiten der Kariesprophylaxe beim Menschen und ihre Untersuchung im kurzfristigen Rattenexperiment, Verlag Hans Huber, Bern und Stuttgart, 1966.

3. Heine, W. Gnotobiotechnik, Verlag M. und H. Schaper, Hannover, 1968

4. Gehring, F. J. dent. Res. 53: 122, 1974.

5. Gehring, F. Dtsch. zahnärztl. Z. 29: 769-771, 1974.

6. Scheinin, A. and Mäkinen, K.K. Acta Odont. Scand. Suppl. 70, 1975.

7. Gehring, F. et al. Acta Odont. Scand. Suppl. 70, 223-237, 1975.

8. Buchanan, R.E. and Gibbons, N.E. Bergey's Manual of Determinative Bacteriology, 8th Ed., The Williams & Wilkins Company, 1974.

9. Nowlan, S.S. and Deibel, R.H. J. Bacteriol. 94: 291-296, 1967.

10. Rogosa, M. et al. J. Bacteriol. 65: 681-699, 1953.

11. Karle, E.J. and Gehring, F. Caries Res. 10: 149, 1976.

12. Karle, E.J. und Gehring, F. Dtsch. zahnärztl. Z. 31: 22-25, 1976.

13. Mühlemann, H.R. Schweiz. Mschr. Zahnheilk. 86: 1339/23-1345/29, 1976.

14. Mühlemann, H.R. and Schneider, Ph. Helv. odont. Acta 19: 76-80, 1975.

15. Rosen, S. et al. J. dent. Res. 47: 358-363, 1968.

16. Gehring, F. and Karle, E.J. Caries Res. 12: 118-119, 1978.

17. Karle, E.J. und Gehring, F. Dtsch. zahnärztl. Z. 33: 189-191, 1978.

Health and Sugar Substitutes
Proc. ERGOB Conf., Geneva 1978, pp. 235-240 (Karger, Basel 1978)

METABOLIC CRITERIA INDICATIVE OF CARIOGENICITY IN PRIMATES

W. H. Bowen

Caries Prevention and Research Branch, National Caries Program,
National Institute of Dental Research, Bethesda, Maryland 20014 USA

There appears to be little doubt that dental caries results from the interaction of carbohydrates with specific microorganisms on the tooth surface. This interaction gives rise to several biochemical activities which, theoretically, at least, should be reflected in the formation of plaque, its chemical composition and accumulation of metabolites.

It is frequently assumed that dental plaque does not form in the absence of dietary carbohydrate. However, it is apparent that in primates, even in the total absence of foodstuffs, plaque develops on tooth surfaces[1]. Animals which receive their entire diet by gastric intubation form dental plaque which differs in several respects from that formed in the presence of glucose, sucrose, casein, or a complete diet[1,2]. Because sugars play an essential role in the pathogenesis of dental caries, it appears reasonable to assume that plaque formed in gastric intubated animals lacks cariogenic potential[3]. All the available evidence indicates that the ability of plaque to form acid from sugar solutions is intimately related to its cariogenicity[4]. Plaque formed in monkeys in the absence of dietary carbohydrate fails to lower the pH of sugar solutions.

The biochemical composition of plaque is also affected by the composition of the diet. The carbohydrate content of plaque is substantially lower in gastric fed animals than in conventionally nourished animals[2,5]

The amount of water soluble extracellular polysaccharide is considerably reduced as judged by biochemical assessment and electron microscopic examination.

Reduction in the carbohydrate content could affect the pathogenic capacity of plaque in one or more ways. The ability of many oral microorganisms to adhere to tooth surfaces will be substantially reduced in the absence of carbohydrate; indeed, it was observed that significantly fewer streptococci, lactobacilli and yeasts are present in plaque from tube-fed animals than in that from conventionally fed monkeys[1,2]. It is also probable that the diffusion limiting properties of plaque will be considerably altered. Recent evidence has shown that less lipoteichoic acid (LTA) is found in plaque formed in the presence of sucrose than in that formed in the presence of glucose[6]. LTA has the capacity to confer a substantial net negative charge on microorganisms and appears to be intimately related to mutan produced by Strep. mutans from sucrose.

Microorganisms in plaque formed in gastric intubated monkeys appear to contain little intracellular polysaccharide as judged by electron microscopic examination[5]. A reduced amount of IPS in plaque results in diminished capacity by plaque to form acid when extraneous sources of carbohydrate are lacking, and probably influences the ability of microorganisms to survive in an inimical environment.

Profound changes are also observed in the inorganic constitutents of plaque when the entire diet is administered by gastric intubation. Plaque formed under such circumstances contains enhanced amounts of calcium and phosphorus. The concentration of these ions appears to be inversely related to caries activity[2,5,7].

Plaque formed in the presence of sugars differs significantly from that formed in the absence of extraneous source of substrate. The ability of plaque to lower the pH of sugar solutions is restored within days following exposure to sugar. Glucose, fructose and glucose, and sucrose

appear to be equally effective in restoring acid producing ability of

dental plaque. pH values as low as 5.0 are frequently recorded in

animals in which plaque was formed exclusively in the presence of sugars.

Plaque formed over several days in the presence of casein only, while the

remainder of the diet is intubated, lacks any capacity to produce acids

from sugar[2]. Extracellular polysaccharide is formed rapidly, the type of

polymer is influenced by the sugar being fed to the animals. For example,

polymers of mannose are found in plaques from monkeys fed exclusively on

glucose and fructose[5,8]. As the concentration of carbohydrate increases

in dental plaque, the content of calcium and phosphorus declines; however,

the critical concentrations at which plaque becomes cariogenic have not

been determined.

The types of acids formed in cariogenic plaque has not received the

attention commensurate with their importance. A series of experiments[9]

was carried out to determine the types and quantities of acids produced

by plaque bacteria in groups of monkeys fed a high sucrose diet, and

monkeys fed a diet in which sucrose was replaced as far as possible by a

mixture of glucose and fructose. The major acids detected in the resting

samples (17 hours after the last intake of food) were acetic, proprionic

and N-butyric with traces of iso-butyric, iso-valeric, lactic, caproic

and succinic. Volatile acids accounted for 88% of the total acids

identified. The group fed glucose and fructose had significantly higher

acid concentrations than the sucrose group.

Following exposure to sugar, more acid was found than that determined

in resting plaques. The acid concentration increased in the sucrose group

from 6.76 to 42.2 u-moles/μl and in the invert sugar from 28.8 to 75.5

u-moles/μl. There was a significant increase in the level of lactic acid.

The concentration of N-valeric acid also increased significantly in both groups. In the invert sugar group there were significant increases in the concentrations of iso-valeric, caproic and succinic. The volatile acids analyzed in the plaque samples following the application of sucrose represented only between 45-55% of the total amount of acid produced. Thus it appears that caries active plaque contains more non-volatile organic acids and more lactic acid than "resting" plaque, which is presumably non-cariogenic.

Differences were not detected in the caries scores between animals fed sucrose and those fed glucose and fructose[10].

All the available evidence suggests that under well-defined experimental conditions biochemical differences exist between cariogenic and non-cariogenic plaque. However, it is unclear whether under less subtle circumstances differences could be detected in the biochemical activities of plaque from caries-active and caries-free individuals. For example, if differences in caries activity were reflections of susceptibility of the tooth surface, biochemical activities of plaque from the two groups would not necessarily be dissimilar. Furthermore, if the reduction in caries activity is associated with a reduced frequency of intake of carbohydrate, differences might not be detected in the biochemical activities of dental plaque, determined at specific times.

Several attempts have been made to determine the influence of either proven or potentially cariostatic agents on the biochemistry of dental plaque in monkeys. The results from some of these studies are presented to illustrate that the effects on biochemical activities in dental plaque of the addition of some cariostatic compounds to cariogenic diets may vary greatly.

The influence of two organic phosphates, viz., calcium glycerophosphate and sodium inositol phosphate on dental caries and plaque composition has been studied in monkeys[11,12]. The addition of either compound to

part of the diet resulted in a significant reduction in the incidence of
dental caries. Several biochemical determinations were carried out on
plaque from the control and experimental animals. It was observed that
the animals receiving glycerophosphate had significantly more phosphorus
in their plaque than the control animals. Differences were not detected
in the carbohydrate or protein content of plaque from the two groups.
No differences were detected in the acid producing abilities of plaque.

Sodium phytate has been shown to be cariostatic in rats and in
monkeys and to have plaque desorbing properties in humans[13]. However,
significant differences were not detected in the plaques from the experimental and control monkeys. The acid producing capacity of plaque from
both groups was similar[9].

The long-term effects of sorbitol on the composition of plaque and
development of caries have been studied in primates. Ingestion of
sorbitol instead of sucrose neither aided the implantation nor supported
the continuance of populations of Strep. mutans in plaque.

Plaque in monkeys had little ability to ferment sorbitol at the
beginning of the experiment; even after two years of daily ingestion of
1 gram of sorbitol, the ability of plaque to ferment sorbitol was not
enhanced. The numbers of microorganisms capable of fermenting sorbitol
did not increase over the two year period.

Significantly less extracellular polysaccharide, both hexose and
ketohexose, was found in plaque from animals fed sorbitol than in
animals fed sucrose. Monkeys fed sorbitol developed few small carious
lesions, whereas those fed sucrose had many large extensive lesions.

In summary, cariogenic plaque has the ability to produce acids,
particularly lactic, from sugars, contains more extracellular and intracellular polysaccharide and less calcium and phosphorus than non-
cariogenic plaque.

REFERENCES

1. Bowen, W.H. and Cornick, D.E.R. Int. dent. J. 20: 382, 1970.

2. Bowen, W.H. Archs oral Biol. 19: 231, 1974.

3. Kite, D.W., Shaw, J.G. and Sognnaes, R.F. J. Nutr. 42: 89-93, 1950.

4. Stephan, R.M. J. dent. Res. 23: 257-260, 1944.

5. Critchley, P., and Bowen, W.H., in Dental Plaque, edited by W.D.
    McHugh, pp. 157-169, E. and S. Livingstone, Edinburgh and London,
    1969.

6. Rolla, G. Personal Communication, 1978.

7. Ashley, F.P. Archs oral Biol. 20: 167-169, 1975.

8. Critchley, P., Saxton, C.A. and Bowen, W.H. Abstract #157, IADR
    British Div., 1972.

9. Cole, M.F., Bowden, G., Korts, D. and Bowen, W.H. Caries Res. (in
    press) 1978.

10. Colman, G., Bowen, W.H. and Cole, M.F. Brit. dent. J. 142: 217-221,
    1977.

11. Bowen, W.H. Caries Res. 6: 43-47, 1972.

12. Cole, M.F. and Bowen, W.H. J. dent. Res. 54: 449, 1975.

13. Nordbo, H. and Rolla, G. J. dent. Res. 51: 800-802, 1972.

14. Cornick, D. and Bowen, W.H. Archs oral Biol. 17: 1637-1648, 1972.

Health and Sugar Substitutes
Proc. ERGOB Conf., Geneva 1978, pp. 241-246 (Karger, Basel 1978)

CLINICAL TRIALS ON SUGAR SUBSTITUTES

A. Scheinin

Department of Cariology, Institute of Dentistry,
University of Turku, SF-20520 Turku 52, Finland

INTRODUCTION

The potential use of sugar substitutes may be viewed in
relation to the generally accepted cariogenicity of sucrose.
Despite this concept, an examination of previous findings in
man shows the relationship between sugar intake and dental
caries to be complex and partly independent of dosage. There
are thus several studies in which little or no difference
between caries scores has been observed in relation to varying
sugar consumption[1,2,3,4,5,6,7,8,9,10]. Consequently, even a
high loading of peroral sucrose has been found to be virtually
unrelated to caries incidence[11].

On the other hand, ample evidence has been presented on the
high cariogenicity of sucrose being associated with the consumption of sugar-containing products between meals. Under
these conditions frequent intake, even in combination with
surprisingly low dosage has resulted in high caries incidence[2,11,12], as also observed in recent clinical trials[13,14,15,16,17].
The contradiction of high sugar dosage being unrelated to
caries scores, and very low consumption leading to a high
increment rate, is thus explained by considering the profound
role of the type and frequency of intake.

EVALUATION OF CLINICAL TRIALS

In view of this background, the reasoning for sugar substitution may be based on the concept of replacing sucrose particularly in foodstuffs proven to be highly cariogenic. The
clinical evaluation of the cariogenicity of specific sugar
substitutes has usually been carried out in comparison to a

control situation, however, for ethical reasons predominantly
without a predetermined frequency of sucrose intake.

So far, the existing trials have covered the replacement of
sucrose with other sugars, polyols or mixtures of these. The
results of these studies are summarized here in terms of
duration, age and number of subjects, compound and vehicle used,
frequency of intake, and caries reduction in comparison to
groups exposed to sucrose with known or *ad libitum* dosage
(Table I).

TABLE I.

CLINICAL TRIALS ON SUGAR SUBSTITUTES

STUDY	SUBJECT NO.	AGE	COMPOUND	VEHICLE		DURATION (YRS)	CARIES REDUCTION (%)	SUCROSE CONTROL
Slack et al. 1964[18]	213 202	11-12	SORBITOL	TABLET	> 3 x ? x	1 2	4 8 1 2 - 2 7	AD LIB.
Møller & Poulsen 1973[19]	174	8-12	SORBITOL	CH.G	3 x	2	1 0	AD LIB.
Frostell et al. 1974[20]	173 113	3-6	LYCASIN[R]	CANDY	REGULAR	1 2	2 5	AD LIB.
Scheinin et al. 1974[13]	35	26.2 ($\bar{x}$)	FRUCTOSE	TOTAL SUBSTITUTION		2	> 3 2	AD LIB.
Scheinin et al. 1975[14]	47	29.1 ($\bar{x}$)	XYLITOL	TOTAL SUBSTITUTION		2	> 8 5	AD LIB.
Scheinin et al. 1975[15]	50	22.0 ($\bar{x}$)	XYLITOL	CH.G	4.5 x	1	> 8 3	SUCROSE 4 x
Bánóczy et al. 1978[16]	404	3-12	SORBITOL	CHOCOLATE	1 x	1	5 4 - 6 2	SUCROSE 1 x
Frostell et al. 1978[21]	70	3-6	GLUCOSE + FRUCTOSE	CANDY	? x	1	3 9	AD LIB.

These trials have been listed in chronological order. The
study of Slack et al.[18] was clearly not conducted to evaluate
the effect of sorbitol. The purpose was to examine the effects
of chewable tablets aimed to stimulate the salivary flow.
These tablets contained i.a. malic acid, dicalcium phosphate
and 84.5 % sorbitol.

After the first study year a 48 % caries reduction was noted
in comparison to an untreated control group. After the second
year the difference between the groups diminished, the overall
reduction (12 - 27 %) being largely due to the effect achieved

during the first year. The authors remarked, however, that the use of the tablets was greatly reduced during the second study year.

The study of Møller and Poulsen[19] involved the use of 3 sorbitol chewing gums daily. The observed reduction in the experimental group was small (10 %) but significant in comparison to an untreated control group.

The "Roslagen study"[20] was carried out in order to ascertain whether substitution of sucrose by Lycasin[R], a hydrogenated starch hydrolysate, could influence the incidence of caries in the deciduous dentition. An overall reduction of about 25 % was estimated, although the observed reduction during the substitution phase varied between 34 and 49 % in children with 3 or less than 3 carious surfaces.

Only 2 clinical trials have compared substitution with monosaccharides in relation to sucrose. In the "Turku studies"[14] an almost complete substitution with fructose in adults resulted in a reduction exceeding 32 %. A similar trend was observed in the "Gustavsberg study"[21]. According to the preliminary 1-year findings a 39 % reduction was measured in the deciduous teeth of children exposed to products sweetened with glucose and fructose. In the "Turku studies", however, the effect was entirely due to a low increment rate of incipient lesions in the fructose group.

A massive reduction, exceeding 85 % was observed when substituting nearly all dietary sucrose for 2 years with xylitol[14]. An almost identical result, i.e. a reduction exceeding 83 % was obtained when substituting sucrose with xylitol in chewing gum only[15]. The substitution rate for sucrose consumed in solid form between meals was 68 % in the xylitol group of the chewing gum study. This implies that about 2/3 of the cariogenic fraction of sucrose was replaced by xylitol.

Recently, a substantial caries reduction was obtained also with sorbitol in relation to partial substitution of sucrose[16]. A reduction of 62 % in terms of DMF teeth and 54 % in terms of DMF surfaces was measured when using 20 g of sorbitol chocolate (sorbitol 8 g) in comparison to an equal intake of sucrose in chocolate. This study was undertaken in institutionalized children, and exposure to chocolate occurred only once per day.

INFLUENCE OF THE DIAGNOSTIC LEVEL

The caries registration in the "Turku studies"[14,15] was
carried out through ranking according to severity into incipient
and advanced classes. The caries incidence, however, included
both categories, the incipient lesions forming the majority of
the cumulative caries increment. Recent assessment[22] of the
clinical and radiographical data, the advanced lesions only
being calculated as decayed and the incipient lesions being
disregarded, yielded a significant reduction (56 - 60 %) for
the xylitol groups of both trials in comparison to the sucrose
and fructose groups. Analysis of these results (Fig. 1)
revealed virtually identical increment levels 1) in the xylitol
groups of both trials (1-year findings), 2) in the sucrose
groups of both trials (1-year findings), and 3) in the sucrose
and fructose groups (2-year findings), respectively. These
closely matching results from two independent series of observations indicating a high level of reproducibility were considered to be due to the facilitated diagnostic level.

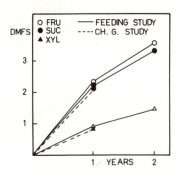

Fig. 1. Mean increment of the
DMFS index in two controlled
clinical trials[14,15] when calculating only the advanced lesions
as decayed and the incipient
lesions as intact surfaces.

DISCUSSION

Clinical trials indicate glucose and fructose to be cariogenic, however, less so than sucrose. In contrast, some
polyols may be considered virtually or completely noncariogenic.

A superficial analysis of the clinical trials on sugar
substitutes shows a significant caries reduction of varying
magnitude in comparison to sucrose. The caries reduction
percentages (Table I) deserve to be treated with reservation.

Already the varying assessment of caries, and differing experimental and control group situations with regard to frequency of intake, are sufficient reasons to consider comparison unjustified. There is thus a definite need for further controlled clinical trials of sufficient duration, preferably through large scale field studies in young, high caries prevalence populations.

The crucial problem, whether a noncariogenic caloric sweetener also possesses anticariogenic properties may not be proved beyond doubt in clinical and experimental caries studies. In the case of some polyols and mixtures of these it seems feasible to devise proper protocols for the assessment of remineralising capacity and cariostatic effects in general. Such design should account for the already known effects of peroral administration to stimulate a number of existing defence mechanisms to caries.

REFERENCES

1. Volker, J. F. J. Amer. Dent. Ass. 36: 23-27, 1948.
2. Zita, C, McDonald, R. E. and Andrews, A. L. J. Dent. Res. 38: 860-865, 1959.
3. Toto, P. D., Rapp, G. and O'Malley, J. J. Dent. Res. 39: 750-751, 1960.
4. Mansbridge, J. T. Brit. Dent. J. 109: 343-348, 1960.
5. McHugh, W. D., McEwen, J. D. and Hitchin, A. D. Brit. Dent. J. 147: 246-253, 1964.
6. Slack, G. L., Duckworth, R., Scheer, B., Brandt, R. S. and Ailianou Maki, C. Brit. Dent. J. 133: 371-377, 1972.
7. Bagramian, R. A. and Russell, A. L. J. Dent. Res. 52: 342-347, 1973.
8. Jackson, D. Brit. Dent. J. 137: 91-98, 1974.
9. Retief, D. H., Cleaton-Jones, P. E. and Walker, A. R. P. Brit. Dent. J. 138: 463-469, 1975.
10. Walker, A. R. P. and Cleaton-Jones, P. E. Lancet II: 765, 1975.
11. Gustafsson, B., Quensel, C. E., Lanke, L., Lundqvist, C., Grahnen, H., Gonow, B. E. and Krasse, B. Acta Odont. Scand. 11: 232-363, 1953.

12. Weiss, R. L. and Trithart, A. H.   Amer. J. Publ. Hlth 50:
     1097-1104, 1960.

13. Scheinin, A., Mäkinen, K. K. and Ylitalo, K.   Acta Odont.
     Scand. 32: 383-412, 1974.

14. Scheinin, A., Mäkinen, K. K. and Ylitalo, K.   Acta Odont.
     Scand. 33: Suppl. 70, 67-104, 1975.

15. Scheinin, A., Mäkinen, K. K., Tammisalo, E. and Rekola, M.
     Acta Odont. Scand. 33: 269-278, 1975.

16. Bánóczy, J., Esztári, I., Hadas, E., Marosi, I., Fözy, L.
     and Szántó, S.   Dtsch zahnärztl. Z. (in press), 1978.

17. Glass, R. L.   IADR Abstract 1978.

18. Slack, G. L., Millward, E. and Martin, W. J.   Brit. Dent. J.
     116: 105-108, 1964.

19. Møller, I. J. and Poulsen, S.   Community Dent. Oral
     Epidemiol. 1: 58-67, 1973.

20. Frostell, G., Blomlöf, L., Blomqvist, T., Dahl, G. M.,
     Edward, S., Fjellström, A., Henrikson, C. O., Larje, O.,
     Nord, C. E. and Nordenvall, K. J.   Acta Odont. Scand. 32:
     235-254, 1974.

21. Frostell et al.   Personal communication, 1978.

22. Scheinin, A.   ORCA Abstracts 1978, Abstr. No 20.

Health and Sugar Substitutes
Proc. ERGOB Conf., Geneva 1978, pp. 247-252 (Karger, Basel 1978)

SETTING CRITERIA FOR APPROPRIATNESS OF VARIOUS CARBOHYDRATE
SWEETENERS

K.K. Mäkinen

Section of Biochemistry, Institute of Dentistry, University
of Turku, SF-20520 Turku 52, Finland

INTRODUCTION

In spite of the fact that many currently known sweet carbohydrates have been investigated in organic chemistry for around a
hundred years, the possibility of substituting them for sucrose
for sweetening purposes has received serious attention only during the last few decades. The concern to replace sucrose is
chiefly based on its suggested "arch criminal" role in the causation of dental caries[1,2]. From the dental point of view this substitution can be considered well-grounded, but it must also be
recognized that apparently only a small part of total sucrose
consumption is responsible for the majority of dental caries lesions. Total substitution only comes into question in limited
clinical situations. Consequently, since the role of sucrose in
the human diet is unlikely to be significantly diminished, the
recommendations for its substitution ought mainly to be directed
to those groups of people which are associated with the major incidences of dental caries. A marginal sucrose replacement would
thus lead to the most significant reductions in the caries incidence.

BIOCHEMICAL CRITERIA

A starting point for setting criteria for the suitablity of
carbohydrate sweeteners is the acceptance of the idea that sweet
taste perception is included in the basic senses, developed during evolution. The following main biochemical criteria should be
considered:

1. The compound should be physiological and nontoxic even when
   consumed in fairly high concentrations. The human body should
   have a high metabolic capacity for the compound.

2. The compound should preferably appear in the normal intermediary metabolism of man. It should thus have normal metabolic
   pathways in the body. Channeling of exogenous sweetener
   through this pathway should not lead to pathological consequences. The functioning of other pathways should be essentially
   unchanged.
3. The compound should be practically or totally nonfermentable
   in the human dental plaque, even in chronic use.
4. The ability of the compound to interfere with the glucose or
   sucrose utilization of cariogenic microorganisms might be an
   advantageous property.
5. Administration of the compound should not decrease the defensive power of innate antimicrobial mechanisms of saliva and
   oral mucosa.
6. The compound should not cause staining or inflammatory changes
   in the oral tissues.
7. The compound should not have too strong effect on the
   apatogenic indigenous oral flora.

The above list includes aspects which belong to microbial
physiology, human intermediary metabolism and toxicology. As the
safety aspects of natural carbohydrate sweeteners will be dealt
with elsewhere, the effects of these sweeteners on oral biology
will be specifically considered here.

FERMENTABILITY IN THE HUMAN DENTAL PLAQUE

Detailed microbiological studies in vitro and in vivo have
shown that the ability of human dental plaque microorganisms to
effectively ferment carbohydrates is to a high extent genetically
fixed according to the physical and chemical conditions which
have prevailed in the oral cavity. The indigenous oral flora has
developed during the consumption of carbohydrates which occur
richly in Nature: glucose, fructose, sucrose, starch and similar
compounds. A prerequisite for effective utilization has thus been
a six-carbon skeleton in the basic monosaccharide units[3,4]. This
situation has apparently dominated in human dental plaque during
an enormously long period regardless of certain variation in the
composition of food. Although the adaptive power of microorganisms is known, it may be considered unlikely that plaque micro-

organisms would automatically start to metabolize preferentially such carbohydrates, for example, which currently are being tested as sucrose substitutes. It would be uneconomical, from the micro-organisms' point of view, to elaborate new transport and enzyme systems for each carbohydrate which might appear in food.

The above views are illustrated by the poor fermentability of five-carbon carbohydrates in human dental plaque, although such compounds have always existed in the diet (for a list of refer- ences, cf. ref. 5). It would appear that as long as the current, easily available and water-soluble carbohydrates with six-carbon structure occur in the diet to the present extent, the small- scale consumption of natural sucrose substitutes with a five- carbon pattern would not justify the assumption of any ready ad- aptation of plaque microorganisms to use the latter ones effec- tively.

Sucrose, glucose and fructose are readily metabolized by den- tal plaque microflora through glycolysis. This metabolism is in the oral cavity characterized by effective lactic acid formation and, depending on the microorganism involved, by the biosynthe- sis of insoluble extracellular glucans or soluble glucans and fructans[6]. Sorbitol and mannitol are readily metabolized by car- iogenic strains of <u>Streptococcus mutans</u> and certain other oral microorganisms[7-9]. Lycasin, maltitol and sorbose are also to a certain extent attacked by dental plaque bacteria. Long-term human studies suggest that the following bacteriophysiological criteria should be considered:

1. The nonacidogenic nature of the sweetener in relation to den- tal plaque should not change in prolonged use. For example, the nonacidogenic nature of xylitol did not change in 4.5-year use. Sorbitol produced acidic plaque in in vitro experiments 5,10.

2. The ability of plaque microorganisms to dehydrogenate or phos- phorylate the compound should not increase in prolonged use. For example, the activity of xylitol dehydrogenase was practi- cally nil in 4.5-year use of xylitol[10].

3. Experiments with labeled carbohydrates should be used to test if human dental plaque microorganisms possesses specific or non-specific recognition sites for the compound involved. This low binding of a carbohydrate should be regarded as a neces-

sary prerequisite for poor suitability as an energy substrate. For example, dental plaque microorganisms contain recognition sites for xylitol to a very limited extent only[11].

4. The compound should not increase the invertase-like or other disaccharase activity in plaque. Normally high invertase activity will be associated with sucrose consumption[12].

CRITERIA RELATED TO SALIVARY GLANDS OR ORAL MUCOSA

The suitability of a sucrose substitute should be tested by examining its effects on the efficacy of oral defensive factors, or on the concentration of compounds needed in the function of these factors. Consequently, the following criteria should be met:

1. The substitute should not reduce the antimicrobial potential of the lactoperoxidase-thiocyanate-H_2O_2 system. The effects on the ecretion and concentration of lactoperoxidase, SCN^- and the formation of H_2O_2 should separately be tested. According to present concepts, dietary sugars differ from each other in their ability to maintain high lactoperoxidase activity[13,14].

2. The substitute should not exert any negative effect on the secretion of immunoglobulins.

3. The substitute should not display any negative effect on other host resistance mechanisms, such as the buffering capacity (metabolism of HCO_3^-), concentration of sialin[15], glycolysis-promoting factors, etc.

Dietary sugars also differ from each other in their effects upon the pH values of oral fluid immediately after stimulation with these sugars. Thus, xylitol rinses (10 %) induce higher initial pH values in the oral fluid than sucrose or plain water, and maintain these pH values longer[16].

OTHER CRITERIA

1. Technochemical criteria (suitability for food manufacturing purposes).

2. Organoleptic criteria.

PERTINENT QUESTIONS

1. In bacteria not belonging to the dominating species in human

mouth, mutants capable of utilizing xylitol as a novel carbon have been detected (for example, Aerobacter aerogenes). This requires the involvement of enzymes of a preexisting pathway. It would be necessary to consider this type of genetic changes in relation to xylitol.

2. It would be necessary to fully elucidate the suggested selectivity of the common sugars (sucrose and sugar alcohols, for example) in their effects on the physiology of the salivary glands. Such a selectivity could be used in a physiological manner to maintain maximal host resistance in saliva.

3. Would the above selective effect of carbohydrates also concern the liberation of gastric hormones which would in turn influence salivary glands?

4. Is it possible that sweeteners (along with other ingredients of the diet) would be to a certain extend absorbed directly through the oral mucosa thereby inducing chemical changes (also via nervous impulses) in the salivary glands? There is some experimental evidence to support these ideas.

Elucidation of these matters would facilitate the classification of carbohydrate sweeteners in human use.

REFERENCES

1. Newbrun, E.   Odont. Revy 18: 373, 1967.
2. Newbrun, E.   J. Dent. Child. 36: 239, 1969.
3. Mäkinen, K.K.   Int. Dent. J. 26: 14-28, 1976.
4. Mäkinen, K.K.   Experientia Suppl. 30, 1978.
5. Mäkinen, K.K.   Proceedings "Microbial Aspects of Dental Caries". Eds. Stiles, H.M., Loesche, W.J. and O'Brien, T.C. Sp. Supp. Microbiology Abstracts. Vol. II: 521-538, 1976.
6. Kleinberg, I.   Advan. Oral Biol. 4: 44-90, 1970.
7. Fitzgerald, R.J. and Keyes, P.H.   J. Amer. Dent. Assoc. 61: 9-19, 1960.
8. Edwardsson, S.   Arch. Oral Biol. 13: 637-646, 1968.
9. Guggenheim, B.   Caries Res. 2: 147-163, 1968.
10. Mäkinen, K.K. and Virtanen, K.K.   J. Dent. Res. 1978. In press.
11. Mäkinen, K.K. and Rekola, M.   J. Dent. Res. 55: 900-904, 1976.

12. Mäkinen, K.K. and Scheinin, A.   Acta Odont. Scand. 33, Suppl.
    70: 129-171, 1975.

13. Mäkinen, K.K., Tenovuo, J. and Scheinin, A.   J. Dent. Res.
    55: 652-660, 1976.

14. Mäkinen, K.K., Bowen, W.H., Dalgard, D. and Fitzgerald, G.
    J. Nutr. 108: 1978. In press.

15. Kleinberg, I., Kanapka, J.A. and Craw, D.   Proceedings
    "Microbial Aspects of Dental Caries". Eds. Stiles, H.M.,
    Loesche, W.J. and O'Brien, T.C.   Sp. Supp. Microbiology
    Abstracts. Vol. 11: 433-464, 1976.

16. Mäkinen, K.K. Proceedings "Sweeteners and Dental Caries".
    Eds. Shaw, J.H. and Roussos, G.G.   Sp. Supp. Feeding, Weight
    & Obesity Abstracts, pp. 193-224, 1978.

CRITERIA INDICATIVE OF CARIOGENICITY OR NON CARIOGENICITY OF FOODS AND
BEVERAGES

Ernest Newbrun

Department of Oral Medicine/Hospital Dentistry, School of Dentistry
University of California San Francisco, CA   94143, USA

INTRODUCTION

   In 1974 at a plaque study conference convened at Airlie House, Virginia,
Socransky facetiously enunciated the First Law of Oral Biology: a plaque
sample will not satisfy anybody--it is either pooled or too small, unrepresent-
ative, too young or too old. On the occasion of the ERGOB Conference on sugar
substitutes I wish to promulgate Newbrun's Second Law of Oral Biology: there
is no single test of cariogenicity of a food or beverage--especially none that
would satisfy a committee! In vitro tests have been criticized because they do
not adequately measure host factors, plaque pH determinations predict acidogenicity but not necessarily cariogenicity. Cariogenicity assessments of foods
fed *ad libitum* to rodents or even primates depend on the animal's food preference. Clinical trials on humans have used populations that are too old or
institutionalized and have even been accused of being unethical. Are there any
acceptable criteria of cariogenicity of foods or beverages?

   Over the years at numerous symposia, workshops and conferences the relationship between diet and dental caries has been explored. Some of these meetings
have resulted in the publication of the proceedings [1-6], many have not.
Usually where the proceedings have been published they have constituted individual position papers or reviews of special areas within the field of diet and
dental caries relationships and have not represented concensus reports. It is
worth examining the reasons for a lack of concensus by dental and food scientists as to what criteria should be used in measuring cariogenicity of a
product.

   Dental caries is a multifactorial disease involving three principal factors:
the host (particularly the saliva and teeth), the microflora, and their substrate (i.e. the diet). A fourth dimension: time, or frequency when considering diet, plays an integral role. An ideal test for measuring cariogenicity
of a food or beverage would take into account all these factors, should have a

sound biological basis, and above all the results should be in accord with
clinical experience and epidemiological findings.

If sugar substitutes are to be used, some criteria of cariogenicity and non-
cariogenicity need to be developed and agreed upon. Some assessment methods
will be briefly reviewed.

BACTERIAL ASSESSMENT

A sugar substitute, which is not readily fermentable in vitro either by
mixed plaque flora or pure cultures of cariogenic organisms, is presumably non-
cariogenic. However, the converse does not necessarily follow: all sugar substitutes or foods that are fermented in vitro need not be cariogenic. For example mannitol which is fermented by *Strep. mutans* to form acid, does not
lower plaque pH in vivo nor does it induce bacterial adaptation unless it is
the only carbon source. Such is not the case in human diets. Another example
would be the dihydrochalcones whose glycosidic moiety, at least theoretically,
is fermentable. In practice, however, because of the intense sweetness of the
dihydrochalcones, the amounts used in a food would be so small that its
glycosidic portion would not significantly alter the inherent fermentability
of the food.

IN VITRO ASSESSMENT OF CARIOGENICITY

As early as 1890, Miller differentiated between the caries-producing capacity of foods based on the amount of acids they formed in saliva[7]. Similar tests
have been used by Bibby and his associates[8-10] and others[11]. These valiant
attempts to rank various foods as to their cariogenicity have several obvious
shortcomings. The in vitro model is rather remote from the real life situation. The salivary flora used as an inoculum is not representative of the
plaque microbiota nor is there a continuous salivary flow. Food clearance is
also thought to be important, so that the amount of particular food retained in
the mouth has been measured and combined with the amount of acid formed into a
"decalcification potential". Subsequently, it was recognized that much food
was retained on mucous membranes and that only food retained on the teeth was
of major importance.

A variation has been to measure enamel demineralization by the amount of
^{32}P dissolved by a food-saliva mixture from radioactive bovine enamel[12].
Another in vitro test is the "Orofax" apparatus in which the test food is
placed on the surface of blocks of enamel, inoculated with plaque suspensions.
Saliva drips over these blocks of enamel which are subsequently examined for
demineralization by polarized light[13]. The results of these in vitro tests indicate that the amount of enamel dissolved is not necessarily proportionate to

the acid produced. Bibby[10] has repeatedly stated that there is no parallel between cariogenicity as determined by his test methods, and the "sugar" content
of the food. What do we know from clinical and epidemiological experience with
humans (e.g. hereditary fructose intolerance). Certainly not all carbohydrates
especially starches, are cariogenic as they are consumed by HFI patients with
relative impunity. Yet according to the in vitro tests described, starchy
foods, like various breads and bagels and even potato chips, cause more enamel
demineralization than chocolates, cookies, cakes and pastries. When such in
vitro tests run counter to extensive clinical and epidemiological experience,
one must conclude that the test model does not really measure cariogenicity
and should be discarded as irrelevant.

PLAQUE pH CHANGES AFTER FOOD AND BEVERAGES

Plaque pH changes have been determined following ingestion of various foods
and beverages either by removing a plaque sample[14,15] or directly by biotelemetry. The advantages of biotelemetry include proper assessment of permeability
of plaque and the ability to continuously follow pH changes at the same plaque
site[17], the disadvantage is one of cost. Edgar et al[15] have ranked various
foods according to their ΣD value, which is the sum of all pH depressions and
depends on the shape of the Stephan curve. It is not surprising that they
found no apparent relationship between the plaque pH changes and the soluble
carbohydrate concentration of the food bolus. The anthrone method employed for
carbohydrate determination measures all soluble starches yet these latter
would not diffuse into intact plaque at the same rate or to the same extent as
the much smaller di- and monosaccharides. The Zürich group has, perhaps wisely, not attempted to rank various foods based on biotelemetric drop of pH;
rather, the criterion has been an all or none type. If the food or beverage
causes a plaque pH fall below 5.7 during a 30 minute interval, it is not "safe
for teeth".

Determination of a products acidogenicity, based on plaque pH changes, more
nearly represents the odontolytic process than other in vitro measurements, but
it is still not a measure of cariogenicity per se. Because man is omnivorous
and consumes a mixed diet, it is pertinent that the sequence of ingesting
different foods at one meal influences the plaque pH pattern[17-19]. Accordingly, one can not predict cariogenicity of a single food based on its acidogenicity alone, as this is modified by the other foods consumed.

ANIMAL TESTING FOR CARIOGENICITY

Rodents have been widely used, and often misused, for testing cariogenicity
of foods. Because of inconsistent results, rodent caries has been dismissed

as having no significance for man[10]. However, if this model is used under standardized conditions (animal strain, age, infection, caries scoring system, etc.)
a similar pattern of caries is found[20]. Furthermore, foods can be tested individually which is impossible in human clinical trials. Most important is the
similarity between results of animal tests and actual clinical and epidemiological observations on humans. Some experiments illustrating the parallelism between sucrose content of a food and its cariogenicity are worth citing[21-23].

Stephan[21] compared the cariogenicity of a wide range of foods and beverages
fed to rats *ad libitum* in addition to their basic diet. Generally, items with
a high sucrose and total sugar content were highly cariogenic and those with no
or low sugar content were noncariogenic (soda crackers, milk, sorbitol),
Table I. The relationship is not perfectly quantitative but the exceptions can
be explained on the marked taste preferences of rats. For example, rats drink
sweetened solutions (sucrose water, cola) very frequently if continuously
available, which accounts for the relatively high caries score. Similarly,
given the opportunity, rats eat apples with great frequency. Conversely, rats
do not like chewing gum as much as humans and probably the same explanation
holds for caramels so that these foods were not as cariogenic as anticipated
by their sugar content. These experiments need to be repeated under controlled feeding conditions to eliminate the frequency and preference factor.

When rats are fed more similar foods, a close parallel between sucrose content and cariogenicity, particularly of smooth surface lesions, is found,
Table II[22]. Similarly, hamsters, fed various commercial cereals, develop
caries proportionate to the sucrose content of the cereal, Table III[23]. One
exception, Life, has a relatively lower cariogenicity, presumably because of
its higher phosphate content.

The sugar content of a food is obviously not the only factor affecting cariogenicity, the physical texture and most important the frequency of ingestion
also are of importance. Nevertheless, proper labelling, disclosing the percent
sucrose of a food, would be a useful guide to consumers and health profession-
als giving dietary advice.

CONCLUSIONS

The present mixed human diet with its high sugar intake gives a high background caries activity. Accordingly, clinical trials to test the cariogenicity
of an individual food (candy, chewing gum, cereal, soft drink) are inappropriate. Sugar substitution in a single item will not significantly reduce
caries. A whole spectrum of foods need to be modified and then tested as a
group. Foods can be satisfactorily evaluated for cariogenicity by well-con-

trolled animal tests. Plaque pH measurement of acidogenicity are suitable for
screening foods which are "safe for teeth," but not for ranking of cariogenicity.

TABLE I. COMPARISON OF CARIES SCORE AND SUCROSE CONTENT
OF HUMAN FOODS FED TO RATS AD LIBITUM [21]

FOOD*	% SUCROSE[24,25]	% TOTAL SUGAR	CARIES SCORE
SUCROSE	99.5	100	62.1
MILK CHOCOLATE	42	55	34.1
DATES	47	84	32.7
10% SUCROSE WATER	10	10	32.3
RAISINS	14	70	30.9
COLA	3	11	29.6
CANDY MINTS (LIFESAVERS)	78	89	24.7
CHOCOLATE SANDWICH COOKIE (OREO)	35	35	23.8
BANANAS	9	20	21.0
APPLES	3	11	19.4
HONEY GRAHAM CRACKERS	16	18	19.2
CARAMELS	64	77	16.0
CHEWING GUM (WRIGLEY'S)	55	59	14.0
FIGS	0.1	73	10.3
SODA CRACKERS	0	<1	0.3
MILK	0	5	0
SORBITOL	0	0	0

*RATS FED DIET 581 (NON-CARIOGENIC) FOR 1 HOUR TWICE A DAY. TEST FOOD WAS
CONTINUOUSLY AVAILABLE.

TABLE II. CARIOGENICITY OF SNACK FOODS
FED RATS AD LIBITUM [22]

FOOD	% SUCROSE	% TOTAL SUGAR	CARIOUS FISSURE LESIONS	CARIOUS BUCCO-LINGUAL LESIONS
MILK CHOCOLATE + RICE CRISPIES	42	50	12.9	43
CHOCOLATE WAFERS	30	35	11.2	30
BISCUIT, WHOLE MEAL FLOUR	20	22	8.0	5
BISCUIT, WHITE FLOUR	14	19	10.6	2
BREAD + JAM	7	15	3.0	1.5
BISCUIT, "SUCROSE FREE"	1	3	2.6	0
BREAD AND CHEESE	0.4	3	3.1	0

TABLE III. INFLUENCE OF COMMERCIAL CEREALS
ON DENTAL CARIES IN HAMSTERS [23]

CEREAL*	% SUCROSE[24]	CARIES SCORE
FROSTED FLAKES	44	17.14 ± 0.36
CAP'N CRUNCH	43.3	14.21 ± 0.24
KING VITAMIN	58.5	14.09 ± 0.27
QUISP	44.9	10.46 ± 0.15
CORN FLAKES	7.8	8.95 ± 0.14
CORN STARCH	0	8.46 ± 0.19
CHEERIOS	2.2	7.66 ± 0.12
LIFE	14.5	6.92 ± 0.12
SPECIAL K	4.4	6.85 ± 0.11
SHREDDED WHEAT	1.0	6.07 ± 0.12

*CONSTITUTED 33% OF TOTAL DIET

REFERENCES

1. Bibby,B.G J. Dent. Res. 49:Suppl., 1970.

2. Blix,G. Swedish Nutrition Foundation III, Almqvist & Wiksell, Uppsala, 1965.

3. Gould,R.F. Advances in Chemistry Series 94, American Chemical Society, Washington D.C., 1970.

4. Shaw,J.H. and Roussos,G.G. Feeding, weight and obesity abstracts, Sp. Supp. Information Retrieval Inc. Washington D.C., 1978.

5. Hefferren,J.J. Am. Dent. Assn., Chicago Ill., 1978.

6. Bibby,B.G. and Shern,R.J. Microbiology abstracts--bacteriology Sp. Supp. Information Retrieval Inc., Washington D.C., 1978.

7. Miller,W.D. *The Microorganisms of the Human Mouth*. pp. 208-209. S.S. White Co., Philadelphia, 1890.

8. Bibby,B.G., Goldberg,H.J.V. and Chen,E. J. Am. Dent. Assn. 42:491-509, 1951.

9. Ludwig,T.G. and Bibby,B.G. J. Dent. Res. 36:56-60, 1957.

10. Bibby,B.G. J. Am. Dent. Assn. 90:121-132, 1975.

11. Katz,S., Olson,B.L. and Park,K.C. Pharm. Therap. Dent. 2:109-131, 1975.

12. Bibby,B.G. and Mundorff,S.A. J. Dent. Res. 54:461-470, 1975.

13. Bibby,B.G. In *Methods of Caries Prediction*. Microbiology abstracts, Sp. Supp. pp. 237-240, 1978.

14. Frostell,G. Acta Odontol. Scand. 27:3, 1969.

15. Edgar,W.M., Bibby,B.G., Mundorff,S. and Rowley,J. J. Am. Dent. Assn. 90:418-425, 1975.

16. Imfeld,T., Hirsch,R.S. and Mühlemann,H.R. Brit. Dent. J 144:40-45, 1978.

17. Mühlemann,H.R. and Imfeld,T. In *Methods of Caries Prediction*. Microbiology abstracts, Sp. Supp. pp. 241-244, 1978.

18. Rugg-Gunn,A.J., Edgar,W.M., Geddes,D.A.M. and Jenkins,G.N. Brit. Dent. J. 139:351-356, 1975.

19. Geddes,D.A.M., Edgar,W.M., Jenkins,G.N. and Rugg-Gunn,A.J. Brit. Dent. J. 140:317-319, 1977.

20. Larson,R.H., Amsbaugh,S.M., Navia,J.M., Rosen,S., Schuster,G.S. and Shaw, J.H. J. Dent. Res. 56:1007-1012, 1977.

21. Stephan,R.M. J. Dent. Res. 45:1551-1561, 1966.

22. Ishii,P., König,K.G. and Mühlemann,H.R. Helv. Odont. Acta 12:41-47, 1968.

23. McDonald,J.L. and Stookey,G.K. J. Dent. Res. 56:1001-1006, 1977.

24. Shannon,I. *Brand Name Guide to Sugar*. Nelson Hall, Chicago, Ill., 1977.

25. Pennigton,J.A. *Dietary Nutrient Guide*. Avi Publish. Co. Inc. Westport, Conn., 1976.

VI. Factors in safety, benefit/risk assessment and legal aspects

Moderator: F. Fairweather, London
Co-Moderator: I. MacDonald, London

Health and Sugar Substitutes
Proc. ERGOB Conf., Geneva 1978, pp. 260-261 (Karger, Basel 1978)

VALUE OF TOXICOLOGICAL TESTING IN CHEMICAL CARCINOGENICITY

D. Schmähl

Institute of Toxicology and Chemotherapy, German Cancer Research
Center, 6900 Heidelberg, Im Neuenheimer Feld 280, Germany

Animal experiments have played and still play a decisive
role for the recognition of chemical carcinogenic effects.
In many cases (e.g. in the case of haloethers, vinylchloride,
cyclophosphamide etc.) it was possible to demonstrate first
in animals the carcinogenic effect that was later observed in
man, too. Arsenic is the only substance that has proved to be
carcinogenic in man without showing a distinctly positive result
in animal experiments. For these reasons, any substance that
acted carcinogenic in animal experiments has to be regarded as
carcinogenic for human beings, too, as long as this has not
been disproved e.g. by epidemiological studies.

For the evaluation of the carcinogenic activity of a chemical
substance and for the examination of the question whether the
result obtained in the experiment is also relevant for man and
can be extrapolated to human conditions, a few important parameters have to be considered:

1. The carcinogenic effect should - if possible - be proved
   in several animal species.

2. The doses necessary for cancerisation should not exceed the
   doses taken in by human beings too much, because otherwise
   the detoxication systems are overstrained and an excessive
   dosage may change the whole metabolism.

3. It should be guaranteed that the "carcinogenic effect" does

not proceed unspecifically but that the carcinogen leads to interactions with the genome.

4. The carcinogenic effect should show clear pharmacological-toxicological correlations and criteria in dose-time and dose-response studies in order to evaluate threshold doses.

5. The results obtained should be reproducible and provide plain and statistically significant data compared to an untreated control.

In consideration of these most essential criteria (detailed elaboration of this problem in "Problems of Dose-Response Studies in Chemical Carcinogenesis with Special Reference to N-Nitroso Compounds", Critical Reviews in Toxocology, CRC Press, Palm Beach, in press), animal experiments have a high degree of prediction value. The negative result of an experiment, too, has a high prediction value if the experimental setup was plain and corresponded to modern criteria. It goes without saying that a negative result never completely excludes a risk for man and a positive result never allows an absolutely evident conclusion on the carcinogenic effect in human beings. In dimensions of relative safety, however, animal experiments have without doubt a high value.

Health and Sugar Substitutes
Proc. ERGOB Conf., Geneva 1978, pp. 262-265 (Karger, Basel 1978)

ADVANTAGES AND DISADVANTAGES OF ARTIFICIAL SWEETENERS AND SUGAR SUBSTITUTES

H. Mehnert

Forschergruppe Diabetes und Krankenhaus München-Schwabing,
Kölner Platz 1, 8000 München 40, Bundesrepublik Deutschland

ARTIFICIAL SWEETENERS

Inquiries conducted amongst a random sample of 500 diabetics
showed that only 84 patients felt no craving for sweeteners
or sugar substitutes (1). The overwhelming majority used
sweeteners; approximately half taking cyclamate (177 patients)
and half saccharine (174 patients). This proves that the old
requirement, according to which diabetics should ideally
dispense with sweeteners altogether, is quite unrealistic. It
is certainly also wrong to claim that most diabetics develop
an aversion to all sweet foods, once their condition has been
diagnosed. The main advantage of artificial sweeteners as
opposed to sugar substitutes is presumably mainly due to the
fact that the former are calorie-free and consequently more
advisable for the obese.

SUGAR SUBSTITUTES

The diminished glucose tolerance encountered in Diabetes mellitus and other catabolic situations ("post aggression conditions"
following surgery, infections, etc.) justifies experimental
and clinical work on those carbohydrates which, under certain
conditions, are utilized more or less "independent of insulin".
The most important sugar substitute or "diabetic's sugar" is
fructose. Its use is extensively described in the literature
(2, 3). The polyols sorbitol and xylitol should also be
regarded as sugar substitutes, since their metabolism in the
mammalian organism undoubtedly resembles that of the carbohydrates and since, on account of their taste, they are sugars
rather than alcohols. A sugar substitute is defined as being

a carbohydrate that produces no, or only slight, hyperglucosaemia; this property clearly distinguishing it from
sugars such as glucose and sucrose.

In metabolically healthy subjects, the intraduodenal or oral
application of fructose has no significant influence on
blood glucose level or on serum insulin concentration. If
such an alteration were to occur, it would be most likely
to appear after the use of fructose, since this is the
most rapidly absorbed of the nutritive sucrose substitutes.
For this reason, xylitol and sorbitol were not subjected
to similar tests. A comparing study using orally administered
glucose and fructose in diabetics produced a significantly
higher rise in blood glucose concentrations following the
administration of glucose. This difference is clearly
demonstrated, both by the individual blood sugar curves as
well as by the overall representation showing alteration
in blood sugar as a percentage of the initial value. It is
worthy of note that the diabetics included in the study
were regularly taking sulphonylurea medication and
receiving their normal dosage of tablets on the day of the
trial. This ensured that the diabetics were under everyday
conditions during the course of the study. The only change
was the replacement of their breakfast by 50 g glucose or
50 g fructose respectively. Both the obviously maximum of
stimulated insulin secretion by the sulphonylurea and the
concentrations of free fatty acids were the same for both
monosaccharides.

Since the utilization of fructose, sorbitol and xylitol
may, under the above-mentioned conditions, be "insulin
independent", these substances should be used in the
diabetic's diet rather than sugars of the glucose type.
The term "insulin independent" may not, as is sometimes
the case, be taken to mean that every single administration
of a sugar substitute to every diabetic will fail to
increase blood glucose and serum insulin level. On the

contrary, each and every administration of a sugar
substitute to a metabolically healthy individual may lead
to hyperglucosaemia and hyperinsulinaemia - and this is
even more the case for every diabetic. The advantages of
sugar substitutes lies in the modest level of these metabolic changes (in comparison to glucose, sucrose and
maltose). Sugar substitutes may be considered as "glucose
with delay" because they are absorbed more slowly than
glucose and are then converted to glucose either gradually
or not at all. Elderly diabetics generally tolerate
considerably larger quantities of sugar substitutes when
these are spread out over the day into 5 - 6 individual
dosages. Our own studies showed that elderly diabetics can
utilize up to 80 g fructose per day without increasing
their blood and urine glucose values (4). In general,
neither patients nor doctors favour such a large amount
of fructose   . The same must apply to sorbitol and
xylitol.

Given the correct dosage, carbohydrate tolerance can be
raised and a stabilization of the metabolic situation of
unstable diabetics may be achieved through the administration of small amounts of fructose, sorbitol or
xylitol. It goes without saying that the latter procedure
comes as a second behind exactly controlled insulin
therapy. However, it is these, usually slim, insulin-
deficient diabetics (frequently children and young adults)
who may be offered a pleasant tasting sugar substitute to
replace the glucose type sugar which they are quite
rightly forbidden to take. The antiketogenic effect of
sugar substitutes is particularly pronounced. This fact
could also be utilized effectively in just this type of
diabetes.

As has been stated above, there is only a small liklihood
of preventing diabetics from taking no sweeteners at all.

The calorie intake inevitable with the administration of
sugar substitutes may interfere with desired weight loss
in elderly diabetics who are frequently obese. On the other
hand, tolerance to sugar substitutes in the rather under-
weight, younger diabetic of unstable type is limited since,
in this form of diabetes (insulin deficiency diabetes)
there is of course a greater tendency of gluconeogenesis
in which sugar substitutes are involved. For this reason,
when calculating carbohydrates and hence calorie balances,
in West Germany not only carbohydrates of the glucose type
(in particular products containing starch), but also sugar
substitutes are taken into account. It is therefore easier
for the physician to enable his patients to enjoy the
limited consumption of sugar substitutes in their authorized
carbohydrate allowance without the risk of additional
uncalculated intake of calories.

REFERENCES

1. Mehnert, H.: Wissenschaftliche Veröffentlichungen der
    Deutschen Gesellschaft für Ernährung, Band 20. Calorien-
    arme und calorienfreie Lebensmittel. Dr. Dietrich Stein-
    kopff Verlag, Darmstadt 1971, 79 - 84.

2. Mehnert, H., G. Dietze and M. Haslbeck: Nutr. Metabol.
    18 (Suppl. 1): 171 - 190, 1975.

3. Haslbeck, M., W. Bachmann and H. Mehnert: Akt. Ernährung
    2, 53 - 57, 1978.

4. Mehnert, H., K. Stuhlfauth, B. Mehnert, L. Wiener and
    A. Hoeflmayr: Münch. med. Wschr. 102, 276 - 279, 1960.

Health and Sugar Substitutes
Proc. ERGOB Conf., Geneva 1978, pp. 266-271 (Karger, Basel 1978)

LONG-TERM STUDIES ON THE POTENTIAL CARCINOGENICITY OF ARTIFICIAL SWEETENERS
IN NON-HUMAN PRIMATES

S. M. SIEBER AND R. H. ADAMSON

Laboratory of Chemical Pharmacology, National Cancer Institute, National
Institutes of Health, Bethesda, MD 20014, USA

INTRODUCTION

The question of the carcinogenic risk to humans of artificial sweeteners is
of scientific, medical, social and economic importance. Cyclamate was banned
by the FDA for use in all foods and drugs in 1970. This action was taken because results of in vivo carcinogenesis studies in rats using combinations of
cyclamate and saccharin indicated an increased incidence of bladder tumors in
the treated animals[1,2]. Since that time, several long-term studies on the
carcinogenicity of cyclamate in animals have produced negative results[3]. Seven
years after the cyclamate ban, in 1977, the FDA proposed a similar ban on saccharin, whereby its use in foods, beverages, some cosmetics, drugs, and animal
feeds would be prohibited. This was primarily the result of a 2-generation study
in rats where an increased incidence of bladder tumors was found in males[4].

However, a number of questions remain as to the actual carcinogenic risk
that these artificial sweeteners pose to human beings. For example, would
these substances also induce tumors in animals when given at levels likely to
mimic human exposure levels, rather than at the many-fold greater doses used in
the rat studies? Were the tumors found in such studies a secondary effect of
the high doses of the chemical used rather than a direct carcinogenic effect of
the chemical itself? Could the tumors have been induced by an impurity in, or
a metabolite of, the compounds? And finally, what is the carcinogenic potential
of these substances in species other than the rodent?

Studies on the mutagenic effects of saccharin were commissioned by the Office
of Technology Assessment in order to provide additional information as to the
possible hazards associated with this compound. The compound was subjected to
a battery of 12 short-term in vitro tests for mutagenicity; 10 of these tests
have been completed, and saccharin possessed clear mutagenic activity in only 3
of them[3].

In addition to the ambiguities of the results of in vivo carcinogenesis
studies in rats and the in vitro mutagenesis data, the problem is further con-

founded by the hazards of extrapolating mutagenicity and rodent carcinogenicity
data into human risk factors. Although carcinogenesis studies in rodents are
relatively fast and inexpensive, there are certain factors which make the results of such studies, either positive or negative, subject to question. The
high incidence of spontaneous tumors noted in some rodent colonies frequently
obscures the carcinogenic effects of the test chemical. The bacterial flora of
the intestine of rodents differs from that of the human intestine; furthermore,
in many instances, rodents metabolize chemicals by pathways markedly different
from those used by the human being. These factors are of particular importance
in the field of chemical carcinogenesis, where many potential carcinogens
require activation to their ultimate carcinogenic species by liver, other
tissues, or by intestinal bacteria.

Thus it is of importance to consider evidence for the carcinogenicity of
chemicals obtained from sources other than in vitro mutagenesis assays or from
the rodent carcinogen bioassay. We have been testing both cyclamate and
saccharin for carcinogenic effects in non-human primates for the past 7-8 years,
and the results of our ongoing studies are summarized below.

MATERIALS AND METHODS

Animals. The present colony consists of approximately 600 animals; 80 of
these are adult breeders which supply the newborn animals for experimental
studies. The monkeys represent 4 species, namely Macaca mulatta (rhesus, 48%),
Macaca fascicularis (cynomolgus, 42%), Cercopithecus aethiops (African green,
8%), and the prosimian Galago crassicaudatus (bushbaby, 2%). The majority of
the animals are housed in an isolated facility which contains only animals
committed to this study, and with the exception of the monkeys in the breeding
colony, most animals are housed in individual cages. Details of maintenance
and management procedures, and the method used to rear neonates have been described elsewhere[5]. Newborns produced by the breeding colony are taken within
12 hours of birth to a nursery which is staffed on a 24 hour basis.

The control population includes untreated breeders and vehicle-treated
animals ranging in age from neonates to older than 16 years. The species com-
prising the control population are rhesus (49%), cynomolgus (38%) and African
greens (13%); 36% of the control animals are males.

A number of clinical, biochemical and hematological parameters are monitored
weekly or monthly, not only to evaluate the general health status of each
animal, but also for the early detection of tumors. The monkeys are observed
daily, weighed weekly, and given a thorough physical examination by the staff
veterinarians every 6 months. Samples of blood are drawn every 6 months for
various hematologic and clinical chemical tests such as SMA-12, CBCs and deter-

mination of serum alpha-fetoprotein and carcinoembryonic antigen levels. All
animals which die or are sacrificed during the course of the study are carefully
necropsied and their tissues subjected to histopathologic examination.

Administration of test compounds. The compounds are administered by the oral
route daily, 5 days every week. For dosing newborn monkeys, the compound is
added to the Similac formula at the time of feeding; when the monkeys are 6
months old, the compounds are incorporated into a vitamin mixture which is given
to monkeys as a vitamin sandwich on a half slice of bread. The sandwhich consists of powdered milk, Parvo (a folic acid supplement), Cecon (a vitamin C
supplement), and molasses. Dosing with the test compounds is initiated within
24 hours of birth, and continues until the animal dies or a tumor is diagnosed.

Chemicals. Sodium cyclamate is the kind gift of Abbott Laboratories, North
Chicago, Ill. 60064 and is used as received. Sodium saccharin ("purified")
is purchased from Fisher Scientific Co., Fairlawn, N.J. 07410, and is used as
obtained without further purification.

RESULTS

Controls. Since the inception of the colony 16 years ago, 4 monkeys have
developed spontaneous neoplasms out of a total of 211 control monkeys, yielding
a spontaneous tumor incidence of approximately 2%. Three of the tumors were
lymphomas, and developed in African green monkeys; the fourth tumor was a
carcinoma of the gallbladder which arose in a 10 year old rhesus monkey.

Cyclamate. Of a total of 12 monkeys that have received cyclamate at 100
mg/kg, 10 are alive and without evidence of toxicity. These monkeys have
received total doses of cyclamate ranging between 377.3 - 1169.8 gm for an
average of 94 months (Table 1). The 100 mg/kg dose in monkeys corresponds,
on an equivalent surface area basis, to a daily intake of 2.3 gm/day/70 kg man;
with an average of 384 mg of cyclamate in a 10 ounce diet drink[6], this is equivalent to drinking about 6 diet drinks per day. The average cumulative dose of
cyclamate ingested by the monkeys receiving daily doses at 100 gm/kg, 730.6 gm,
is equivalent to the ingestion of about 15,000 diet sodas by a 70 kilogram man.

Table 1:   Summary of Surviving Cyclamate-Treated Monkeys

Dose	No. of Monkeys		Av. Total	Av. Months
(mg/kg)	♂	♀	Dose (gm)	Treated
100	5	5	730.6	94
500	6	3	4714.5	95

Eleven monkeys have received cyclamate at 500 mg/kg, and 9 are alive at present. The average total dose of cyclamate ingested by these monkeys was 4714.5 gm (range 3721.0 - 6998.4 gm), and they have been dosed for an average of 95 (range 93 - 96) months. The 500 mg/kg daily dose of cyclamate ingested by this group of monkeys corresponds, on an equivalent surface area basis, to a daily intake of 11.6 gm/day/70 kg man; this is equivalent to drinking about 30 diet drinks per day. The average cumulative dose of cyclamate ingested by the monkeys receiving daily doses at 500 mg/kg, 4714.5 gm, is equivalent to the ingestion of about 95,000 diet sodas by a 70 kilogram man.

Since the inception of the cyclamate study, 2 monkeys at each dose level have died (Table 2). The 2 monkeys in the 100 mg/kg group died within 4 months of initiation of the study, and had received relatively small amounts of compound. No evidence of tumor was found at necropsy or after histological examination of tissue from these monkeys. In both cases, however, there was histopathologic evidence of damage to the kidneys, although this damage cannot be directly attributed to cyclamate intake. One of the 2 deaths in the 500 mg/kg group was accidental, and although the animal had received more than 90 gm of cyclamate, no specific abnormalities were found in any tissue. The other monkey that died in the 500 mg/kg group had received a total of 1851.0 gm of cyclamate over the course of 84 months. Histopathologic examination of kidney tissue taken from this monkey revealed the presence of vacuolar degeneration of the collecting tubules of the kidney. No lesions were found in any other tissue examined.

Table 2:   Summary of Dead Cyclamate-Treated Monkeys

Dose (mg/kg)	Monkey #	Species & Sex	Total Dose (gm)	Months Dosed	Findings at Necropsy
100	767J	Cyno, ♂	1.6	4	fatty degen. of kidneys
	775J	Cyno, ♂	0.8	2	fatty degen. of kidneys
500	789J	Gr, ♂	91.9	28	no specific abnormalities
	790J	Rh, ♀	1851.0	84	vacuolar degen. of kidneys

Saccharin. Two groups of 10 monkeys each have been receiving oral doses of saccharin at 25 mg/kg, 5 days every week (Table 3). The initial group of monkeys (Group I) have received an average total dose of saccharin of 176.5 gm (range 107.8 - 244.6 gm) for an average of 89 months (range 87 - 91). A second group of monkeys (Group II) was entered on study less than one year ago, and has

received to date an average total saccharin dose of 6.1 gm (range 3.9 - 8.8 gm).
The 25 mg/kg dose corresponds, on an equivalent surface area basis, to a daily
intake of 5 cans of diet soda (containing 120 mg of saccharin per can[7]) or 15
packages of Sweet 'N Low® (40 mg of saccharin per package[8]) per day. The average cumulative saccharin dose in the Group I monkeys (176.5 gm) corresponds to
a total intake of approximately 11,000 diet drinks or 34,000 packages of Sweet
'N Lo® by a 70 kilogram man. Since the inception of the saccharin study almost
8 years ago, none of the animals have died, and there has been no evidence of
toxicity in any of the animals thus far.

Table 3: Summary of Saccharin-Treated Monkeys

Group	No. of Monkeys ♂	♀	Av. Total Dose (gm)	Av. Months Dosed
I	4	6	176.5	89
II	5	5	6.1	10

DISCUSSION

We have found no evidence that cyclamate is a carcinogen, although in 3 of
the 4 monkeys necropsied to date there was some evidence of damage to the
kidney tubules. Saccharin also has not provided any indication of a carcinogenic effect in 2 groups of 10 monkeys each receiving the compound at 25 mg/kg.
One group has been treated with this compound for longer than 7 years, and no
deaths have as yet occurred.

Our negative results are in agreement with those of Coulston[9], who tested
cyclamate and saccharin for carcinogenicity in several small groups of monkeys.
He administered cyclamate orally to 3 monkeys at 200 mg/kg/day for 6 days
every week and no tumors developed during the 6 - 7 years of treatment. Similarly, no tumors developed in 14 monkeys given oral doses of sodium saccharin
over a period of about 5 years.

Although ours is the largest study yet reported on the carcinogenic potential
of artificial sweeteners in non-human primates, nevertheless the number of monkeys employed is small in comparison to the number of rodents conventionally
used in carcinogenesis bioassays. However, the use even of relatively small
numbers of non-human primates in carcinogenesis testing has some advantage over
the use of rodents in such tests. For example, results of rodent carcinogenesis
testing are frequently obscured by the high incidence of tumors observed in con-

trol animals; in one rodent colony, this incidence was 26% for control mice and 46% for control rats[10]. In contrast, the tumor incidence in our control colony during the past 16 years has been about 2%. Moreover, monkeys are phylogenetically closer to man than are rodents, and certain of their metabolic pathways resemble those of humans more closely than do those of rodents[11]. This latter consideration is of particular importance in chemical carcinogenesis studies, where metabolic activation of a pre-carcinogen to its ultimate reactive species is frequently required. The relatively longer life span of monkeys makes it possible to administer test compounds at doses equivalent to estimated human exposure levels; it also provides a more reasonable estimate for the latent period for tumor development following exposure to potential carcinogens than is possible with rodents. Thus, although carcinogenesis testing in non-human primates is expensive, time-consuming, and frequently precludes the use of large groups of experimental animals, such tests may provide a more accurate estimate of the carcinogenic risk of a compound for human beings, and are a valuable supplement to the rodent carcinogen bioassay.

REFERENCES

1. Jukes, T.H. J. Am. Med. Assoc. 236: 1987-1989, 1976.

2. National Academy of Sciences, Sweeteners: Issues and Uncertainties.
    Washington, D.C.: National Academy of Sciences, 1975.

3. Office of Technology Assessment. Cancer Testing Technology and Saccharin.
    Washington, D.C.: Office of Technology Assessment, 1977.

4. Health Protection Branch, National Health and Swlfare Department, Canada.
    Toxicity and Carcinogenicity Study of Orthotoluenesulfonamide and Saccharin.
    Project E405/405E. Typescript, 1977.

5. Adamson, R.H. in Medical Primatology, 1972 (Proc. 3rd Conf. on Exp. Med.
    and Surg. in Primates, Part III), edited by Goldsmith, E.I. and Moor-
    Jankowski, J. pp 216-225, S. Karger, Basel, 1972.

6. Barkin, M., Comisarow, R.H., Taranger, L.A. et al. J. Urol. 118: 258-259,
    1977.

7. Cohen, B.L. Science 199: 983, 1978.

8. Batzinger, R.P., Ou, W.-Y.L. and Bueding, E. Science 198: 944-946, 1977.

9. Coulston, F., McChesney, E.W. and Goldberg, L. Fd. Cosmet. Toxicol. 13:
    297-300, 1975.

10. Weisburger, J.H., Griswold, D.P., Prejean, J.D. et al. Recent Results in
    Cancer Res. 52: 1-17, 1975.

11. Smith, R.L. and Caldwell, J. in Drug Metabolism - From Microbe to Man,
    edited by Parke, D.V. and Smith, R.L. pp 331-356, Taylor and Francis, Ltd.
    London, 1977.

Health and Sugar Substitutes
Proc. ERGOB Conf., Geneva 1978, pp. 272-276 (Karger, Basel 1978)

EVALUATION OF RESULTS OF ANIMAL DATA WITH RESPECT TO EXTRAPOLATION

R.Kroes

Central Institute for Nutrition and Food Research, P.O.Box 360,
Zeist, The Netherlands

INTRODUCTION

Since laboratory animal experiments are still the cornerstone in the
assessment of safety of compounds it is of extreme importance that results are
evaluated in the right way. Especially long term carcinogenicity experiments
offer a wide variety of possible results which need a more detailed
mechanistic consideration before a compound can be designated as a carcinogen
or as "safe". One of the best examples of the difficult problems involved in
the interpretation of results are the carcinogenicity studies carried out with
cyclamate and saccharin. It is the aim of this presentation to present some
possibilities to reach a better, more balanced judgement of results.

DEFINITION

If a carcinogen is defined as a compound which is able to induce
development of cancer, it must be emphasized that this definition is only
based on the biological result, and not on the actual mechanism of action.
This means that complete carcinogens (i.e. compounds acting on the genes of the
organisms, the so-called genotoxic compounds) as well as compounds acting
through a different (indirect) mechanism (e.g. hormones, immunosuppressants,
cocarcinogens, promotors) come within this definition. In the evaluation of
experimental results it is of great importance to determine whether a compound
is a complete carcinogen or an indirect acting agent. If a compound is
classified as a complete carcinogen, the extrapolation and risk assessment for
man should be based on the concept that the determination of a threshold, if
at all possible, is different from that for indirect acting agents for which
treshold can be established and therefore a no risk situation for man can be
defined.

INTERPRETATION OF RESULTS

In the following discussion, it is assumed that the results of experiments
in relation to evaluation and interpretation which will be discussed, are
derived from well designed studies carried out according to internationally
accepted guidelines. If experiments have been carried out under conditions
inappropriate for this type of study or when several basic standards in
protocol or conduct cannot be met, results of such experiments may at the most
be regarded as additional information, but can never be accepted as definite
evidence susceptible to risk-benefit analysis.

In the case of carcinogenicity studies the possible carcinogenic action of
a compound may appear from, among others, the following theoretical
possibilities:

a. one or more types of malignant tumors develop and the type of tumor is rare
   in the animal species used
b. normally occuring benign tumors are replaced by malignant tumors in the
   same organ or system
c. a shortening in latency period of malignant tumors
d. an increased incidence of one or more types of malignant tumors
e. an increased number of malignant tumors per animal
f. one or more types of benign tumors develop and the type of tumor is rare
   in the animal species used
g. an increased number of one or more types of benign tumors
h. a shortening in latency period of benign tumors
i. any type of combination of the possibilities mentioned above.

When one considers these results it seems reasonable to make some
distinctions in the interpretation of results. In the cases a and b the
indication that a compound giving such results is a complete carcinogen seems
quite strong, but even than more information will still be required to reach
a proper judgement. For example if in a given experiment thyroid carcinomas are
obtained, it is possible that these tumors did develop as a result of nodular
thyroid hyperplasia induced by a hormonal imbalance, rather than as the result
of a direct effect of the compound or its metabolites on the cells of the
organ.

Results as described under c - h, or combinations of these possibilities
(i), may be considered as a possible indication of carcinogenicity but never
as a definite proof of genotoxic action. In all these cases more information
is an absolute necessity, before a judgement can be made. Thus, evidence of
genotoxicity through various appropriate assays provides essential collateral

data.

The same can be said when results as described under a - i are obtained in an experiment where a combination of a known carcinogen and a compound is given to experimental animals and in which the dose of the known carcinogen was set at such a level that tumorformation could not be expected when the carcinogen was given alone. An example of such a type of experiments is the work of Hicks et al 1975 (1), with NMU and saccharin or of Cohen et al (2) with FANFT and saccharin or tryptophan.

When experiments have been carried out under extreme circumstances (i.e. unreasonable high doses, imbalanced diet, unphysiological temperature or environment) results may only indicate that the compound tested can be suspected for carcinogenicity.

Compounds tested locally (subcutaneously, intraperitoneally, by implantation or instillation) and leading to tumor formation at the site of application, should only be suspected for carcinogenicity, pending analysis of the system.

Though in the cases a and b as described earlier the evidence for genotoxic action seems likely, it is evident that in all the other cases mentioned above the compound tested can be regarded as either genotoxic of as an indirect acting agent. Since a definite conclusion can usually not be derived from the results, further investigation seems justified. It seems recommendable in such cases to carry out another long term experiment in another species, and to investigate the possible genotoxic action of the compound in short term assays such as mutagenicity tests, DNA repair tests or in vitro cell transformation tests, with and without metabolic activation. When in these short term tests no indications are obtained for genotoxic action it seems justified to conclude that the carcinogenicity of the compound can be attributed to a different mechanism of action such as - non specific or specific irritation

- hormonal imbalances

- cocarcinogenic or promoting action

- suppression or hyperstimulation of the
immunesystem

CLASSIFICATION

It is therefore suggested to introduce the following different classes of "carcinogens":

Class I: complete carcinogens and initiators, which act on the genes and have therefore an irreversible effect

II: compounds acting through a different known mechanism as compared to the mechanism stated under category I

III: compounds suspected for carcinogenic action. All compounds which bear suspicion for carcinogenicity on the basis of results of an animal experiment or of short term screening tests belong to this group. Further investigation is necessarry to determine whether the compound belongs in one of the preceding categories.

IV: compounds suspected for carcinogenic action which have been investigated extensively and for which on the basis of results a genotoxic action can be excluded, but for which on the same time a <u>known</u> different mechanism of action cannot be proven.

EXTRAPOLATION

Class I

As stated earlier it seems justified to assume that for genotoxic carcinogens (class I) a true threshold does not exist. Since the megamouse approach can not shed any more light on this problem, it must be assumed, and excellent papers have been published relative to this concept (3, 4), that on a theoretical basis the possibility exists that even one molecule may have (a very little, but still possible) chance to transform one cell in an organism. Thus, the lower the dose the lesser the chance. It is on this basis that it seems justified, if a risk benefit analysis for the use of a compound is at all necessary, to calculate the risk on the basis of a mathematical model which is based on the principle that the dose is directly proportional to the incidence of tumors at a given life time. This means that a certain "tolerable" tumor-incidence in man will be accepted as a risk, only when certain benefits from the use of a compound outweigh this risk.

Class II

Compounds in this class act through a different (indirect) mechanism. For these compounds it will be possible to establish a no effect level for the first step in the process of cancer causation. When the first step will not occur it is evident that following steps in the cancer causing process do not take place. Thus, for this class a threshold does exist. Compounds belonging to this class must be regarded and handled in the same way as other toxic compounds when an acceptable daily intake (ADI) for man is calculated.

Class III

Compounds belonging to this class should in principle never be considered for extrapolation. If due to whatever circumstances a compound must be considered for extrapolation such a compound should be considered as belonging to class I, untill a proper classification of such a compound can be made.

Class IV

As for class II, compounds belonging to this category do not act directly on the genes, but their different mechanism is not known, though extensive research on this matter has been carried out. It is suggested to consider these compounds in the same way as those belonging to class II, although it may be recommended to use a larger safety factor in the establishment of the acceptable daily intake for man.

CONCLUDING REMARKS

In this presentation it is recommended that a system of classification of carcinogens will be used which is based on their mode of action. The classification of the compounds determines the way of extrapolation in establishing a safe dose for man.

The concepts and thoughts put forward in this presentation have been developed in a Committee of Dutch scientists, asked to advise the Government how tho handle carcinogens and to give some general rules for extrapolation and risk assessment. As a member of this Committee I have the pleasure to introduce these thoughts to this audience, in the hope to get critical remarks, suggestions and valuable additions to this important problem.

REFERENCES

1.   Hicks, R.M., Wakefield, J.St.J. and Chowaniec, J.   Chem.Biol.Interactions 11: 225-233, 1975.

2.   Cohen, S.M.   Personal communication, 1978

3.   Crump, K.S., Hoel, D.G., Langley, C.H. and Peto, R.   Cancer Res. 36: 2973-2979, 1976.

4.   Emmelot, P and Scherer, E.   Cancer Res. 37: 1702-1708, 1977.

Health and Sugar Substitutes
Proc. ERGOB Conf., Geneva 1978, pp. 277-280 (Karger, Basel 1978)

REGULATORY ASPECTS OF THE USE OF SUGAR SUBSTITUTES IN DENMARK
AND NORWAY.

E. Poulsen

National Food Institute, Institute of Toxicology,
DK 2860 Søborg, Denmark

The attitude towards sugar substitutes in the two scandina-
vian countries, Denmark and Norway, is similar in certain
respects and different in others. In both countries the most
commonly used sugar substitutes - some of which are artificial
sweeteners - are legally considered as food additives.

In Norway (1), as in the other Nordic countries, the positive
list system for food additives is used.

The following sweeteners are allowed in food products:
saccharin, sorbitol and xylitol.

Saccharin can be used in the following products: fish-half-
preserves, 400 mg per kg; soft drinks and squash, 100 mg per kg;
carbondioxide-containing soft drinks, 50 mg per kg; chocolates
and sweets, 500 mg per kg and in special vitamin preparations,
120 mg per kg. At the moment (June 1978) there are no plans
for new regulations in this field, but it is possible that the
industry will propose to take saccharin out of fish-half-pre-
serves.

Sorbitol and xylitol are allowed in chewing gum and sweet
pastills.

In addition cyclamate is permitted in special commodities
for use of people with diabetes, as for example in soft
drinks, icecream, chocolates and as a powder for sweetening
purposes.

In Denmark the following sugar substitutes are permitted
as food additives (2):

Cyclamate (sodium and calcium salts), which can only be
sold in the form of tablets. These tablets can be purchased
in the shops normally selling foodstuffs. This legislation

was introduced after the ban on cyclamate in the USA. In the
report of the 21. session of the FAO/WHO Expert Committee on
Food Additives (3) cyclamate has been allocated a temporary
Acceptable Daily Intake of 4 mg per kg b.w.. This might lead
to a reevaluation of the permitted use, although a more widespread use as a food additive in Denmark does not seem likely.

Xylitol is permitted only for the use in chewing gum. The
presently available toxicological data are not considered
sufficient for extended use.

Mannitol and sorbitol can be used both as sugar substitutes
and as stabilizers due to their water retaining properties.
Both substances are included in the EEC directive (Council
Directive of 18 June 1974, on the approximation of the laws
of the Member States relating to emulsifiers, stabilizers,
thickeners and gelling agents for use in foodstuffs). In the
Danish positive list of food additives both mannitol and
sorbitol are classified as stabilizers for their use in
mayonnaise, marmelade and fine bakers wares and for sorbitol
also in icecream and sherbet. Due to their laxative properties a maximum allowed concentration of 50 g per kg foodstuff is fixed. The only exception is that in confectionary
the combined concentration of glycerol, mannitol and sorbitol
must not exceed 100 g per kg. Lower concentrations are permitted in fish roe (30 g per kg) and in soft drinks (0,5 g
per liter).

Sorbitol is permitted as a sweetener in amounts according
to good manufacturing practise in chewing gum and in lozenges.
It is further permitted in preparations for domestic use as
a sweeting agent (20 g per kg).

Saccharin - and its sodium and calcium salts - is permitted
both in the form of tablets, powder and solutions for domestic
use as well as in foodstuffs. The range of foodstuffs in
which it is permitted is wide and include all the groups of
foodstuffs outlined for sorbitol above. Saccharin is also
permitted in soft drinks. A survey of the use in 1977 based
on information from the industry has, however, indicated that
most of the use in foodstuffs (up to 90%) was in soft drinks
and soft drink concentrates, especially in the cheaper types

mainly consumed by children.

At its 21. session in 1977 the FAO/WHO Expert Committee on Food Additives (3) and later in 1977 the EEC Scientific Committee for Food (4) both recommended a lowered temporary ADI of 2.5 mg per kg b.w. of saccharin. The EEC committee further recommended special considerations in relation to saccharin intake in pregnant women and small children and clear labelling. In Denmark it was decided - from July 1978 - to lower the con- centration in soft drinks to 75 mg per liter. The permitted concentration in non-beverages was, for the time being - left unchanged at 400 mg per kg foodstuff. It was, however, stressed that new toxicological and epidemiological information might change the situation.

In Scandinavia the artificial sweeteners are legally food additives, not drugs as in some countries. In Norway cycla- mate can be used in foodstuffs especially manufactured for people with diabetes. This is not the case in Denmark, where a foodstuff must not be labelled e.g. "for diabetics". The use of the wording "sugar-free" will, however, be tolerated. It is not legal to sell a foodstuff as especially suited to people with a certain disease. It is the Danish view that the substitution of sugar with an artificial sweetener (e.g. saccha- rin) not necessarily in all respects make the foodstuff sui- table for a diabetic. It is felt that it is possible from the range of foodstuffs normally available on the Danish mar- ket to compose a diet suitable for a diabetic person (5).

Concerning labelling the use of an artificial sweetener shall be indicated by use of the term "artificial sweetener" on the label. If saccharin is added the word "saccharin" must be used.

REFERENCES

1. Dahle, H.K. Institute of Food Hygiene, The Veterinary University of Norway, Oslo, Pers. comm., June 1978.

2. List of Approved Food Additives (The Positive List) The National Food Institute, Søborg, Denmark, October 1977.

3. Evaluation of Certain Food Additives. (Twenty-first Report of the Joint FAO/WHO Expert Committee on Food Additives). WHO Technical Report Series No. 617, Geneva, 1978.

4. Reports of the Scientific Committee for Food. Fourth Series. Commission of the European Communities. Brussels 1977.

5. Funch, J. Tidsskr. f. Sukkersyge 36: 11-13, 1976.

Health and Sugar Substitutes
Proc. ERGOB Conf., Geneva 1978, pp. 281-287 (Karger, Basel 1978)

SCIENTIFIC BASIS FOR REGULATORY DECISIONS ON SACCHARIN

Morris F. Cranmer, Jr.

13924 Rivercrest Drive, Little Rock, Arkansas 72212

When the Food and Drug Administration proposed a ban on
saccharin as a food additive on the basis of recent animal and
human research that related its consumption to the development
of urinary bladder cancer, the intense public and scientific
response against the FDA proposal led Congress to initiate the
present 18-month moratorium and delay of the ban during which
time additional assessments of the research and deliberations
over the fate of saccharin have ensued.

FDA examined 12 human epidemiological studies of artificial
sweetener consumption and bladder cancer risk. Only one reported
that saccharin usage had significantly increased the risk for
bladder carcinoma and this investigation was criticized for
defects in methods and analyses by an accompanying editorial
and subsequent review by qualified scientists. The remaining
studies, as well as newly completed work, disclosed no association
between saccharin and malignancy. However, the FDA has concluded
that such epidemiological studies lack sensitivity for detection
of relatively weak carcinogens and "that at the present time,
there is neither enough evidence to accept nor to reject the
hypothesis that use of artificial sweeteners, specifically
saccharin, increases the risk of bladder cancer in humans."

The application of mutagenicity testing by FDA to evaluate
saccharin is based on the premise that most cancer-inducing agents
are mutagenic, that is, they alter the genetic material of cells.
However, mutagen tests have yielded conflicting results due, in
part, to variable contamination of many commercial preparations

of saccharin with mutagenic impurities. The Office of Technology
Assessment of the United States Congress commissioned several
reputable laboratories to perform additional studies on a
relatively pure form of saccharin. Results suggest that either
the majority of mutagenicity studies do not relate to the carcinogenicity of saccharin in the rat feeding experiment or that
factors other than saccharin contribute to the development of
malignancies in animals studied by the Canadian investigators.

Single generation animal feeding experiments utilizing rats,
mice, hamsters, and monkeys for periods of 24 months or more and
at doses of as much as 7.5% have failed to link saccharin ingestion
to urinary bladder cancer. A 5% dietary intake approximates
2500 mg/kg/day, which is roughly equivalent to 1000 soft drinks
containing saccharin daily.

The only positive animal cancer experiments were experiments
in which the second generation was exposed via the mother to
doses equivalent to a pregnant woman drinking 1500 soft drinks
a day, during suckling, and throughout remaining life to saccharin.
However, the number of animals involved was relatively small,
and no meaningful dose-response effect for cancer could be constructed, since effects of intakes less than 5% were not examined.
Secondly, conditions in two of the experiments would preclude a
fair evaluation of carcinogenic potential of saccharin according
to guidelines formulated by the National Cancer Institute.

Cigarette smoking is a definite etiologic factor in the
development of bladder cancer in humans. Although an association
between coffee drinking and bladder cancer has been observed,
this trend is not strong. In these same investigations, no trend
or association between the malignancy and saccharin could be
found. Thus, among three popular habits in the U.S., cigarette
smoking, coffee drinking, and the use of saccharin, the artificial
sweetener appears to constitute the lowest risk for the development of bladder cancer.

Since the quality of life of many individuals with diabetes
mellitus has benefited from the availability of saccharin, the

American Diabetes Association began a review of all relevant
scientific data in July 1977. The American Diabetes Association
concluded that much more research of broader scope and greater
detail is needed before the saccharin controversy can be resolved.
This opinion has been shared by the American Cancer Society and
other eminent groups. A comprehensive appraisal of the experimental data through May 1978 has been submitted to FDA by Morris
Cranmer and is available under Freedom of Information for
approximately $80.00.

Has the needed research been done or is it being done?

The Calorie Control Council independently launched an extensive program of research into the possible harmful effects of
saccharin and has subsequently expanded its program in response
to questions raised via several meetings conducted by the Toxicology Forum and is to be commended for its efforts.

The Congress added $1,000,000.00 to FDA's research budget for
relevant low dose animal studies. The NCTR was established to
conduct just such studies. Instead, FDA has decided to largely
commit these funds to epidemiological studies which has been
widely criticized as too complicated to prove successful. Research
is not yet underway by FDA at NCTR on the real problem, low doses.

The FDA epidemiological study hopes to gain some insight into
the possible relationship between saccharin and bladder cancer.
The Federal Drug Administration and National Cancer Institute
are undertaking the joint study comparing the lifestyles of
3,000 patients with bladder cancer diagnosed during 1978 and
6,000 matched controls from the same geographical regions.
Participants on the study will be drawn from New Jersey, Connecti-
cut, Iowa, New Mexico, Utah, and the metropolitan areas of Detroit,
San-Francisco-Oakland, New Orleans, and Atlanta. The study will
take 18 months, and although the findings will not be completed
before the congressional ban on saccharin expires, some preliminary results should be available by that time.

Are there medical benefits of saccharin other than calorie
reduction? The "hyperkinetic behavior syndrome" also known as

hyperkinesis or "minimal brain dysfunction"(MBD), has been
identified as one of the most common problems among school-aged
children in the United States. The major symptoms are an increase
of purposeless physical activity and a significantly impaired
span of focused attention, and poor powers of concentration.[1]
These children demonstrate diminished ability to experience
pleasure and frequent refractoriness to disciplinary measures of
any sort.[2]

There have also been observed relationships between the
occurrence of hyperactivity in children with regard to nutritional
status,[3] and an interest in the consumption of specific foods
and food additives.[4] Although there has been a great deal of
interest since the Feingold hypothesis, there has been no
conclusive evidence to show a strong cause and effect relationship between the ingestion of food coloring or other additives
and hyperkinesis.[5]

Metabolically induced hyperactivity has also been linked to
abnormal carbohydrate metabolism. A recent study by Langseth
and Dowd reported abnormal glucose tolerance test in 75 percent
of 265 hyperkinetic children. Four predominant types of abnormal
glucose tolerance curves were seen. The majority of these were
characterized by low flat curves 37 percent and 13 percent represented peaks and rapid declines. These are similar to some of
the findings noted in hypoglycemia and reactive hypoglycemia of
adults. Another 10 percent of the abnormal curves exhibited a
high initial peak and a slow recovery. These curves are similar
to those found in pre-diabetic children. These authors suggest
that since hypoglycemia is a potent stimulus for an increased
production of epinephrine, and the characteristic nervousness
or hyperkinetic behavior observed in these children is not unlike that seen in hypoglycemia, and many hyperkinetic children
may indeed be undiagnosed hypoglycemics. It seems reasonable
that some of the marked behavioral abnormalities found in hyperactive children could in many ways result from inadequate fuel
stores. It is known that a child is affected much more by short
periods of fasting than a adult. Even normal children are at a

much greater risk to hypoglycemia than adults. Although this
mechanism is not worked out, it is suggested that marked
increase in glucose utilization with diminished gluconeogenic
reserves is one of the contributory factors.

To date there have been no comprehensive studies on the food
habits and nutrient intake of hyperkinetic children. However,
two studies have suggested that there is a relationship between
sugar intake and the cause of hyperkinetic behavior in susceptible
children.[6,7] In the average American diet, 40-50% of the calories
come from carbohydrate, and it has been estimated that in
children over half of this carbohydrate is in the form of
sugar.[8] It is reasonable to hypothesize that hyperkinetic
children consume an even greater amount of sugar due to
their high consumption of the so-called "junk" food. If they
are sensitive to sugar because of abnormal carbohydrate
metabolism, this could explain why some responded to the
Feingold diet. The following is one example of how sugar intake could affect and perhaps make worse the behavior of hyperactive children. If these children are in a hypoglycemic state,
such as in the morning and for breakfast all they want is a bowl
of sugar-coated cereal, this will result in an immediate rise
in blood sugar which stimulates high levels of insulin and is
then followed by a rapid fall in blood glucose which results
again in hypoglycemic state. If the adrenergic system is working
properly the hypoglycemia should stimulate the production of
epinephrine and a rise in blood glucose may follow. If not, the
hypoglycemic state will persist which could account for some of
the behavioral problems seen in these children. Consumption of
sugar, especially before a meal, could have another adverse effect
on the child by suppressing the appetite, then the child will not
be hungry enough to eat a well balanced meal and the hypoglycemic
state will be worsened, along with his total state of nutrition
with respect to vitamin and mineral intake.

If the findings of Langseth et al[9] can be confirmed by more
comprehensive endocrine-metabolic studies, it is conceivable
indeed, that sugar and other low molecular carbohydrates may prove
to be a major contributory factor in today's number one para-

psychiatric childhood disorder. By the same token, reducing similar carbohydrates in these hyperactive children may be expected to have beneficial effects on hyperkinetic behavior. Most children would not permit all sugar products to be taken away from them and would probably react in a violent manner even worse than when in a hyperactive state. An alternative would be to substitute as much of the sugar products in the diet with a product that would not affect the insulin and glucose levels and at the same time produce a satisfying sweet taste. The non-nutritive sweeteners would be one possible substitute.

It would be of benefit for the sugar substitute not to cause a depression in appetite, since this was a contributing factor in the hypoglycemia if the sugar was taken before a meal. In the case of saccharin, this has been shown to be true. On the basis of the preceeding discussion it can be concluded that the use of non-nutritive sweeteners could be beneficial in the treatment of hyperkinetic children. Questions remaining to be answered include: (a) Do hyperkinetic children have abnormal glucose metabolism? (b) Do hyperkinetic children consume an excess of ingested calories in the form of simple sugar? (c) Would substituting non-nutritive sweeteners in the place of sugar result in a reduction in the hyperkinetic behavior of these children?

In conclusion, it seems to this observer that in the U.S. the FDA continues to pursue the doctrine of absolutes and has not been as responsive as possible to the wishes of the consumer or Congress. Millions of dollars of precious legislative and bureaucratic time has been squandered on trying to argue a solution to a scientific problem. In a real sense, most knowledgeable cancer researchers and epidemiologists consider saccharin vs FDA to be a bureaucratic game and a non-issue health hazard. The medical community is more concerned over the control of obesity, dental caries, diabetes and hyperkinesis. Perhaps the cruelest hoax of all is that the American people now speak of saccharin and cancer in the same breath, as cigarettes or asbestos and cancer. This delusion of relative importance dilutes concern and attention from the real causes of cancer and for this there can be no excuse.

REFERENCES

1. Laufer, M.W. and Denhoff, E. Hyperkinetic Behavior Syndrome
    in Children. J. Pediat. 50: 463, 1957.

2. Wender, P.H. Some Speculations Concerning a Possible Bio-
    chemical Basis of Minimal Brain Dysfunction. Ann. NY Acad.
    Sci. 205: 18, 1973.

3. Hoffman, M.S. The National Aspect of Learning Disabilities.
    Presented at the 7th Annual Convention of Texas Association
    for Children with Learning Disabilities, Dallas, Texas, 1971.

4. Feingold, B.F.J. Hyperkinesis and Learning Disabilities
    Linked to the Ingestion of Artificial Food Colors and Flavours.
    J. Learning Disabilities 9: 19, 1976.

5. Kolbye, A. First Report of the Preliminary Findings and
    Recommendations of the Interagency Collaborative Group on
    Hyperkinesis. Bureau of Foods, Food and Drug Administration,
    1976.

6. Crook, W.G. Learning Disabilities and Hyperactivity in
    Children Due to Foods. Presented at the International Food
    Allergy Symposium, Toronto, Canada, 1976.

7. Rapp, D.J. Double Blind Study in Relation to the Role of
    Foods and Dyes to Hyperactivity. Presented at the Internatio-
    nal Food Allergy Symposium, Toronto, Canada, 1976.

8. Stare, F.J. Sugar and Sugar Substitutes in Preventive
    Medicine and Nutrition. Nutri. Metabol. 18 (Suppl. 1):
    133, 1975.

9. Langseth, L. and Dowd, J. Glucose Tolerance and Hyperkinesis.
    Fd. Cosmet. Taxcol. 16: 129-133, 1977

VII. Summaries of Panel Discussions

SUMMARY AND DISCUSSION OF SESSION I: THE REASONS FOR SUBSTITUTING OR NOT
SUBSTITUTING SUGAR

K.G.M.M. Alberti and H. Keen

University of Newcastle upon Tyne and Guy's Hospital, London

The first session examined the role of sucrose as a nutrient and the
evidence that it contributes to disease states in man, and if it does whether
this justifies the use of alternative sweetening agents.

The moderator introduced the main speakers for the session by posing a
series of questions which it was hoped the subsequent presentations and
discussion around them would help to solve. He felt that it was important to
categorise the different ways in which sucrose might be harmful, so that one
could be rational in one's recommendations and at the same time balance the
gains of decreasing sucrose intake against the possible hazards of the
nutritive and non-nutritive substitutes. He also pointed out that any
nutrient taken in excess, from water to protein, from vitamins to sodium,
could be harmful.

The first question concerned the role of sucrose as a non-specific
calorie source. Simply as a seductive and readily available source of food
energy it could contribute to excessive calorie intake and so to obesity.
Much sucrose is consumed in coffee, tea, soft drinks and sweets. Did this
matter? Was it a cause of obesity?

The second question concerned the role of sucrose as a provider of glucose.
Could this do harm? Was it atherogenic or was it only in the diabetic where
one was trying to avoid swift surges in glucose in the peripheral circulation
that sucrose ingestion was to be avoided? The third question was whether
sucrose itself was specifically harmful. In certain situations, such as
sucrose deficiency, where sucrose could then act as an osmotic agent in the gut
there were obvious problems. Similarly sucrose was definitely implicated in
the development of dental caries, a point to be developed later by
Dr. Marthaler. Much more controversial, however, were the asserted
associations between sucrose intake and heart disease, and sucrose intake and
diabetes mellitus.

Drs. Campbell and Renold were to discuss the relationship between sucrose intake, and obesity and diabetes mellitus.

The panel and discussants also needed to consider whether substitution was desirable, and if it was thus considered, what the substitute should be. Dr. Moskowitz was to discuss the psychological and taste factors involved, while Dr. Clements would discuss the role of polyhydric alcohols in causing or preventing the development of neuropathy and/or vascular disease in diabetes.

Dr. G.D. Campbell opened the formal presentations. In presenting his information on Sucrose in Human Nutrition, he noted particularly the importance of the context in which high sugar intakes occurred. The African sugar cane cutters of Natal, for example, consumed 114 kg sugar yearly. Their daily food energy intake lay between 5,500 and 6,300 Calories but they "worked it off" without developing obesity or diabetes. The African worker could cut and carry as much as 9 tons of cane per day. He went on to discuss patterns of eating and diabetes prevalence in urban and rural Zulu people. Over 4% of the urban blacks were diabetic compared with 0.1% of the rural population, despite sometimes quite low calorie intakes in the former. Differing levels of physical activity in town and country life probably accounted for some of this diabetes gradient, but so also, in his view, did the use of refined and processed cereals by town dwellers compared with rough, home-ground cereals consumed by the peasantry. It appeared to take about 20 years of exposure to urban conditions before the excess diabetes incidence became fully established.

Dr. Campbell showed a figure comparing many human and animal groups which he felt supported his assertion that diabetes incidence rose with falling caloric intake. Nevertheless, among diabetes prone human groups in Natal, propaganda to restrict sugar intake coincided with an apparent fall in South African sugar consumption and he felt that this was evidence of the considerable impact that individual anti-sugar activity could have. One could not ignore the economic problem of the surplus production of sugar. He suggested that a fall in world sugar prices coincided with attacks on alternative sweeteners. However, alternative uses for sugar, perhaps as a fuel source for internal combustion engines, might solve the problem of surpluses.

He was followed by Dr. A.E. Renold who discussed the relationship between Obesity and Diabetes, emphasizing the importance of over-eating in the genesis of obesity and the diabetogenic effect of overweight in genetically predisposed persons. Sugar substitutes clearly had a place in the avoidance of obesity. Both the diabetic and the obese states arose from varied mechanisms (i.e. were heterogeneous) so their relationship was likely to be

complex. Vague had early pointed out that adipose tissue was an active
metabolic organ; and the distribution of adiposity into android and gynoid
patterns and the number as well as the size of fat cells were all among the
determinants of the metabolic outcome in the obese individual. The metabolic
effects of obesity were set against a strong genetic background, and genetic
factors had surprisingly turned out to be a major determinant for the appearance of non-insulin dependent diabetes in man. The strength of the
hereditary factor was especially noteworthy in insulin-independent diabetes
in the young (MODY). The interaction of nutritional factors in the environment
with the genome requires further explanation. There was no reason to suppose
that sucrose, or carbohydrate generally, was more adipogenic or diabetogenic
than other nutrients. Essentially adipogenesis depended on the balance
between food energy intake and total energy expenditure. The increased per
capita income in French Polynesia, for example, had led to an increase in total
calorie and sucrose intake with an associated explosive rise in frequency of
inappropriate hyperglycaemia. In one small island, however, where food intake
had also changed, the frequency of diabetes remained low - it was present in
only 3 of the 300 inhabitants aged 20 years or more living there. Unlike other
populations, this small island group still had much hard physical work to do.
They shared the 'Polynesian hyperuricaemia' with the main islands. He concluded
by admitting that he was unable to conceive any obvious mechanism which would
make sucrose a specially potent cause of diabetes, other than by promoting
weight gain.

In the discussion which followed these two papers, Dr. Campbell drew
attention to an important factor in promoting adiposity, diminished physical
activity. His students had made a careful observational study of the activity
of the obese, diabetes-prone Natal Indian population, and had demonstrated their
extraordinarily slow pace of physical movement. Dr. John Yudkin (London)
pointed out the limitations of the epidemiological approach to nutritional
factors and disease - so many factors were associated with each other that
there was always the danger of selecting spurious relationships and assuming
causality. Direct experimental studies of nutrition in man and animals
suggested that sucrose ingestion had specific effects, not mimicked by starches.
Sucrose administration initiated a series of changes, including deterioration
of glucose tolerance; increased circulating insulin; a rise in plasma
11-hydroxycorticosteroids and uric acid; insulin resistance; elevation of
plasma lipids; and, in rats, retinal and renal glomerular basement membrane
thickening, and increase in the glycosyltransferase enzyme responsible for
glycoprotein synthesis. All these together, he suggested, were an indictment

of the use of sugar. Questioned about the quantities of sugar used to provoke
these changes, Dr. Yudkin claimed that they fell within the range of 'normal'
sugar intake. Dr. Renold cautioned against the equating of some experimental
situations with the 'free-living' situation. Carbohydrate intake (though not
necessarily sucrose) was probably inversely related to diabetes rates as
Himsworth had noted 40 years ago. Ethnic variation in response to the same
stimulus was also important. While the Polynesian responded to a Western diet
with a rise in serum uric acid, the Pima Amerindian responded with a fall.

In answer to a question from Dr. Hildick-Smith of New Brunswick, U.S.A.,
Dr. Campbell stated that 6% of cane cutters had dental caries or peridontitis
compared with 99% of African gold miners, of whom 24% have false teeth. The
abrasive action of sugar cane chewing, the absence of sticky foods and the
frequent use of toothpastes were probably responsible. Dr. Muehlemann (Zurich)
asked whether the high water intake of the cane cutters might be the reason for
their clean mouths and further requested information about sugar eaten by
Marathon runners. Dr. Campbell replied that up to 7 litres of water were drunk
and noted that in cane cutters, rectal temperature might rise as high as 40°C.
They chewed 4-6 kg sugar cane daily. Marathon runners doing the 80 km from
Durban to Pietermaritzburg train on Coca Cola and consume up to 13 litres of
Coca Cola containing almost 1.8 kg of sucrose!

Dr. Keen (London) then commented that populations which ate more sucrose
were heavier on average than those that consumed less; this correlation did not
hold true within populations, at least within the inhabitants of the advanced
countries. Nor was there any obvious link within countries between sugar
consumption and a diabetic pattern of glucose tolerance. In the Whitehall
Survey in London there was, in fact, a low order (p = -0.07) but significantly
(p < 0.01) inverse correlation between blood sugar levels and total sugar consumption
assessed by three day dietary questionnaire in about 1500 randomly selected
male Civil Servants aged 40+. In the Israeli Civil Service Prospective Study
total calorie and added sugar intake at baseline showed no correlation with the
new appearance of diabetes among 10,000 men followed - in fact, in each age
group they had consumed slightly (but not significantly) less sugar than those
who remained non-diabetic. These findings could be explained by the unexpected
but highly significant inverse relationship between total food intake and
specifically sucrose consumption, and body mass index, a measure of adiposity,
a relationship which ran across the whole range of adiposity and of food intake
and which had been found by others. In reply to a question from Dr. Koenig
(Netherlands) about the apparently low sugar intake of the Israeli men, Dr.Keen
explained that this was added sugar consumption. Dr. Renold questioned the

role of physical exercise in maintaining low weight in the face of high energy
intake, especially in societies where economic factors and physical need played
little part in determining food intake. Dr. Keen agreed that it was important
but considered that variation in metabolic, rather than physical work done, was
a major determinant of energy flux. Dr. Renold mentioned experimental obesity
in animals and drew attention to the importance of the genetic background on
which the 'obesity' genes were superimposed. Obese animals ate more while
gaining excess weight, but less when it had been achieved.

   Dr. Campbell challenged Dr. Keen's assertion that sugar intake had nothing
to do with the genesis of diabetes, suggesting that 'indirect' sugar intake
(i.e. taken in foods) rather than 'added' sugar had not been considered, a
suggestion which Dr. Keen denied. Clearly, if everyone ate substantially less
sugar, or anything calorific for that matter, they would be less obese and
there would be less diabetes. Dr. Yudkin had questioned obese people after
successful weight loss and had been impressed by how much surreptitious extra
food they admitted to having taken while overweight. Such self-deception by
reducing the admitted food consumption, might have been responsible for Dr.
Keen's 'inverse relationship' between food intake and fatness. This was unlikely in Dr. Keen's view since his studies had been conducted not in patients
attending obesity clinics but in large normal population samples among which
very obese people were rare. Furthermore, the inverse relationship held across
the whole range of body weight, it was not just limited to 'obese' and
'normals'. Dr. Hugill (London) stated that sugar surpluses were nothing like
as massive as Dr. Campbell had suggested and denied any link between sugar
prices and anti-artificial sweetener campaigns. Alternative uses for sugar,
as a fuel for example, were being effectively developed and were likely to be
economically competitive.

   Following these controversial subjects Dr. H.R. Moskowitz of New York led
an interesting discussion on Psychological Correlates of Sugar Consumption.
Moskowitz started by emphasizing the characteristics of sweetness perception
and of acceptability. With sucrose perception increases linearly with
concentration while acceptability peaks at 9% (w/v) and then falls again.
With artificial sweeteners to achieve the same degree of acceptability a
higher degree of sweetness is required. Similar acceptability characteristics
can also be achieved with salt solutions (with a peak at 0.9% w/v). Dr.
Moskowitz also emphasised that although the human taste system cannot distinguish between the sweetness of sucrose and those of artificial sweeteners,
sucrose has effects on taste perception of other foods and this property is
not shared by the artificial sweeteners. He then went on to give evidence

that the inverted "U" curve of sweetness acceptability of normal subjects is
lost or shifted to the right in the obese meaning that acceptability is still
obtained for extremely sweet solutions which would be unpalatable to the nonobese. This is also found in the prepubertal. Acceptability can be modified
by abstinence or alternatively by over-exposure so that repeated exposure to
sucrose rich foods can act as a form of aversion therapy.

Dr. Neal (New Jersey, U.S.A.) asked if there were any clear explanations for
cultural differences in sweetness acceptability. Thus baclava and very sweet
coffee are widely accepted in Turkey but considered too sweet in many other
Western countries. Apparently, however, there are no good studies available of
these differences.

Dr. Baume (Geneva) then raised the question of the small group of people
who have an almost pathological craving for sweets. Was it possible that they
were conditioned in childhood?; but again there was little hard data forthcoming
in explanation.

The question was also raised as to whether there was a further fall off in
the sucrose concentration required for peak acceptability in the elderly
(Dr. Ericson, Umea, Sweden). Dr. Moskowitz replied that the elderly find foods
less sweet but there was almost certainly a multifactorial basis to this as the
elderly also suffer a loss in physical sensory perception. Finally Dr. Yudkin
pointed out that hedonics matched consumption in that peak sucrose intake
occurred in teenagers.

The discussion then moved on to the topic of polyhydric alcohols. Dr.
Clements began by reviewing the formation of sorbitol within cells and emphasised that although high plasma glucose levels induced increased intracellular
sorbitol formation, it was only in the lens that this had an osmotic effect.
Otherwise it was difficult to show pathological effects. He continued with a
review of myoinositol pointing out that persistent hyperglycaemia, as in
diabetes mellitus, caused a decrease in intracellular myoinositol concentration
and an increase in urine myoinositol excretion. Myoinositol is necessary for
nerve phospholipid formation and it has been suggested that a decrease in
neuronal myoinositol results in, or contributes to, the neuropathy found in
diabetes mellitus. He showed data showing that in the diabetic the distribution space of myoinositol was greatly decreased. It was also possible to show
experimentally that myoinositol feeding could improve the impaired nerve
condition velocity of diabetic animals, but interestingly the effect was much
greater on sensory than on motor nerves.

In the discussion, the moderator asked whether there was any relation at all
between sucrose, fructose and sorbitol feeding on the one hand and intra-

cellular sorbitol or myoinositol content on the other. Dr. Clements reported
that there was no relationship. Incubation of aorta pieces with different
concentrations of sorbitol and fructose caused no change in intracellular
polyol content. This was obviously important in relation to the choice of
dietary sugars. Professor Mehnert (Munich) then asked whether diabetic patients
with neuropathy given myoinositol showed any subjective improvement in neuropathy. Dr. Clements replied that some patients on both low and high myoinositol diets had shown symptomatic improvement! However, three patients on the
high diet had shown improvement of ankle jerks while four on the low diet
stopped the diet because of increase in neuropathic pain.

The final part of the session was led by Dr. Marthaler (Zurich) on the
epidemiological aspects of sugar and oral health. He began by pointing out
that the association between sucrose ingestion and dental caries was much
more clearcut than the associations discussed in the earlier parts of the
session. He also stressed the importance of population studies rather than
anecdotal reports. The association of sugar eating and caries was recognized
already in the 1930's, when it was found that subjects on "primitive" diets
had a much lower occurrence of caries. The bipartite relationship of sugar
and dental plaque was also emphasised. Removal of the plaque alone is not
enough to prevent caries. Much of the more recent evidence in studies of
children in particular was also reviewed. Striking epidemiological evidence
was presented: for example, sugar consumption in 20 year olds in Ethiopia is
extremely low and caries is almost unknown, while in Iceland sugar consumption
and the incidence of caries are both high. Dr. Marthaler then reviewed the
situation concerning fluoridation, showing the overwhelming weight of evidence
in favour of fluoridation in the prevention of caries. He finally emphasized
the need for oral hygiene although this is of little benefit when sucrose
intake is high.

Dr. Scheinin (Turku, Finland) opened the discussion with the comment that
Finland leads the juvenile caries league table presumably due to the high
consumption of hard candies. He also wondered (a) whether one could not
distinguish between glucose and sucrose plaques, and (b) whether intensive
oral hygiene programmes were helpful as one could not get into deep fissures -
perhaps intensive dietary counselling was of more use. Dr. Marthaler replied
first that caries starts at the entrance to the fissure, not in the depths;
and second that intensive fluoridation, dietary counselling and oral hygiene
taken in combination were needed. Dr. Newburn (San Francisco, USA) then
pointed out that Dr. Campbell's data on cane-cutters (6% caries compared with
98% in gold miners) was in sharp contradistinction with the published data

e.g. from Cuba. He felt that studies that did not employ trained dentists as observers were invalid. Dr. Campbell thought that his observers were well-trained and the differences could be explained by different living standards between Cuban and South African cane-cutters. Dr. Fejerskov (Aarhus, Denmark) stated that the Tanzanian cane-cutters also had a low incidence of caries but agreed strongly with Dr. Newburn regarding the need for trained observers. There was then a lively discussion on the fluoride intake of cane-cutters in different parts of the world, with Dr. Bowen (Bethesda, USA) making the important point that a high fluoride intake should not be regarded as a license for uncontrolled sugar consumption.

Dr. Keen then raised the twin points of (a) genetic influence on susceptibility to develop caries and (b) the nature of the organisers involved with the possibility of vaccination programmes. Little information was forthcoming on (a) but useful comments on (b) were made by Dr. Bowen (Bethesda, USA). He pointed out that Streptococcus mutans was strongly implicated in cross-sectional studies but that longitudinal studies at The London Hospital had now shown that Streptococcus mutans appeared only after the lesion had developed. Finally it was stated that Actinomyces may be implicated in root caries.

In summary, have the questions posed at the beginning been answered? There is general agreement that sucrose, if eaten in excess of normal daily requirements, must lead to obesity. The harm lies in the ease with which sucrose hyperphagia can be achieved due to the pleasant taste and the convenient foodstuffs available. It should also be emphasised that many people who apparently have excess sucrose intakes compensate unconsciously by decreasing intake of alternative caloric sources and maintain a stable body weight. Looking at the converse situation we also have the interesting information that people already established as obese have a lower sucrose, and total caloric intake, than nonobese individuals. The evidence on whether sucrose acted specifically to increase dental caries was clearcut but the possible associations between sucrose and diabetes must still remain controversial and, with respect to a causal relationship, unproven. Changes in tissue polyols were presented as a possible important component of the multifactoral aetiology of diabetic complications, but are probably unrelated to dietary polyol intake. It is possible that a high sucrose, and hence glucose, intake may cause changes in tissue polyhydric alcohol levels, but this remains to be proved. Finally we were presented with potentially exciting data relating to the perception of sweetness in children and in the obese, with the possibility of altering this psychotherapeutically, or in the long term, pharmacologically.

Many questions remain to be answered. Is sucrose consumption harmful to
tissues other than teeth if obesity is avoided? Is sucrose intake really
related to ischaemic heart disease? Does it matter if we produce nations of
the edentulous like the middle-aged Scotsmen of social classes four and five?
Can we educate people to moderate their input of sucrose and avoid alternatives?
Hopefully these questions will be answered in the future.

Health and Sugar Substitutes
Proc. ERGOB Conf., Geneva 1978, pp. 299-301 (Karger, Basel 1978)

SUMMARY AND DISCUSSION OF SESSION IIa: ABSORPTION, METABOLISM
AND SAFETY OF SUGAR SUBSTITUTES; NON-NUTRITIVE SWEETENERS

P. Shubik and G. Zbinden

Eppley Institute for Research in Cancer, University of Nebraska,
Medical Center, 3632 So. 102nd Street, Omaha, Nebraska 68105, USA
and
Institute for Toxicology, Federale Institute of Technology and
University of Zurich, Schorenstrasse 16, CH- 8603 Schwerzenbach

SUMMARY OF THE DISCUSSION

The session dealt essentially with the two most widely used
non-nutritive artificial sweeteners, cyclamate and saccharin.
Both compounds have been subjected to very extensive toxicological and metabolic investigations. This is explained by their
great socio-economic importance. In addition with both substances
some animal toxicity experiments have indicated the possibility
of an induction of bladder cancer.

CARCINOGENICITY OF CYCLAMATE

Extensive recent work failed to confirm an earlier study which
suggested that the sweetener might induce bladder cancer in rats.
This issue was, therefore, not further persued.

CARCINOGENICITY OF SACCHARIN

There was general agreement among the panel members and various
discussants that saccharin is not a classical genotoxic carcinogen. Experimential evidence shows that the compound is not metabolized, does not bind covalenty to DNA and is not mutagenic in
most in vitro and in vivo test systems.

The possibility that the bladder tumors reported induced with
saccharin could be said to have resulted from a secondary
"promoting" or "cocarcinogenic" effect was discussed in depth.
3 of the papers dealt with the problem experimentally. Dr.
Jacobs reported that saccharin gave rise to enhanced bladder
carcinogenesis in rats pretreated with the carcinogen FANFT.

Tryptophan had a similar effect. In contrast Schmähl reported that no tumor enhancement occurred when saccharin followed pretreatment with BBW. Lastly Althoff reported an inability to reproduce the study of Hick's in which intravesical instillation of the carcinogen NMU was followed by oral administration of high doses of saccharin or cyclamte.

These findings were discussed in depth, and it was generally concluded that they were of considerable interest - particularly those reported by Dr. Jacobs. However, it was felt particularly important to establish the specificity of these effects and to learn something of the dose requirements.

It was noted that results so far reported cannot be equated with "promoting" effects previously reported in mouse skin since the effects decreased if the interval between the two treatments is increased. It was deemed premature to label these observations with a specific term or to extrapolate these results to man. These findings, once again, emphasize that saccharin is not a classic carcinogen.

In this respect several questions related to the problem of microcrystalluria and bladder stone formation as a causative factor in the development of bladder tumors were asked. O-toluene sulfonamide, a common impurity in saccharin, is a carbonic-anhydrase inhibitor and leads to an alkalinization of the urine. However, in the Canadian toxicity study there was no correlation between bladder stone formation and bladder tumor incidence. There was also no evidence that the saccharin treatment might have induced an inflammation of the bladder mucosa.

The findings of Dr. Renwick that with high dietary levels of saccharin (5% and more) the pharmacokinetic behavior of the compounds is drastically changed, received great attention. It was pointed out that most studies in which a possible promotor effect of saccharin was investigated, were done only with one high dose. It is essential, however, that such experiments also include groups of animals treated with lower doses that do not lead to excessive accumulation of saccharin in the tissues. Moreover, the use of several dose levels will permit the establishment of a dose-effect relationship which is essential for a rational evaluation of a carcinogenic or a co-carcinogenic effect.

A discussant also pointed out that administration of large doses of saccharin leads to saturation of tubular secretions in the kidney. As a consequence, a competition with other substances being secreted by the tubules develops. This leads to significant metabolic alterations. Thus, the comparison of saccharin-treated animals with untreated animals (whose tubular secretion is unimpaired) is not justified, since the two populations differ not only with regard to saccharin treatment but are wastly different in their metabolism of a number of endogenous substances.

The paper of Stoltz reported the presence of a mutagenic impurity in saccharin. It was pointed out that this could still account for effects seen particularly if saccharin had a secondary modifying effect. It was observed that the quantitiy of impurity present would necessitate a potent agent that would at the least have to be one third as potent as aflatoxin.

In discussing Dr. Kessler's epidemiological findings which were essentially negative, the question was asked, how the author explained the positive findings of a recent Canadian study. Dr. Kessler pointed out that his study was done before the recent publicity about the danger of artificial sweeteners started. He feels that in the present situation of public concern a reliable epidemiological evaluation is not possible any more. He furthermore indicated that all his findings were consistent with each other, while the Canadian data contain several inconsistencies that are difficult to explain (e.g. saccharin appears to increase bladder cancer risk in males but decreases it in females, saccharin taken in tablet form increases risk, saccharin in food does not). Therefore, Dr. Kessler has greater confidence in his own findings.

Health and Sugar Substitutes
Proc. ERGOB Conf., Geneva 1978, pp. 302-320 (Karger, Basel 1978)

SUMMARY AND DISCUSSION OF SESSION II b: ABSORPTION, METABOLISM
AND SAFETY OF SUGAR SUBSTITUTES; NUTRITIVE SWEETENERS

H. Mehnert, Munich, and E. R. Froesch, Zurich

Forschungsgruppe Diabetes und Krankenhaus München-Schwabing,
Kölner Platz 1, 8000 München 40, Bundesrepublik Deutschland
and
Dept. für Innere Medizin, Klinik Universitätsspital, Stoffwechsel-
labor, Rämistrasse 100, 8091 Zürich, Schweiz

Since restriction of glucose and sucrose from different diets
should be recommended, nutritive sweeteners such as fructose,
sorbitol and xylitol are particularly left for consideration.
Additionally, some newer products like Palatinit and hydrogenated starch hydrolysates are also of interest. All these
substances have been involved both in the contributions given
by the speakers and in the discussions from the panel and the
auditorium, as well. Of course, it was not possible to give
complete answers for all questions of "Absorption, Metabolism
and Safety of Nutritive Sweeteners". One could only touch a few
important and sometimes controversial points hoping to stimulate
further discussions during this meeting and elsewhere.

The first two papers by van den Berghe and Jakob could be
discussed together since the experimental approach used by both
was similar. Van den Berghe and Jakob discussed mainly the
acute metabolic fate and the effects of fructose,sorbitol and
xylitol in the perfused rat liver or during rapid intravenous
infusion in man. Their interesting contributions do not allow,
of course, to decide the problem of orally applicated nutritive
sweeteners in man. They even cannot answer the question which
kind of parenteral nutrition with carbohydrates is preferable.
However, results gained under extreme conditions are helpful in
trying to predict possibilities and limits, indications and
contraindications of any kind of therapy.

At first, Bässler gave his comment from the floor: "I am trying
to relate Dr. Jacob's liver perfusion system to oral biology.
You have used in your system a xylitol concentration of 10 mM.
Since we know very well the pharmacokinetic data of xylitol for
man, we can easily calculate how much we have to infuse intravenously in order to reach a plasma level of 10 mM: It is a
little above 1 g/kg/h. We know further that this rate is far
above the maximal turnover rate of the human body for xylitol,
which is somewhere between 0,3 and 0,4 g/kg/h. The well
established and recommended upper limit for safe intravenous
xylitol application is 0,25 g/kg/h, e. g. less than a quarter
of your dose. Let us go one step further and consider the oral
use of xylitol. Here the rate of absorption from the gut is the
limiting step. It can be estimated to about 0,1 g/kg/h. So,
between your system and the situation in practical dietary use
there is a factor of at least 10. That means, you have performed
pharmacological experiments. By no means I want to deny the
importance of these experiments, because they indicate critical
points that have to be observed during practical use. With this
in mind I can answer your questions regarding human physiology
and pathophysiology as far as dietary use of xylitol is concerned:
There is a slow and sustained glucose production from xylitol
which can be of benefit for dietary treatment of certain
diabetics; there is no accumulation of lactic acid; there is no
depletion of adenine nucleotides; because the absorption is so
slow, there is diarrhoea if you take too large single doses and
this effect makes it impossible to cause metabolic effects of
the kind observed in experiments with liver perfusion."

Another statement was given by Froesch involving problems of
parenteral nutrition: "The need for glucose substitutes for i.v.
feeding originated from the clinicians' and biochemists wish
to be able to administer carbohydrates to diabetics without
making it difficult to control blood sugar with extra insulin.
Fructose, sorbitol and xylitol are almost quantitatively taken
up and phosphorylated by the liver and they reach the hepatic

glycogenolytic pathway independently of insulin. Thus, the first
steps in their metabolism are, indeed, insulin-independent. Moreover, the activity of the enzymes which are responsible for
fructose (fructokinase and hepatic aldolase), sorbitol and
xylitol (L-iditol dehydrogenase) metabolism are insulin-independent in contrast to glucokinase which is induced by insulin and
the activity of which is markedly decreased in the insulin-
deficient diabetic. In contrast, fructokinase, fructose-1-
phosphate aldolase, aldosereductase, sorbitoldehydrogenase and
xylulosekinase which are responsible for the first steps of
fructose, sorbitol and xylitol metabolism are entirely insulin-
independent. In this way, the removal of fructose, sorbitol and
xylitol from blood and their funneling into the glycolytic
pathway is guaranted independently of insulin. There is a further
characteristic for all these substrates which contrasts again
with the properties of glucose. Glucose metabolism in the liver
is not primarily controlled by the rate of phosphorylation of
glucose but much more so by the activity of phosphofructokinase
i. e. by the enzymatic step by which fructose-1,6-phosphate is
phosphorylated to fructose-1,6-diphosphate. This enzyme is inhibited by high concentrations of citrate and ATP, that is to
say when alternate substrates such as free fatty acids or ketone
bodies are oxydized by the liver. Whenever citrate and ATP levels
increase, glucose metabolism is inhibited at the step of the
conversion of fructose-6-phosphate to fructose-1,6-diphosphate.
Under such conditions, glucose is primarily diverted to glycogen
synthesis and will be stored in the liver in the form of
glycogen. If, on the one hand, phosphofructokinase is blocked
and, on the other hand, the endocrine and metabolic setting
does not favour glycogen synthesis, glucose-6-phosphate is
simply dephosphorylated and again released as glucose by the
liver. In this respect, the metabolism of fructose, sorbitol
and xylitol is entirely different. Since the enzymes which
funnel these substrates into glycolysis are not under any endocrine control, since they do not depend on concomittant oxidative
processes in the liver cells and since phosphorylation of all of
these substrates is not reversible as in the case of glucose,

these substrates are phosphorylated and must be converted subsequently to something else. There are several possible metabolic fates: they can be released from the liver as glucose or converted to glycogen if the endocrine setting favours glycogen synthesis. They can also be released as lactate and pyruvate or else they can be converted to triglycerides and released into the blood in the form of very low density lipoproteins. There are some rare metabolic disorders in which the administration of fructose or either one of the glucose substitute polyalcohols leads to acute lactic acidosis. The two most prominent examples are glycogenosis type I and fructose-1,6-diphosphatase deficiency. In these two disorders gluconeogenetic substrates can not be converted to glucose, and in the case of fructose-1,6-diphosphatase deficiency they can not go further than fructose-1,6-diphosphate. In such patients an acute intravenous load of fructose, sorbitol or xylitol leads to a rapid increase in the lactate levels in plasma and to severe and sometimes lethal lactic acidosis. Now, it is perfectly clear that we can not extrapolate from these rare metabolic disorders to patients in need of parenteral nutrition. However, we do recognize that there are potential dangers in the administration of large amounts of fructose, sorbitol and xylitol by the intravenous route. Particularly, in severely ill patients with tissue hypoxia, polytraumatism, severe burning, renal and/or hepatic failure the chances are that these substrates are rapidly converted to lactic acid and that lactic acidosis can result. The same holds true for diabetic ketoacidotic coma where ketotic acidosis may be succeeded by lactic acidosis if fructose, xylitol or sorbitol are administered in early therapeutic stages.

It is said, that the administration of these glucose substitute sugars leads to a positive nitrogen balance whereas the same goal can be achieved with glucose only if insulin is administered concomittantly. This may, indeed, be so in insulin-deficient states. However, we should recognize that any catabolic situation can be managed with glucose and insulin alone if the latter is given in sufficient quantities. In most intensive care units allover the

world the routine procedure of treating polytraumatized catabolic
patients consists of the infusion of glucose, amino acids, fat
emulsions and insulin, if needed. If glucose is substituted by
xylitol, fructose or sorbitol less insulin may be needed because
the conversion of the substrates to glucose is relatively slow.
However, one runs the unpredictable and unforseeable risk of
lactic acidosis, a complication that is never encountered if one
uses glucose and insulin. Furthermore, insulin is the major anabolic hormone which almost all tissues need to overcome a catabolic situation and to reach an anabolic state. In contrast, sorbitol, fructose and xylitol as such can not be utilized by any
tissue except the liver with or without insulin.

The rapid infusion of fructose and, to a lesser extent, also of
xylitol leads to a transient depletion of liver ATP. The rate-
limiting enzyme of uric acid production in the liver is AMP-
deaminase which is inhibited normally by physiological concentrations of inorganic phosphorus and GTP. The dramatic fall of
inorganic phosphorus following i.v. fructose, sorbitol or xylitol
administration due to rephosphorylation of ADP to ATP in the
mitochondria results in a release of the inhibition of AMP deaminase and finally in an increased production of uric acid. So far
we have delt with the acute effects of fructose, sorbitol and
xylitol on liver metabolism and its dangers."

Van den Berghe also made a strong point that the i.v. use of fructose should be forbidden for two reasons: 1) several cases of
lethal lactic acidosis have been reported in severely ill patients
and 2) several patients with known or unknown hereditary fructose
intolerance died after surgery because of parenteral nutrition
with fructose.

Förster interpreted the adverse effects of glucose substitutes in
another way: "The results shown by Dr. van den Berghe and by Dr.

Jacob do not constitute conclusive evidence for the existence of
real side effects of sugar substitutes in man. These in vitro results of xylitol in perfused rat liver and of the parenteral
application of fructose in mice cannot be extrapolated to the
situation caused by the oral administeration of sugar substitutes
in man. Furthermore, a correlation between physiological effects
and the pathophysiological significance of the so-called side
effects of these substances administered intravenously in high
doses for experimental purposes have not been established until
now.

The increase in uric acid production due to the rapid intravenous
administration of the glucose substitutes shown first by us in
collaboration with Mehnert (Klin. Wschr. 45, 436, 1967 and Klin.
Wschr. 48, 878, 1970) is the unique metabolic effect not shown
by glucose. Following the high dosed rapid intravenous infusion
of the respective substances to human volunteers, an increase in
serum uric acid concentration amounting to 1.5 - 2.0 mg/100 ml
is repeatedly found. However, the long term intravenous infusion
of these glucose substitutes in higher doses (up to 124 g/kg bw.
per 48 hours) causes merely a small increase in serum uric acid
excretion, too. Until now the induction of a gouty attack caused
by sugar substitutes has never been demonstrated. The effect
caused by the oral administration of the sugar substitutes is
negligible as it has been shown by us (Z. Ernährungsw. 10, 394,
1971). This connection of carbohydrate metabolism with purine metabolism seems to me to be a curious biochemical effect without
any pathophysiological significance.

Lactic acid acidosis is often said to be caused by the high dosed
infusion of sugar substitutes, especially in addition with ethanol.
However, the few cases published until now are often very poorly
documented and therefore are inconclusive and, additionally, it
is not clear if the same effects were not also caused by glucose.
Following the high dose intravenous infusion of glucose or

glucose substitutes in volunteers there is a small increase in
lactic acid concentration. Fructose is most effective, sorbitol
and glucose show equal effects and xylitol is without any effect.
These small increases in lactic acid concentration in the range
of 1 mmol/l should be called lactic acidemia but not lactic acid
acidosis. Furthermore, the terminus technicus lactic acid acidosis has to be defined more clearly. The single report of a
so-called lactic acidosis caused by xylitol is based on the
increase in lactate of 1 to 1.5 mmol/l during eight hours high
dosed application (Thomas et al., Med. J. Australia 1, 1242,
1972). The few case reports on lactic acid acidosis following
fructose administration were accompanied by a lactate concentration of 6 - 10 mmol/l; this is the border range for the lactic
acidosis accepted by most authors. Until now not a single case of
increase in lactate concentration following sorbitol was reported.
However, glucose was shown in several cases to cause a worsening
of a real lactic acid acidosis. Therefore it is concluded that
lactic acid acidosis is only found following high dosed intravenous infusions when a contraindication (i. e. the preexisting
tendency to lactic acid acidosis) exists for glucose administration. The danger of lactic acid production is, however, without
any importance during the oral administration of glucose or of
sugar substitutes because of the very small quantities of the
substances used.

The increase in uric acid production was thought to be due to an
alteration in the concentrations of ATP and of adenine nucleotides in the liver caused by the administration of the glucose substitutes. However, this effect was until now exclusively found
following a short term high dosed fructose application. The reported effects of sorbitol and xylitol (one paper each) are not
completely reproducible in animal experiments. Furthermore,
following the long term high dosed intravenous fructose administration a normalization of the concentrations of ATP and of
adenine nucleotides in the liver was found by several authors
within a short time. The early effects of fructose not shared by

xylitol and sorbitol (and also not by glucose) are due to the extremely high capacity of the liver for the phosphorylation of
fructose. Therefore, the temporary alteration of the steady state
of the respective nucleotides in the liver is normalized within
a short time. As a decrease in the adenine nucleotides is not
found following the administration of sorbitol and xylitol, this
cannot be the single effect of the glucose substitutes evoked on
purine metabolism. It seems to be generally accepted now that
there is an additional effect on de novo synthesis of purines
caused by an increased concentration of ribosephosphate.

The increase in triglyceride production is the next side effect
connected often exclusively with the application of the glucose
substitutes. The high dosed intravenous infusions of glucose and
of the glucose substitutes fructose, sorbitol and xylitol in
human volunteers during 48 h cause an increase in serum triglyceride concentration of a comparable order of magnitude. The
differences are merely in the time of the appearance of the increased triglycerides. The effect is seen first during the administration of the polyols xylitol and sorbitol, the sugars
fructose and glucose being effective merely at the end of the
experimental period. Therefore, the increase in triglyceride
concentration seems to be at least a mere quantitative problem
and not a qualitative one. Triglyceride synthesis in the liver
is caused also by glucose. The high dosed infusion of glucose,
lasting for 72 h, leads to a severe fatty liver in the experimental animal. The triglyceride concentration of 100 mg/1 g fresh
weight (i. e. 10 ml/100 g) is indicative for an increase of triglycerides in the liver by a factor of 10 - 50 as compared to the
normal concentration of triglycerides. The glucose substitutes
without doubt also lead to fatty liver in equal doses. Therefore,
the results of studies using high dosed infusions with volunteers
and with the experimental animal show that an increase in hepatic
triglyceride production and in the induction of fatty liver is
not restricted to the high dosed sugar substitutes, it is characteristic for the high dosed intravenous glucose administration,
too.

In our further investigation we have performed intravenous infusions in volunteers of fructose, xylitol and sorbitol in a dose of 0.25 gm/kg/bw per hour for 48 hours (Dtsch. med. Wschr. 99, 1300, 1974). The volunteers therefore received 800 - 900 g of the sugar substitutes within 48 hours. Additionally, a double dose of fructose was infused in volunteers (i. e. 800 gm/day). In polytraumatized patients we performed also the continous intravenous infusion of fructose or sorbitol in a dose of 0.5 gm/kg bodyweight per hour (i. e. 700 - 850 g/day) for weeks. In one case we can document a time of 10 weeks, during this time the patient received 800 gm of fructose per day by the intravenous route. In none of the cases with 700 - 800 gm of fructose or sorbitol per day we have discontinued the infusions because of the existence of so-called side effects (Infusionstherapie 3, 228, 1976).

In polytraumatized patients glucose causes hyperglycemia, and, therefore, it is not suited for parenteral application. The glucose substitutes (fructose, sorbitol, xylitol) are tolerated without insulin by these patients, despite of a high dosage. There are clear cut advantages of the glucose substitutes in respect to glucose in these patients.

If these results are taken into consideration (i. e. intravenous application of 800 gm of fructose or sorbitol in severely ill patients and in volunteers), it is impossible to imagine that a few grams of sugar substitutes taken by the oral route would cause serious side effects. Furthermore, the uncomplicated intravenous application of fructose and sorbitol as well as of xylitol (400 - 800 gm per day) is documented. Reports concerning serious side effects of these substances (i. e. lactic acidosis, hyperuricemia, hepatic failure) are often cited, however, these cases are not published. Therefore, it is questionable, if they exist."

Mehnert: "Regarding the still very controversial questions of

parenteral nutrition I like to make a few concluding remarks since
afterwards we should spend our time in discussing the problems of
oral application of nutritive sugar substitutes, definitively. In
my opinion advantages and disadvantages of fructose, sorbitol and
xylitol given intravenously depend on the correct dosage, e. g.
the application of reasonable amounts in an appropriate manner.
Therefore, Froesch, van den Berghe and Jacob gave very interesting
contributions in order to avoid dangerous complications due to an
overdosage of fructose, sorbitol and xylitol. However, in many
catabolic (and particularly polytraumatized) patients any kind of
parenteral nutrition may be harmful in a hypoxic state of peripheral tissues, at least. Should we expect that infusions of
mainly peripherally utilized glucose are less dangerous than the
application of substances predominantly metabolized by the liver?
Where are well-documented cases of lactic acidosis due to fructose, sorbitol or xylitol given in reasonable amounts with the
right indication? Are the potential dangers of insulin in the
wrong hands - additionally given to glucose - less important than
the possibility that the extremely rare cases with hereditary
fructose intolerance will be undiagnosed treated with fructose or
sorbitol? Obviously, we cannot solve the problems of parenterally
infused sugars and polyols, today. However, the first part of the
discussion gave us some help for the following part, at least.
Actually, we now should discuss the oral application of the sugar
substitutes."

Froesch pointed out that the acute and chronic oral ingestion of
sucrose substitutes is an entirely different matter: "The question
whether or not sucrose may have causally anything to do with obesity was delt within the first session of this meeting. It is a
fact that people of many ethnic groups living a hard life for a
minimum of food were slim. In these populations there was no
diabetes, no obesity and no hyperlipidemia. Sucrose usually
became available together with improved overall nutrition. It is,
therefore, extremely difficult to assess the special role of the
fructose moiety in sucrose with regard to diabetes, obesity and

hyperlipidemia. The data in the literature related to the problem
whether fructose is particularly harmful with regard to hypertriglyceridemia are very controversial. The experimental data depend
on which animal model was used. Also in men it is not at all clear
whether sucrose as such has any clear cut effect on triglyceride
levels in long term studies provided that the comparative diets
were isocaloric. However, there can be no doubt, that obesity,
diabetes and hyperlipidemia are particularly frequent in those
populations which were rapidly transferred from their natural
environment into the western civilization including among all the
goodies sucrose. Whether or not sucrose has any special effect on
eating habits or on triglyceride concentrations has not become
clearer during this meeting, unfortunately!"

Mäkinen pleaded for the use of xylitol instead of sucrose. The
main advantage of substitution of sucrose by xylitol obviously
is its failure to promote caries. Furthermore, Mäkinen showed
convincingly that the use of up to 100 g of xylitol by normal
volunteers over a period of 6 years did not result in any detectable toxicity or metabolic abnormalities. These normal subjects
tolerated xylitol perfectly well and all biochemical tests performed on them yielded normal results. Whether or not this long
term study will ever have practical implications is not certain
because of the prize development in this technological field. It
appears that the production of xylitol remains much more expensive than that of sucrose. Its use as a sweetener in bakery,
chocolate etc. appears to be prohibitive for economic reasons
whereas its use in the fabrication of chewing gum, candy and
lollipops etc. may be very valuable for the prevention of caries.
It appears now that the use of xylitol will be limited mostly to
the production of chewing gum, candies and lollipops.

The further discussion was also colourful and interesting. Jacob
fully agreed with Bässlers comments cited above and made it again
clear that his liver perfusion experiments were an experimental

tool to demonstrate the metabolic effect of large concentrations
of xylitol on the liver. The reducing power of 200 g of xylitol
is about equal to that of 30 g of ethanol. That is to say that
the reduction of the cytosolic NADH/NAD ratio is about the same
when 200 g xylitol or 30 g of ethanol are metabolized. The
question then is whether 30 g of ethanol per day are safe. Since
it is impossible to absorb 200 g of xylitol per day from the gut
it would appear that from this point of view, the use of xylitol
in an amount of 50 to 100 g per day should be safe.

Van den Berghe raised the point that xylitol should be expected
to increase hepatic alpha-glycero-phosphate concentrations and,
therefore, that it should increase triglyceride formation in the
liver and the secretion of very low density lipoproteins.

The moderators countered that the absorbable amount of xylitol is
not above 100 g so that the overall xylitol absorption cannot
possibly raise the level of triglycerides to any great extent.
Furthermore, in the moderators' opinion oral application of fructose may increase triglyceride levels only in rare cases when there
is a genetic defect of triglyceride metabolism, e. g. possibly in
type IV hypertriglyceridemia. However, one has to mention new
work both from Bierman and coworkers and Schlierf who have shown
that in familial hypertriglyceridemia, formerly believed to be
carbohydrate-induced, triglyceride levels are in fact not higher
on a high than on a low carbohydrate diet. This disease should
no longer be called carbohydrate induced hypertriglyceridemia but
rather calorically induced hypertriglyceridemia. In normal persons
and in most diabetics fructose does not increase triglyceride concentrations, at all. In the same way Mäkinen did not find a clear
cut relationship between xylitol feeding and hypertriglyceridemia.
Since xylitol is not absorbed in large amounts by the gut it does
not lead to hypertriglyceridemia.

This questionable effect of fructose was also commented by Bässler:

"With regard to the question of hypertriglyceridemia after fructose a study of Dr. Bierman's group in Seattle is of considerable interest (J. L. Turner, E. L. Bierman, J. D. Brunzell, A. Chait: Effect of dietary fructose on triglyceride transport and glucoregulatory hormones in hypertriglyceridemia in man. Am. J. Clin. Nutr. 1978, in press). The authors used patients with pre-existing hypertriglyceridemia because it seems reasonable to assume that subtile alterations in triglyceride metabolism attributable to fructose would be magnified in amplitude in patients with elevated plasma triglyceride levels. The persons have been subjected to four dietary periods of at least 2 weeks. In two of the periods, the isocaloric formula diet contained 45 % of calories as carbohydrate, 40 % as fat, and 15 % as protein. For the other two periods, the formula contained no fat, 85 % of calories as carbohydrate, and 15 % as protein. During one of the periods with the fat-containing diet and one with the fat-free diet, substitution was made with fructose for 20 % of the carbohydrate calories, that was 33 - 46 g fructose with the 45 % carbohydrate diet and 90 -154 g fructose with the 85 % carbohydrate diet. Neither in the fat-free nor in the fat-containing diet fructose caused any elevation of plasma triglyceride levels. - Considering long-term effects of fructose it should be referred to the Turku-studies. There was no change of plasma triglycerides over a period of two years at a mean daily intake of 70 g of fructose. There was also no difference between the sucrose and fructose group, although the individuals of the fructose group received twice as much fructose as those in the sucrose group."

Pirard mentioned that in Belgium sorbitol was prohibited for oral use because of Gabbay's data according to which intracellularly formed sorbitol is causally related with microangiopathy and, furthermore, because sorbitol leads to hypertriglyceridemia. This is obviously a most unfortunate misunderstanding of valid scientific data by government agencies which cannot distinguish between the fate of orally or intravenously administered sorbitol and the effects of hyperglycemia which leads to the intracellular formation of sorbitol which than may have undesirable effects on small

and large vessels. Van den Berghe told the audience that Belgian
scientists have taken steps to reverse that ruling regarding the
use of sorbitol in food stuffs.

Schlatter cautioned that xylitol should be available in food only
under strictly limited and controlled conditions. Adverse effects
of xylitol on the adrenal glands and the bladder have been reported. Admittedly, 20 % of the total caloric intake in these instances was in the form of xylitol, an extremely high percentage
which cannot be reached in nutrition for men. According to Mäkinen the dose of xylitol administered in these animal studies is
equivalent to 600 g per person per day, a huge dose.

Förster emphasized that following the oral administration of the
sugar substitutes merely one side effect has to be considered:
"This side effect is the laxative effect of the sugar substitutes
and especially of the polyols. The so-called diabetic diarrhoea
is often caused by the uncontrolled dietetic use of sorbitol as a
sugar substitute . In healthy volunteers diarrhoea is caused by
a single dose of 15 - 25 gm of sorbitol, by 20 - 35 gm of xylitol
or by 80 - 120 gm of fructose. On the other hand it is impossible
to induce diarrhoea by glucose (or by galactose) in the healthy
subject, even if very high doses up to 400 gm are used. Therefore,
by the laxative effects of the sugar substitutes a kind of self
limitation of the oral uptake in the diet is exerted. In fact it
is not realistic to use more than 50 - 80 gm of these substances
per day. The polyols should not be used for the sweetening of
beverages, because greater amounts are needed for this purpose.
On the other hand xylitol for the next time will remain too expensive to be used in greater amounts."

Siebert also discussed van den Berghe's paper and gave some newer
aspects of the fate of sorbitol: "Besides data on α-D-glucopyra-
nosido-1,6-sorbitol, one of the components of Palatinit, we also

performed experiments with free sorbitol which, in comparison
with fructose, leads to much higher specific radioactivities in
triglyceride fatty acids from adipose tissue and liver choleste-
rol, but diminished incorporation into triglyceride glycerol and
liver glycogen when ingested orally in trace amounts (E. Schnell-
Dompert und G. Siebert, unpublished observations). These differences disappear totally after intraperitoneal administration;
the working hypothesis of incomplete absorption of sorbitol, microbial fermentation in the upper large intestine, and absorption
of intestinal degradation products of sorbitol as volatile fatty
acids is finally proven by the finding that the acetate pool of
the liver - measured by acetylation of sulfanilamide - has a
manyfold higher specific radioactivity after oral sorbitol than
after fructose.

The sharply enhanced formation of H_2 gas, analysed in the respiratory air, after oral uptake of sorbitol in man demonstrates
beyond doubt that bacterial colonic fermentation of unabsorbed
sorbitol occurs in human beings. It is actually pyruvate in the
upper large intestine which is formed on microbial degradation
from sorbitol and leads to the release of H_2 and in some persons
also of CH_4 in the exhaled breath.

Other actions of sorbitol, after prolonged   feeding at 10 - 15 %
levels in synthetic diets to rats, include less isotope incorporation from sorbitol into triglycerides of subcutaneous adipose
tissue, a decrease of body fat - i. e. increased lean body mass -
and a lowered level of plasma insulin, observations which, taken
together, demonstrate clearly that not all ingested sorbitol is
metabolised via fructose but partially through the symbiotic cooperation of microbes with mammalian systems."

Hill fully agreed with the interpretation of Sieberts' data
according to which most of the sorbitol is not absorbed as such
by the gut but rather as short chain fatty acids which are fur-

ther degraded by bacteria in the gut and which are, therefore, not calorigenic.

Newbrun raised the question whether the increased salivary lacto-peroxidase activity after oral xylitol was specific or not. Mäki-nen could'nt make it quite clear whether the increased activity of lactoperoxidase was specific for xylitol or whether it was just one of many xylitol effects such as an increase of amylase, sialoprotein and some other less specific enzymes not related to dental caries. Guggenheim stated that increased lactic peroxidase by itself has no protective effect on teeth since it is not the rate limiting step in the protection against caries.

Hoogendoorn mentioned that an increase in salivary flow may, by itself, have a protective effect. Mäkinen made it finally clear that the increase in lactoperoxidase was by no means the only pro-tective effect of xylitol against caries but that the main pro-tection came from the fact that 1) xylitol was not metabolized by bacteria and 2) that a change of the bacterial flora in the oral cavity occurred. All these changes together have an anticarioge-nic effect.

Siebert presented a very interesting paper on Palatinit which is split in the small bowel to glucose and sorbitol. The rate of in-testinal cleavage of Palatinit into its constituents is about 1/15 of that of saccharose. Therefore, digestion of Palatinit in the small intestine is incomplete. Only small amounts of Palati-nit are excreted in the urine and it appears that undigested Pa-latinit and sorbitol reach the colon where they are converted by bacteria to short chain fatty acids. Accordingly, the energy yield of Palatinit is only between 50 and 75 % of that of isoca-loric amounts of saccharose in growing rats. In men only about 40 % of Palatinit seems to be absorbed as carbohydrate and used by the organism. The conclusion of the authors who have the grea-

test experience in this field was that Palatinit is of interest
as a sugar substitute because its calorigenic effect is much
lower than that of sucrose, while it remains metabolically compatible and safe. Siebert also mentioned that sorbitol is less
calorigenic than sucrose because part of the sorbitol also reaches the colon and is metabolized by bacteria to short chain
fatty acids.

Leroy gave an interesting contribution on hydrogenated starch
hydrolysates which can be considered as starch which was more or
less predigested according to the degree to which starch was previously hydrolysed. Accordingly, the ingestion of hydrogynated
starch hydrolysates leads to an almost comparable increase of
blood glucose and insulin as that obtained with starch alone. Only when very strongly hydrogynated starch hydrolysates were used
a less pron-ounced peak of hyperglycemia was noted. It is too
early at this stage to say anything more about the future of these
hydrogenated starch hydrolysates.

The last paper by Hill was on microbial metabolism in the lower
gut. Hill made a strong point that it is very difficult to change
the flora in the gut except maybe by the use of potent antibio-
tics. Following the ingestion of lactulose and probably also
large amounts of sorbitol the stool pH falls below 6. One result
of the stool acidification is that many compounds reaching the
colon remain undegraded because many enzymes of the intestinal
bacteria have a pH optimum greater than 7. The possible side effects of this failure of the intestinal flora to degrade these
components are not known. Hill also made a point that lactulose
and sorbitol administered in large amounts for therapeutic purposes lead to flatulence and diarrhoea leading to complaints by
many patients who believe that they were poisoned. Since stool
bulking has clear cut advantages these polyalcohols may be useful in the treatment and prevention of colonic diseases such as
diverticulitis, constipation and hemorrhoids. The questions

raised by Hill regarding what the main products of the metabolic degradation of sugar substitutes by the gut flora are remained unanswered. His third question regarding caloric restriction may have been answered to some extent in that sorbitol and Palatinit seem to be less calorigenic than sucrose, fructose or glucose and that they, therefore, may be of some use as sugar substitute in the diet of obese and diabetic persons. They do provide the necessary bulk for food ingredients which one does not achieve with artificial sweeteners. Sorbitol has been widely used for the production of so-called "diabetic" chocolate for many years without any apparent side effects for these patients.

Additional information on the diarrhoea producing effect of Palatinit was given by Siebert. Palatinit occupies a position between fructose and sorbitol. Accordingly between 50 and 80 gms of Palatinit can be taken per day without causing loose bowels, flatulence, discomfort and diarrhoea.

Important questions remaining to be solved regard the fate of the polyalcohols in the colon. Even though we do not have any evidence that sorbitol, xylitol and Palatinit cause anything more than discomfort, flatulence and diarrhoea we should eventually know what products are formed in the gut and what their fate is.

Mehnert: "It does not seem to be useful to give a further summary of the whole discussion, since the main problems have been summarized before. However, let me mention four points, at least, hoping both the panel and the audience will agree:

1. The possibilities of parenteral nutrition with fructose, sorbitol and xylitol are still under discussion.

2. There is no reason to believe that the oral intake of sugar substitutes in reasonable amounts induces harmful metabolic effects.

3. All these substances should not be a source of undesirable calories. Therefore, they have to be calculated in the diet.

4. Gastrointestinal side-effects particularly due to high doses
   of slowly absorbed sorbitol, xylitol and Palatinit should be
   avoided."

Health and Sugar Substitutes
Proc. ERGOB Conf., Geneva 1978, pp. 321-326 (Karger, Basel 1978)

SUMMARY AND DISCUSSION OF SESSION III:

PRACTICAL PROBLEMS IN SUBSTITUTING SUGAR IN VARIOUS FOODS

Donald A. M. Mackay and Pierre M. Vincent

Life Savers, Inc., 40 West 57th Street, New York, N. Y. 10019

Roquette Freres, 4, Rue Patou, 59022 Lille Cedex, France

The Moderator opened the session by reminding the audience that hopes for substantial replacement of sugar in the dietary had to be founded on a clear understanding of the role of a sweetener and the necessary distinction of sweetness and bulk properties of a sweetener, whether in sucrose, sorbitol or saccharin. Sucrose had both; sorbitol had some sweetness but was valued mainly for bulk; saccharin had only sweetness.

The purpose of sugar substitution had also to be kept in mind. Dentists were concerned about substances that could be metabolized in the mouth to give acid products; dieters were concerned about substances that could be metabolized anywhere in the body if they produced sufficient calories; diabetics should also be concerned about avoiding calories, and particularly about avoiding consumption of substances leading to glucose in the blood; and doctors concerned about the heart no longer seemed sure what to avoid.

The purpose of substitution, and hence the labelling and description of "non-sugar" products, had always to be considered with the means of substitution. Artificial sweeteners were important in that their concentrated sweetness permitted the use of water (usually) as the bulking agent in products designed to avoid calories, or acidogenesis in the mouth, or glucose in the blood, or perhaps lipogenesis in the arterial wall. Foods for which artificial sweeteners were unavailable, or foods which in any case could not utilize water as the bulk replacement phase for sugar, had to face the much more critical problem of finding a bulk substitute for sugar. Not only had this new bulking agent to avoid that particular metabolic property (dental, diabetic, caloric) that was the critical cause of dissatisfaction with sugar, but its other possible metabolic consequences had to be considered. However, the most important practical consideration for a safe, pharmaceutically functional substitute for sugar was often that its bulk properties also permitted its function as a food component. Most scientists outside the food industry failed to realize that considerations for sugar substitution also included substitution for physical functionality in foods, and if not functionality,

at least compatibility. It could be asserted that <u>even if sugar did not taste</u>
<u>sweet, sugar would continue to be a major ingredient</u> in many food products.
A large part of the problem was that long-time sugar usage had led to
inventiveness in exploitation of sugar's unique properties, leading to unique
food products in which the physico-chemical functionality of sugar had been
advantageously employed to create that food.

The Moderator said he had a list of forty properties of sugar, any one of
which conceivably could create a need for sugar in food quite apart from its
taste. Admittedly, some were highly specialized uses, or even trivial, but
were none the less determining factors in the choice of sugar as a food ingredient. In confectionery, sugar solutions could be boiled down to form the
plastic masses needed for high speed processing; or reacted with fat and
proteins to give characteristic flavor and texture of caramel and toffees; or
pulled or aerated or spun for novel textures. In bakery, sugar was needed
for its leavening action, or to give desirable texture, moistness and anti-
staling properties, or for creation of desirable color and flavor. Other uses
were as a diluent, or wetting agent, or flow agent, or tabletting agent, or for
icing, or for liquefiable centers, or for dissolving other ingredients, or as
aids in co-drying, or spray drying, or agglomeration. Humectant and pre-
servative properties were also very important.

It was pointed out that three of the four polyol contributions had been
made by the manufacturer of that product. Only the sorbitol paper had been
given from the more critical point of view of the user; this fact should be
allowed to permit a fairer comparison with the other bulking agents as
described by their manufacturers.

The formal program began with short abstracted presentations on the
practical considerations of using xylitol, Lycasin, sorbose, Palatinit,
saccharin and cyclamate in place of sugar, and was then opened to a joint
discussion of all papers.

The first question to the panel was on economics. What were the prices
of the substitutes? No answer was immediately forthcoming. Eventually a
factor of two to three was tentatively suggested for sorbitol and Lycasin,
and some price reduction for xylitol was foreseen when resolution of regulatory issues permitted large scale production economies.

Mr. Voirol (Xyrofin) was also asked by Dr. Muhlemann (Zurich) about
the hygroscopicity of xylitol. In handling, storage and bulk shipment it was
superior to sugar, he said, but this lack of humectancy also meant it could
not replace sorbitol in toothpaste.

Dr. Beereboom (Pfizer) introduced a new sugar substitute by describing a new Pfizer product called polydextrose. Made by catalytic condensation of glucose, it contained completely random glycosidic linkages very stable to enzyme action. Detailed metabolic studies in rats, dogs and man using C^{14} labels had shown only 1 calorie/g. for caloric utilization. The product was bland and needed an artificial sweetener. It was very water soluble and behaved like sugar in boiling down to give hard candies. It made a very good ice cream, with a fat sparing action needing only 2% fat. All toxicity studies were completed, using sucrose as a positive contro. Up to 18 g/kilo/day had given no problem in rodents with either substance. Polydextrose was tolerated well (between sorbitol and xylitol) and did not interfere with absorption or utilization of other dietary constituents. In answering Dr. Roussos (NIDR) he added it was quite resistant to oral bacteria, gave no significant drop in the plaque pH test, and caused no caries in rat feeding studies.

Dr. Roussos then inquired about a Searle product, similar to Palatinit, called glucosylsorbitol. Dr. Schiewek said this was a B-linked product containing many 1-2, 2-3 and 4-5 linkages and was not a uniform product like Palatinit which contained only a mixture of two stereoisomers. Polydextrose was also not uniform, being a mixture of many compounds.

Dr. Guggenheim (Zurich) returned to xylitol, asking why xylitol jam does not need preservatives since the fruit contains fermentable sugar. Mr. Voirol reflected his puzzlement. He did not know, but it was a fact that xylitol jams were more stable than the sucrose type. Research on this antifermenting action of xylitol was now under way.

Some questions referred to health issues for xylitol, and to the kind of studies needed by the medical community to make xylitol freely available on the market in a variety of foodstuffs, but were deferred for answer in a later session. The Moderator pointed out that there was a very small number of foods in which any sugar substitution by polyols had achieved economic importance, and in fact only sorbitol in confectionery (and only in chewing gum at that) could be cited as a successful story of sugar replacement in foods. Why hadn't this success spread to the rest of the food supply?

Mr. Lynch (ICI) thought the answer was in high cost of polyols, and also in the variability of their equivalent sweetness at use levels, particularly in complex food systems. Mr. Voirol agreed that 13 g. xylitol was needed to replace 9 g. sugar in coffee, but much less was needed to sweeten low pH drinks, compared to sucrose. The Moderator suggested, however, that economics were not that critical to sugar substitution, provided it was possible for the manufacturer to describe his product in terms to draw attention to its virtue and sell it. He felt the determining factor in the narrowness of present sugar substitution in foods was that only in confections was it possible to make a 100% substitution of polyol for a 100% sugar product and call attention to it. If the public wanted it, the food manufacturer would supply it, and the polyol manufacturer would eventually get his price. Dr. Doty (Xyrofin) felt the answer lay more in the eventual medical determination of the good and bad points of all sweeteners, and whether the dental, or non-glycemic or hedonic properties were judged to be most important. Dr. Muhlemann (Zurich) suggested the partial substitution of foods with polyols like xylitol was a way to ease into gradual consumption and build tolerance without side effects, and felt it was fortunate that candy pieces were so small individually that the ADI was not going to be exceeded if confections were the only source of the polyol. Other questioners again raised the need for a medical consensus on safety of sugar substitutes, and suggested the reason for partial substitution perhaps lay here. A wide body of agreement had been reached in dental circles, but in medical ones there was still a very few negative comments and reservations which needed to be cleared up.

The Moderator pointed out that the audience contained great expertise of all types, and if such a body could not agree on a course of action for sugar substitution, then regulatory authorities in various countries would not have the assurance to devise the regulations to permit food manufacturers to use sugar substitutes to make certain foods, and also to permit them to make the marketing efforts to bring certain food claims to the attention of the public. If market forces could not be used to bring about sugar substitution, then by fiat was presumably the only other way. The dental success of sorbitol in chewing gum was partly a flavor story, and partly the result of strong professional dental support in the U.S.A. of the description "sugarless" for sorbitol gum, although it was now necessarily qualified by the statements, "does not promote tooth decay" and "contains calories". If any group wanted to achieve the objective of the increased use of sugar substitution, the way had to be cleared for the manufacturer of the food to sell the food, and for the manufacturer of the sugar substitute to supply him. Manufacturers either of the food or the sugar substitute were seen to be in self-serving positions, and were thus quite ineffective in dealing with the regulatory authorities who decide product categories and permitted label or advertising statements. In view of the diversity of technical opinion, as for example expressed at this conference, it was hardly surprising that the

regulatory bodies had also failed to develop their own unanimous positions.
He concluded by apologizing if this call to putting our own house in order
had offended members of either the audience or the panel.

Dr. Guggenheim (Zurich) said he appreciated the need for advertising
to develop a new substitute, and for medical people to define their viewpoint
on sugar substitutes. However, academic people had also the right to ask
manufacturers not to put false claims on their product just to sell it better,
or at least to use data which were reproducible in different laboratories. He
also felt more progress would result if manufacturers united in a common
cause instead of fighting each other.

Mr. Rockstrom (Bastad) pointed out that only Switzerland had set rules
in this area for companies to follow, and hoped other countries would follow.
He also recited the early history of Lycasin, and stressed its success was
the result of cooperation of a candy company, with the Swedish Starch Association, and eventually with the University Dental Faculty. He felt that if
this conference could aim to broaden the use of claims, such as those in
Switzerland, this would be a big step forward in wider use of sugar substitutes.

The discussion then moved to nomenclature and terminology. What was
the English equivalent of "zahnschonend"? Was the reference to safety too
strong? The Moderator suggested many food manufacturers would have to
be able to use claims like kind or protective to teeth, and would certainly
welcome the methodology that would permit this, and encourage the development of this type of product. At the moment, in reference to the U.S.
situation, "sugarless - does not promote tooth decay" was the only permitted
statement. Any other statement had to be very carefully considered to avoid
drug claims.

Dr. Muhlemann (Zurich) as author of "zahnschonend", said "safe for
teeth" was the translation he used, though he had long considered the need
for better semantics. He did not like "does not promote tooth decay" because he felt this implied a clinical study with supporting data. He preferred
the use of pH telemetry for measurement of acid in dental plaque, as this
did not claim to evaluate cariogenicity but only acid production, though he
assumed a clinical correlation would show the equivalence. Only in the case
of xylitol had the clinical study been done, and also animal studies, to show
equivalence, but who could afford to do this, product by product?

It was wrong, he added, to suggest "protective for teeth" was a possible
meaning of "zahnschonend". There had been discussion that xylitol might
be protective, but there was no evidence he had seen with the plaque pH

method that would support it. "Not harmful to teeth" might be the best
suggestion. The situation was complicated by the possibility of acid erosion,
besides fermentation, on teeth not covered with plaque. A very acid product
would not be "kind to teeth". "Safe for teeth" - to be on the safe side -
could also be considered. "Sugarless" was a term he preferred to leave for
discussion in a later session.

The Moderator paid tribute to Dr. Muhlemann's long experience in this
field, and noted he had not meant to offer "protective" as a translation, nor
"does not promote tooth decay" as anything but a statement which may be
made in the U.S. about an inherent property of a product's ingredients
apart from the product itself. In view of time pressure, it was appropriate
to close the session at this point, he said, and did so, after thanking the
members of the panel for their several contributions and the audience for
many stimulating questions and comments.

Health and Sugar Substitutes
Proc. ERGOB Conf., Geneva 1978, pp. 327-335 (Karger, Basel 1978)

SUMMARY AND DISCUSSION OF SESSION IV: NEW SWEETENERS

E. Newbrun and G.A. Crosby

Department of Oral Medicine and Hospital Dentistry, School of Dentistry,
University of California, San Francisco, CA 94143, USA, and Dynapol, Palo
Alto, CA 94304, USA

The title of "New Sweeteners" for this session of the conference is not
quite accurate; perhaps "Old New Sweeteners" or "New Old Sweeteners" might be
more appropriate. The sweetness of the dihydrochalcones was discovered in
1963[1], of Aspartame in 1969[2], of Acesulfame-K in 1967; the latter was not
reported until 1973[3]. Talin is a mixture of thaumatins which were first
isolated in 1971[4]. Many of the other sweeteners of natural origin date back
for decades and some for centuries. So why "new sweeteners"?

Perhaps the answer is that most of these substances have not been official-
ly approved as food additives and are new in the sense that they are still
awaiting introduction into the commercial market. Another reason, at least
in the USA, lies in the slow, step-by-step development and testing required
for food additives. For example, although several limited-usage additives
have been approved in the USA since 1969, only a few have been approved for
widespread use. They are: FD and C Red No. 40, 1971[5]; *tertiary*-butylhydro-
quinone (TBHQ), 1972, an antioxidant stabilizer used in cooking oils (Eastman
Kodak); and Aspartame (Searle), 1974[6]. The Food Additive Petition for
Aspartame was subsequently stayed (December 5, 1975) on the basis of the
Bureau of Foods review.

Zienty[7] recently estimated that it takes about 10 years from discovery to
marketing of a new food additive. This time span includes optimization of
synthesis, short term toxicology, process development, cost, and application
studies (about 4 years), followed by intensive safety, pilot plant, and
engineering studies (year 4-7), and then complete toxicology studies and
preparation and filing of petition with the Food and Drug Administration (FDA)
(year 7-9). If accepted, regulation would be issued (year 8-10), during
which time capital appropriation and plant construction would take place;
and finally, the new additive would be marketed (year 11-14). Zienty estimates the cost of all these procedures at $10 million; clearly, a new

sweetening agent must have a large market to justify such an investment.

If these estimates are correct, then much of the time lag in the development of a new sweetener is not directly due to governmental delays in handling petitions by the FDA, but to regulations intended to ensure consumer safety.

The "new sweeteners" to be discussed in this session are by no means all-inclusive of the known new sweeteners (such as chlorosucrose analogues, aldoximes, and thiophenesaccharin) but include those products closest to acceptance.

In conducting this session we will diverge slightly from the sequence on the printed program. The respective panelists will review their work on Aspartame and the dihydrochalcones, followed by an open discussion. After a short recess we will hear about Acesulfame-K, Talin, and some of the natural sweeteners, and will then have another open discussion period.

Dr. L.D. Stegink introduced his paper on "Aspartame Metabolism in Human Subjects" with several noteworthy comments that do not appear in the published proceedings. The audience was informed that three questions have arisen in the United States regarding the safety of Aspartame. The first of these concerns the presence of the dicarboxylic acid, aspartate, formed by the metabolism of Aspartame in the intestinal mucosa. Aspartate and glutamate, another dicarboxylic amino acid, have been associated with hypothalamic neuronal necrosis when given in large amounts to neonatal rodents. The second question clearly involves the other amino acid released from Aspartame, phenylalanine, and the ability of phenylketonuric heterozygotes to metabolize this compound. The third question relates back to the aspartate content: that is, whether the infant who might consume Aspartame could adequately handle the amino acids released from the sweetener.

Dr. Stegink pointed out that a sensitive animal species is required for study of these questions. The neonatal rodent is acutely sensitive to glutamate and aspartate. Even so, grossly elevated levels of amino acids must be reached before lesions are found in the neonatal rodent. Either of the two amino acids requires threshold levels of at least five times normal, or about 50-60 µmol/dl. Below these levels, no lesions are noted. Contrary to an earlier report, the neonatal primate is not sensitive to the dicarboxylic amino acids. These animals did not develop lesions when fed Aspartame at a level of 2 g/kg.

The paper published in these proceedings adequately documents the selection of 34 mg/kg of body weight as a pharmacological dose representing the 99.9th percentile of projected ingestion. Thus a level of 100 mg/kg represents an

abusive dose and would be equivalent to the consumption of 100 liters of
Aspartame-sweetened beverage at one sitting. In adults, ingestion of Aspartame at a level of 100 mg/kg does not produce any change in blood plasma
levels of aspartate. Phenylalanine is not metabolized as rapidly as aspartate
and thus shows a relationship between blood plasma levels and dose levels.
Yet even at dose levels of 200 mg/kg the plasma phenylalanine did not go
beyond 48 μmol/dl in the adults. In Dr. Stegink's opinion, this level is
high but tolerable and does not represent much of a risk. At all dose
levels of Aspartame studied (up to 100 mg/kg), one- and two-year-old infants
seem to be comparable to adults.

In conclusion, Dr. Stegink feels that Aspartame is rapidly metabolized by
both infants and adults, and that there is no significant accumulation of
the amino acids in plasma even under acute abuse doses.

Dr. Robert Horowitz covered a number of the points found in his published
paper on dihydrochalcone (DHC) sweeteners as well as adding several interesting comments on the ability of the tasteless flavone, neodiosmin, to interfere with the perception of bitterness. This masking effect also appears to
be a property of the sweet dihydrochalcones. Thus, neodiosmin, at a concentration of only 10 ppm, raises the taste threshold of the bitter flavanone
naringen by three- or fourfold, and the threshold of the intensely bitter
triterpenoid limonin by fourfold. Sucrose, even at a concentration of 3%,
has little effect on the taste thresholds of these bitter substances. Dr.
Horowitz reported that investigators at the USDA Laboratories in Berkeley,
California, have examined the effect of adding small amounts of the intensely
sweet neohesperidin DHC (neo DHC) on the taste of grapefruit juice.[8] At an
added concentration of only 12 ppm of neo DHC, 76% of the taste panel liked
the grapefruit juice, as opposed to only 33% of the panel liking pure grapefruit juice. Neodiosmin was reported to have a similar effect on orange
juice containing various levels of added limonin, and to reduce the offtaste
of saccharin.

Dr. Horowitz concluded his presentation with some general comments on
dihydrochalcones. The DHCs are typical examples of a large group of plant
products known as flavonoids. Although neo DHC and naringen DHC do not
occur naturally, in terms of chemical structure they can be considered merely
as the open chain, reduced analogues of the widely occurring flavonoids,
neohesperidin and naringin, respectively. As a group the flavonoids are
generally regarded as innocuous, and are believed to be metabolized to
carbon dioxide and various aromatic acids. But perhaps of most importance

is the fact that since flavonoids occur in all higher plants, they have always been, and will continue to be, a common constituent of the diet.

The first round of questions on both papers was initiated by the Panel.
Question for Dr. Horowitz. Could you comment on whether the petition filed with the FDA for approval of neo DHC is being affected by the unknown identity of the metabolite of neo DHC?
Dr. Horowitz. The FDA has not requested any metabolite data (from us) thus far, but this should come later.
Comment by Dr. H. Blumenthal of the audience (FDA, Washington DC). Regarding neohesperidin DHC, the FDA has been waiting for more data. When it comes before us, we will evaluate it. With regard to metabolism studies, we do ask for these studies and we evaluate them within the full context of the other data. If we feel we still need more data, then we will ask for it.
Question for Dr. Stegink. Could you tell us the percentage of the population that are phenylketonuric (PKU) heterozygotes. Would children and adults unknowingly afflicted with PKU be subject to any risk from Aspartame?
Dr. Stegink. The incidence rate is one in 10,000 to 20,000. Aspartame is scheduled to be labeled as "containing phenylalanine." Further, the amount of phenylalanine ingested with the normal protein of the diet is perhaps on the order of ten times the amount available from a daily dose of Aspartame at 6-8 mg/kg. This would not increase the risk to undiagnosed children.
Question for Dr. Stegink. Could you perhaps comment on the breakdown product of Aspartame that is called diketopiperazine, and its possible safety.
Dr. Stegink. We have not done many studies on that compound. The diketopiperazine can form spontaneously from any dipeptide, including Aspartame.
Dr. H. Blumenthal (FDA). Toxicity data on diketopiperazine was submitted to the FDA. The compound was not totally innocuous, but it could be evaluated and an effect level set where we would not expect any deleterious effects. However, at high doses it did produce benign uterine polyps in female rats.
Question for Dr. Horowitz. Since grapefruit and orange juice are protected in the United States by a standard of identity, would not this prevent the addition of taste modifiers like neo DHC to these products?
Dr. Horowitz. I do not know the answer to that. Neodiosmin does occur naturally in seville oranges. I am not sure what would be needed in the way of clearance.
Dr. Blumenthal. With reference to standards of identity, if a standard is set and someone wishes to change it by adding a new ingredient, they would have to petition for such a change.

Questioning was then opened to the audience.

Question for Dr. Horowitz. I wonder whether the long lasting sweetness of the dihydrochalcones would cause people to oversweeten everything and become accustomed to much higher and longer lasting sweetness levels?

Dr. Horowitz. It might be that one would actually use less because of the long lasting effect. Perhaps the taste would carry through so that one would not want such high levels of sweetness.

Question for Dr. Horowitz. Do these compounds (DHCs and flavones) also have a modifying effect on the perception of salt and acids?

Dr. Horowitz. To the best of my knowledge there is no such effect.

Question for the Panel or audience. It was reported last year that Aspartame, when added under in vitro conditions to 4.5% sucrose solution, would depress plaque formation[9]. Has anybody an idea about the mechanism of this observation?

Dr. Bowen of the audience (NIDR). I cannot comment on the assay as such, but we have done some studies where we have added Aspartame to sugar diets fed to rats and much to our surprise we found lower levels of caries in the animals given the Aspartame.

Dr. Newbrun. Aspartic acid and glutamic acid are known to be decarboxylated by plaque microflora, producing an amine and CO_2[10]. The amine could have a neutralizing effect on acids in the plaque. Presumably Aspartame could be broken down by oral microorganisms to corresponding amines.

Dr. D.A. Mackay. There are also reports that saccharin inhibits the growth of plaque microflora in vitro[11,12].

Dr. Newbrun. We should clarify some issues which have arisen concerning Aspartame, which was originally approved by the FDA. The approval was then withdrawn based on some questions of animal husbandry practices and the reproduction and teratology studies conducted on the animals. Dr. Bost of G.D. Searle has offered to comment on the current status of the review now in progress on Aspartame studies.

Dr. R. Bost. In December 1975, the FDA questioned the validity of some of the animal research supporting the safety of Aspartame. These studies had been submitted with our food additive petition to the FDA. In an attempt to resolve this situation, both the FDA and G.D. Searle agreed to have a third party validate a number of the animal studies termed "critical" by the FDA. This third party review began in August 1977, and has included four long term animal studies, among others. We were recently informed by the third party that their final report would be completed and submitted to G.D. Searle in late November or early December. We expect that the report will support the

validity of the Aspartame studies, and we plan to distribute the report in
early to mid-December, 1978, to regulatory agencies and deliberative bodies
throughout Europe, the US and Canada. We are hopeful that the regulatory
process will proceed with all deliberate speed.

The session on "New Sweeteners" continued with a discussion by Dr. H.-J.
Arpe on Acesulfame-K. One point of interest was presented in addition to the
information appearing in the published paper. Hydrolysis of Acesulfame-K
under chemical conditions follows two different paths from a common intermediate, depending on the pH. Above pH 4 the major unstable hydrolytic
product is the salt of acetoacetic acid, while acetoacetamide is formed below
pH 4. Ultimately, acetone and carbon dioxide are produced by both routes.
The sweetener is stable under use conditions of 8°-25°C and pH 3.5-8 for up
to 50 weeks.

Dr. Arpe also added that carcinogenicity studies have now been carried
through 104 weeks with no signs of carcinogenic activity. The two-year
feeding studies in rats should be finished in November 1978.

Questions were raised by the Panel. Would you comment on the use of the
fluoroisocyanate for the production of Acesulfame-K instead of the more
readily available chloroisocyanate.

Dr. Arpe. We have better yields--up to 80%-85%--with the use of the fluorine
compound.

Question for Dr. Arpe. What are the results of preference tests comparing
saccharin with Acesulfame-K in food systems?

Dr. Arpe. We have hardly any aftertaste with our sweetener. Test panels
have preferred our sweetener.

Question for Dr. Arpe. In your paper you state that "the risk of a N-nitroso
group being introduced into the Acesulfame-K under conditions prevailing in
the organism is very small compared to other nitrogen-containing compounds."
Could you clarify what you mean by a very small risk?

Dr. Arpe. This study was conducted at an institute in Heidelburg. They
tried to produce a nitrosamide from Acesulfame-K and found they had to use a
pH of 1, otherwise they could not find anything. At pH 1 they could only find
traces of nitrosamide. The conditions in the body are above pH 1 and therefore suggest this statement.

The last two presentations, first by Dr. J.D. Higgenbotham on Talin and
the other by Dr. G.E. Inglett on sweeteners of natural origin, closely
followed the published papers and will not be repeated in this summary.

Dr. Higgenbotham did add that the two major proteins in Talin, proteins T_1
and T_{11}, are both sweet but differ slightly in sweetness intensity. T_1 has
been found to be 2500 times more potent than sucrose relative to 8% sucrose,
while T_{11} is 2700 times sucrose. A mixture of the two proteins was determined to be 3000 times more potent than sucrose.

Dr. Inglett's talk brought together a discussion of many types of intensely
sweet materials occurring in nature, and served to greatly broaden the scope
of this session on "New Sweeteners".

Questions to the Panel and audience on the last two papers:

Question for Dr. Higgenbotham. Could you comment on the taste of Talin and
the effect of taste modifiers?

Dr. Higgenbotham. Most people would describe Talin's taste profile as being
a slight delay in perception of the sweet taste, followed by a gradual
increase in sweet taste and then a lingering sweet aftertaste. We found
this depends on the purity of the material and the system you test it in.
There is a long aftertaste in water, especially with the first taste. There
is also a delayed onset, but it is easy to incorporate other sweeteners,
such as xylitol, to bridge the gap. The aftertaste of Talin can be somewhat
masked by fruit flavors. Additives, such as glucuronic acid, reduce the
aftertaste, but also reduce the sweetness, so they are not very effective.

Question for Dr. Higgenbotham. You referred to a modified Talin for long
stability. Do you want to comment on that?

Dr. Higgenbotham. This is the subject of a patent application. I can tell
you it is a very simple combination of Talin with another protein, a
recognized food additive, and citric acid, which is there to adjust to the
correct pH, which is around 2.7. Co-drying Talin with this other protein
at the appropriate pH gives an extremely stable mixture. The protein
combines with the active sites in Talin without masking its sweet taste
and prevents the normal degradation due to oxidation.

Question for Dr. Higgenbotham. Will Tate and Lyle go through all the
necessary testing to seek approval of Talin?

Dr. Higgenbotham. We have done quite a bit of testing. This includes the
LD_{50}, in which we were not able to find an LD_{50} level even feeding over
20 g/kg. We have also done a 13-week semi-chronic study in rats, with no
adverse effects. Also, teratologic, allergenic, and mutagenic experiments
have been conducted. We have not yet gone on to the long term carcinogenic
study. Meanwhile, the United Kingdom Ministry is looking at present data on
Talin to see if it could be allowable as a food additive.

Question for the Panel. Can someone on the Panel comment on the amount of material needed to go through the full series of safety tests.

Dr. Crosby. We are now in the process of carrying out safety studies on several new polymeric, nonabsorbable food additives. We have produced about 600 kg of one of these products for this purpose, and are now completing the preparation of the same quantity of the other product.

Question for Dr. Higgenbotham. Is there any structural similarity between thaumatin and monellin? In the case of monellin there is a single free sulfhydryl (SH) group which is essential for sweetness. Is this shared by thaumatin?

Dr. Higgenbotham. Thaumatin has no free SH groups. It has no cysteine, only cystine. It has seven crosslinked cystine molecules, which account for its very great stability.

Question for Dr. Inglett. Have you made any attempts to reveal the mechanism by which monellin produces its sweetness?

Dr. Inglett. No. We have not done any studies relating structure and sweetness. Studies at the Monell Research Institute show that the tertiary structure of the molecule is essential for sweetness. It was thought that there might be some sequences of Aspartame in monellin. However, a closer look at the structure of monellin reveals no links between phenylalanine and aspartic acid. They are there, but not together.

REFERENCES

1. Horowitz, R.M. and Gentili, B. U.S. Patent 3,087,821, 1963.

2. Mazur, R.H., Schlatter, J.M. and Goldkamp, A.H. J. Am. Chem. Soc. 91: 2684-2691, 1969.

3. Clauss, K. and Jensen, H. Angew. Chemie 85: 965-973, 1973.

4. Wel, H. van der, in Olfaction and Taste, edited by D. Schneider. Proceedings 4th International Symposium, pp. 226-233, 1971.

5. Furia, T.E. (ed.) in Handbook of Food Additives, 2nd Ed., p. 589, CRC Press, Cleveland, Ohio, 1972.

6. Federal Register 39 (145): 27317-27320, 1974.

7. Zienty, F.B. in Conference on Foods, Nutrition and Dental Health, sponsored by Research Institute, American Dental Association, Chicago, Ill. (in press).

8. Guadagni, D.G., Maier, V.P. and Turnbaugh, J.H. J. Sci. Food Agric. 25: 1199, 1974.

9. Olson, B.L. J. Dent. Res. 56: 1426, 1977.

10. Hayes, M.L. and Hyatt, A.T. Arch. Oral Biol. 19: 361-369, 1974.

11. Linke, H.A.B. Z. Naturforsch. 32C: 839-843, 1977.

12. Grenby, T.H. and Bull, J.M. 25th Congress ORCA, Abst. No. 16, p. 61, 1978.

Health and Sugar Substitutes
Proc. ERGOB Conf., Geneva 1978, pp. 336-347 (Karger, Basel 1978)

SUMMARY AND DISCUSSION OF SESSION V: SUGAR SUBSTITUTES IN ORAL
HEALTH - METABOLIC CRITERIA INDICATIVE OF CARIOGENICITY

B. Guggenheim and H.R. Mühlemann

Department of Oral Microbiology and General Immunology and
Department of Cariology, Periodontology and Preventive Denistry
Dental Institute, University of Zurich, 8028 Zurich, Switzerland

The moderator, Dr. H.R. Mühlemann, opened the session by
introducing the panelists to the floor. He then defined "dental
caries" and its pathogenesis, explaining plaque formation beginning
with a clean tooth surface. Further, he explained the special
role of sucrose in the etiology of dental caries, and characterized
its role in the colonization of plaque streptococci and the
importance of acid formation from fermentable carbohydrates
by plaque microorganisms. In this respect, he offered some
definitions which characterize the fermentability of carbohydrates
and sugar substitutes: Carbohydrates (mono-, di-, tri-,
oligo-, and polysaccharides) and sugar substitutes which are
readily and rapidly fermented by plaque microorganisms are
acidogenic. The same compounds, if they are very slowly fermented
and do not lower the pH below 5.7 as measured by the pH-telemetry
system, are hypoacidogenic. The term non-acidogenic may only be
applied to food items, carbohydrates, and sugar substitutes
if they are completely unfermentable. The moderator summarized
the papers written by the members of the panel and stressed
the fact that there was unanimous agreement that lowering the
pH in plaque is an important parameter indicating an association
between food constituents and dental caries. Tooth decalcification
without acid production does not seem to occur.

The moderator opened the panel discussion with the following
questions: (i) Are all sugars cariogenic? (ii) Should we aim
to replace sucrose totally in food, or shhould we seek to eliminate
it from certain items? (iii) What is the role of the frequency
of sugar consumption? (iiii) Would it be enough to eliminate

sugar only from snacks consumed between meals?

Dr. König took up the last question and replied that it is not necessary and would be impossible to substitute all sucrose. Teeth may very well cope with the acid generated during a limited period of about 20 minutes after main meals. He felt that it is much more important to eliminate sucrose from between-meal-snacks. In rats, it is possible to study well the effect of frequency of consumption by programmed feeding, provided that the rats accept the food items offered. Dr. König warned, however, that the palatability of human foods to rats is unpredictable. The acceptance of each compound or food item to be tested must be controlled because "you can lead a horse to water but you can't make it drink."

"What is the importance of the concentration of sucrose in snacks?" was the next question pesented to the panel by the moderator.

Dr. Mäkinen replied that it is not the concentration which is the most important criterion but rather the physical form in which sugars are consumed. The most dangerous products whould be sticky toffees and lozenges even if salivary flow was somewhat stimulated by mastication and sucking.

Dr. Bowen commented that it is wrong to speak of "cariogenic" food items rather,one should speak of the "cariogenic potential" of the food. Thus, if one eats a certain food only once a day, it is unlikely that dental caries will result. It is the frequency, as has been mentioned, that is most important. Within the range of foodstuffs used by man, there is only one which has been shown to be cariogenic in man and that is chewing gum. On the question of retention of sucrose, Dr. Bowen presented old data from Dr. Volker which showed that there are enormous differences in the oral clearance of sucrose from a broad range of food items, as measured by the content of sucrose or reducing sugar in oral fluid. He suggested that sugars in products like chewing gum, which have prolonged retention times have a greater cariogenic potential compared to products in which sugar clearance is more rapid.

Dr. Scheinin felt that the situation was more complex than
dentists might believe. Frequently, it has been stated that
the only requirement necessary to reduce dental caries would
be to reduce the total amount of sucrose consumes. However,
it can be shown that consumption of as little as 10 g per day
can be highly cariogenic. There is ample evidence in the
literature of little or no relationship between caries incidence
and total sugar consumption. On the other hand, a large number of
reports clearly show the profound role of the frequency of
sucrose intake. The seeming findings contradiction between these
can be resolved when the results of the Vipeholm-study are
considered: This study was carried out immediately after the
war with institutionalized persons in a medical hospital in
Sweden. When patients received 40-50 g of sucrose with main meals
only, the caries increment was less than 0.5 DMF surfaces in two
years. In a second group, about 300 g of sugar was provided with
main meals, and a large quantity of the additional sucrose was
dissolved in the form of soft drinks. This led to only a minute
increase in DMF surfaces. In contrast, however, another group of
subjects receiving an additional two toffees, 4 times per day
between meals, had a DMF increment of about 3.5 surfaces. One
should of course be able to achieve the reverse result, i.e.
a caries reduction of the same order of magnitude, by replacing
the sucrose in the between-meal-snacks with sugar substitutes.

Dr. Newbrun, commenting on the issues raised by Drs. König
and Scheinin, stated that there cannot be any arguments that fre-
quency-of-use is one of the most important factors determining
the cariogenic potential of a food. However, it is certainly
not possible to distinguish between purely snack items, where
sugar should be replaced, and foodstuffs eaten only at table
meals. Food consumption habits have changed rapidly in the
last decades, e.g. ice cream formerly consumed mainly as a
desert, is now a typical between-meal-snack. Although it is
possible to define snacks, as ready foods not consumed at
main meals, it is, however, impossible to state that any
food item usually consumed at table meals has no cariogenic

potential simply because it is consumed at such meals. Government
agencies and the food industry is interested in regulations so
we should establish some criteria by using common sense, because
it is impossible to design and carry out clinical experiments
which include the whole spectrum of available foods and all
conditions of their use. With respect to the amount and frequency
of sucrose consumption in humans, there are not enough data
available. It was shown, however, that rats monoassociated
with Streptococcus mutans reached a maximum caries incidence
at a 3% of level sucrose in their diet. In the human, we can draw
only a hypothetical curve defining the relation between amount
and frequency of sucrose consumption and dental caries. It
is clear that this will not be a linear function but rather
a S-type curve. The inflection points of this curve will be
determined by the frequency of consumption and not by the total
amount. With regard to human testing of food, Dr. Newbrun
was concerned that too many clinical trials were carried out
at "saturation level of sucrose" where one could not see any
caries increment.

The moderator asked Dr. Newbrun if the sucrose contained in
between-meal-snacks, especially in confectionary products, should
be termed dietary sucrose and whether or not a more definitve
terminology would be appropriate.

Dr. Newbrun replied that we should aim for full declaration
of amounts of sucrose as well as of other mono-, di- and
oligosaccharides in all food items because these carbohydrates
have a cariogenic potential. In practical terms, however,
sucrose and starch are the main carbohydrates consumed. Based
on observations in hereditary fructose-intolerant persons,
Dr. Newbrun stated that starch does not have the same cariogenic
potential as other fermentable sugars.

Adding to the discussion of the specific role of sucrose in caries
etiology, the co-moderator (Dr. B. Guggenheim) stated that
the animal experiments mentioned by Dr. Newbrun issued from a
single laboratory only and should not be generalized until
they had been reproduced elsewhere. Furthermore, he expressed

the view that sucrose consumed with main meals, in even very low
amounts, would provide plaque with the necessary diffusion
limiting properties necessary for caries induction. Additional
consumption of other fermentable carbohydrates between meals
could then be extremely noxious.

The moderator asked the panel if the term "sugarless" should apply
only products devoid of sucrose or should be enlarged to include
all fermentable carbohydrates.

Dr. Scheinin stated that to his knowledge there were no clear
regulations in Scandinavia, but that he would be in favor of
an extended definition.

The discussion was then focused by the moderator on the methods
currently used to predict the cariogenic potential of carbohydrates and sugar substitutes. The moderator asked Drs. de
Stoppelaar, Birkhed, and Imfeld, who have published on this
issue, for comments.

Dr. de Stoppelaar answered that the first investigation which
should be done to evaluate the potential cariogenicity of a
sugar substitute would be to test, whether or not the compound
could be used as an energy source for growth of selected strains
of oral bacteria. If it could not be used, there should be little
chance that dental plaque could metabolize such a substance.
The second property which should be evaluated is the formation
of acids by standardized resting cells suspensions of selected
oral microorganisms. Working with pure cultures of course has
limitations when compared to the mixed flora present in
dental plaque.

Dr. Birkhed commented that the system used in Malmö was simple and
could be used, in contrast to pH-telemetry, in a standardized
form by many laboratories and industry all over the world. Although
the use of pooled plaque might be a weakness, because caries
develops in limited areas only, nevertheless, it is still a
better system for screening purposes than pure cultures.
A further limitation is the fact that base-line values for differen
subjects may vary considerably. However, by calculating the mean

pH drop this defect may be largely overcome. It might even be possible to indicate the largest pH difference which could still be considered "safe for teeth."

The moderator asked Dr. Birkhed whether or not he believed his system would also be useful for testing also food or not only pure compounds.

Dr. Birkhed replied that the method can also be used with the final products.

The moderator addressed Dr. Imfeld and invited him to point out the advantages of the pH-telemetry system in comparison to the methods decribed by Drs. de Stoppelaar and Birkhed.

Dr. Imfeld replied that the main advantage of pH-telemetry was the information one obtains on the effect that the texture of a product has on acid formation under conditions most like natural consumption. Telemetry is, however, not an economical system for testing pure compounds. Of course, a snack containing 70-80% fermentable carbohydrate will also lead to a long lasting pH drop in the telemetry system because of oversaturation of the plaque with fermentable sugars. However, it may be used to determine if the amount of a certain compound, which is not rapidly fermented, may be reduced beyond a critical level to yield a product which is at least hypoacidogenic. A further advantage is the discrimination between the acid reaching the surface of the electrode covered by plaque and placed in an interdental tooth surface, and the large amount of acid diffusing into the oral fluid. In contrast, the pooled plaque sampling method is not able to make this important distinction because plaque is sampled and homogenized together with saliva and food remnants. The most important diffusion properties of plaque are lost in such a system. A further important feature of the telemetry system is the fact that it allows the discrimination of dietary acids and acids formed by plaque microorganisms by glycolytic pathways. In addition, the clearance of fermentable food constituents can be monitored continously, a feature which is of course not possible with the plaque sampling method.

The moderator then directed the discussion to animal experimen-
tation. In as much as rodents cannot consume diets containing
large amounts of polyol because the animals rapidly develop
severe diarhea, such compounds have to be applied topically
together with a diet of low sucrose content. These experiments
have been done in order to desperatly demonstrate the caries-
and plaque-reducing effect of these polyols. The moderator
showed results of several unpublished animal studies demonstrating that the findings were not reproducible. Even when a significant effect was observed, it was of a rather modest order
of magnitude compared to controls (disinfectants). Thus, it
may be concluded that such experiments are of little value
because similar effects can be demonstrated by the topical
application of any inert solution.

Prof. Scheinin questioned the concept outlined by Prof. König,
that feeding of polyols to rodents is not a valid method for
evaluating their cariogenicity. He made the point that
lifetime feeding studies with up to 20% of sorbitol have
been successfully carried out.

Dr. Bowen, refering to his primate model, stated that the use
of wire telemetry with antimony electrodes which allow the
simultaneous measurement of the plaque pH of 4 tooth surfaces
was a very effective tool for caries prognosis. Refering to
sorbitol and cyclamate, he stated that such measurements
were validated in long term studies by feeding these compounds
to monkeys for a 2-3 year period without the development of
any caries. Furthermore, no adaption of the plaque flora to
sorbitol was observed because the fermentability of sorbitol
by the plaque of these animals was not enhanced at the end
of this 3 years exposure. Dr. Bowen was, however, worried
about pH determinations in general because they measure only
one aspect of the pathogenesis of dental caries, although,
admittedly, a most important one. If one accepts the critical
pH to be 5.5, or with Dr. Mühlemann being on the safe side,
pH 5.7, and labels a product "safe for teeth", are we not then

in danger of indorsing a product which may be used repeatedly during the day. May not this enhanced consumption not be more dangerous than the limited intake of a product which could lower the pH to e.g., 5.5, and which would certainly not receive the indorsement "safe for teeth"?

Dr. van Houte, invited by the moderator to answer this tricky question, state that he is not a physical chemist, but that he felt, nevertheless, that Dr. Bowens last statement was not correct. The critical pH is the point at or below which biologically significant demineralization starts to occur. If this point is not reached no demineralization will occur. The problem is, however, to determine this point exactly. It is of practical importance to know whether this point is at pH 5.8, 5.5 or elsewhere. Collegues of Dr. van Houte who are physical chemists have indicated that this point might be as low as 5.0.

Dr. Birkhed expressed the view that there is no true value for a critical pH. The critical pH varies between different subjects, because of differences in the solubility products of phosphorus and calcium in oral fluid and because of solubility differences between enamel and dentin. We cannot, therefore, indicate a definitive critical pH, we can, however, state that the lower the pH in plaque the higher the risk of decalcification. Dr. Birkhed suggested, therefore, a ranking of products according to their behaviour in pH-based measurements.

The co-moderator intruding into the discussion at this point stated that one of the most important drawbacks of all pH systems had not been mentioned. This is the fact that starch, which gives rise to pronounced pH drops in all systems, cannot be considered to have a cariogenic potential. This statement is based on the following observations: (i) Hereditary fructose-intolerant subjects consuming starch unlimitedly are virtually cariesfree. (ii) Caries incidence in Europe during the last world war was reduced considerably when sucrose but not starch consumption was cut back drastically. (iii) Subjects in the Turku sugar study, who formed part of the xylitol group, consumed far

large amounts of cooked starch than xylitol. On the basis
of point iii, 3 manufactures of starch products could claim
that their products have been proven to be non-cariogenic in
this clinical trial, although e.g. confectionary products
and pastries containing starch and being sweetened with xylitol
could never pass any test based on pH measurements.
As a consequence, any pH test on a product containing starch
is useless. Furthermore, this stresses the point made by Dr. Bowen:
that there are other important factors involved in the pathogenesis
of the disease besides the pH drop measured in these systems.
One of these factors, unpardonably neglected in caries research,
is certainly the diffusion-limiting properties of dental plaque.

Dr. Carlsson explained the parameters involved when a microorganism tries to use a sugar or polyol. In order to metabolize
the carbohydrate, first it has to be transported into the
cell. Two transport systems are involved: the phosphotransferase system and the permease system. Usually, both systems
are not constitutive and are specifically induced by their specific
"sugars". After induction, the sugar is transported into the
cytoplasm. Enzymes necessary for further metabolism are then
induced to introduce the compound into the glycolytic pathway.
This process requires energy in form of ATP or a hydrogen
gradient across the bacterial membrane. Hydrogen ions pumped
out of the membrane using ATP as energy source, form a gradient
which can transport sugars by the permease system. If glucose
is present, other sugars are usually not metabolized, because
glucose is transported by a phosphotransferase system which
is constitutive, blocking the permease systems for other
"sugars". On this basis Dr. Carlsson did not agree with the
statement of the moderator that adaption to sugar substitutes
does not exist. More carefully expressed, there is a low risk
that plaque bacteria could use sugar substitutes as main
carbon and energy sources.

The moderator addressed Dr. Scheinin and asked him whether
he would be prepared to make some comments on which sugar
substitutes could be recommended.

Dr. Scheinin considered this question unfair because, having worked for more than 8 years with xylitol, he considered himself biased. Nevertheless, he stated that there is a definite need for controled, critical studies in general, and the results of the Turku sugar study especially should be verified by other investigators. Such studies should be carried out on a young, homogeneous population with a high incidence of dental caries. Ethical problems in relation to a proper control must, of course, be adequately met.

A general discussion was then opened by the moderator.

Dr. Chilton (University of Pennsylvania) stated that, despite laboratory studies each sugar substitute to be introduced on the market has to prove its efficacy and safety in clinical trials. One of the main problems which clinical research is faced with is the fact that sucrose can for ethical reasons, no longer be used as positive control. As alternatives,Dr. Chilton proposed two possibilities: one, the cohort control and the other, might be called a temporal control. The cohort control examines an age- and sex-matched group of individuals which is not under the influence of the study for the entire experimental period. The temporal control compares the caries prevalence of the experimental group with the caries prevalence of a matched,negative control group from one and the same collection. The negative group receives the test product sweetened by compounds which are believed to have no, or a very modest, cariogenic potential. At present, it is most essential to reexamine the methods of clinical trials to achieve any progress.

Dr. Mackay (Life Savers, New York) offered two clarifications on points previously discussed by the panel: first, a comment on the critical pH, and second some remarks in the regulatory area. As Dr. van Houte well knows, the physical chemistry of calcium phosphate is extremly complicated. One has only to look at phase diagrams to see that there is a very narrow area at low solubilities where the conversion from one form of calcium phosphate to the other occurs. One can only say that lowering

the pH in a calcium-phosphate-solution would gradually change
the proportions of mono-, di- and tribasic calciumphospate.
Around pH 5.1, precipication of apatite occurs. Although
apatite is not completely identical to enamel, one might say
that around pH 5.1 the reverse would occur and enamel would
slowly start to dissolve.

With regard to the regulatory area, sobitol and mannitol are
considered in the US as Gras substance, while xylitol is
only permitted in special dietary products. Sorbitol may regularly
be included in products. If one, however, wants to make a statement
about a product containing sorbitol, e.g. to call it "sugarless",
this automatically puts the product in a group of "special
dietary products" and one has to declare what kind of "special
dietary product" it is. One may, for instance, claim: "Does
not promote tooth decay". The word "sugarless" has, however,
been considered to be misleading because it implies that such a
product would be free of calories. Nevertheless, the term
"sugarless" has been kept because it is backed by the American
Dental Association. The term "not harmful to teeth" is really
the same statement, and it is futile to fight over semantics.
It would be much more useful to remember what the objectives of
dental research in this area are. If you talk about sorbitol
adaptation, raising criticism on rather minor points in the
description of a product, dental research prevents industry
to market such products. If a group of eminent researchers sitting
in a hall in Geneva, are trying to prove that a clearly
hypoacidogenic product like sorbitol may still cause caries,
this will not help to solve the problem.

The moderator stated that the term "sugarless" will not be
accepted in Europe because is is misleading. We shall also,
in the future, try to introduce the term "not harmful to
teeth" for all products which will not lower the pH in vivo
below pH 5.7.

Dr. Mäkinen felt sorry that the discussion had not reached
any depth on the actual topic "metabolic criteria indicative
for cariogenicity".

The co-moderator, after summarizing the session, explained
that a discussion of this large topic could not be achieved
in the time permitted because too many subtopics had been included.
As a consequence far too large a panel was invited to this
session. Nevertheless, by retrospectively analysing this
session, the co-moderator felt that, the given the circumstances,
a valuable discussion had been achieved.

SUMMARY AND DISCUSSION OF SESSION VI: FACTORS IN SAFETY,
BENEFIT/RISK ASSESSMENT AND LEGAL ASPECTS

F.A. Fairweather and I. MacDonald

Department of Health and Social Security, Friars House,
157-168 Blackfriars Road, London SE1 8EU, England
and
Department of Physiology, Guy's Hospital Medical School, London
SE1 9RT, England

Discussion following paper by H. MEHNERT

YUDKIN, J. May I ask if there might be some long term effects of
consuming fructose, etc. as I have found in my experiments in man and
animals that after a few weeks on a fructose diet the fasting blood glucose
levels and more markedly, the fasting insulin levels were raised.

MEHNERT, H. I feel that the replacements for glucose that I have
suggested are sufficiently small as to have minimal long term effects and
furthermore the alternative carbohydrates I have used were practically non-
insulinogenic.

MACDONALD, I. I should like to enquire if sucrose would be preferable to
glucose in the diet of diabetics as it is only half as insulinogenic as glucose,
weight for weight, and has less side effects [such as intestinal hurry]
compared with fructose.

MEHNERT. H. I feel that I prefer fructose to sucrose because unlike
sucrose it is not insulinogenic and in any event the amount of fructose
recommended [60 - 80 g/day] has no side effects. However, I only
recommend fructose if the patient has a desire for sweetness.

ABDELLATIF, A. asked why the free fatty acid concentration in the blood
fell in the patients on fructose and xylitol and MEHNERT, H. gave two
reasons for this:-

1. the action of fructose and xylitol decrease free fatty acid levels

2. the patients in the study discussed were on sulphonylurea therapy.

Discussion following papers by SCHMAHL, D , SIEBER, S. M. , and KROES, R

POULSEN, E. In my opinion if a compound has been in use for many years and carcinogenesis is found in only 1 species then it would perhaps be wise to persuade the regulatory body to delay making a decision. If on the other hand, there is some doubt about the safety of a new compound then it would be wise to advise the regulatory body that more research be undertaken before making a decision. In reply to this SCHMAHL, D. reminded us that saccharin had been in widespread use for 70 years, during which time there had been 14 epidemiological studies on its effects in man and no harmful findings resulting from its ingestion had been reported.

SCHLATTER, C. The value of Dr. Sieber's work on saccharin in monkeys is questionable, because:-

1. the dose levels given are low, and

2. the studies have lasted only 7 years and were neither long time or lifetime for this species.

For this reason I feel that the only conclusion that could be drawn from Dr. Sieber's work is that saccharin and cyclamate are not strong carcinogens.

SIEBER, S. M. I agree with this but may I remind you that my paper is an interim report on part of a lifetime study [up to 30 years in a monkey].

CLAYSON, D. Whilst the work of Dr. Sieber is interesting I should like to question the value of non-human primates in this study with relation to human carcinogenicity testing because of:-

1. the lack of adequate numbers,

2. their relatively long life span, and

3. their differing genetic origin.

SIEBER, S. M. I am of the opinion that the advantages of non-human primates over rodents include the facts that

1. rodents have a high incidence of tumours in control animals, and this is not so in monkeys

2. the metabolic pathways in monkeys bear a closer resemblance to those in man than do those in rodents, although this is not important with saccharin.

CLAYSON, D. May I ask for clarification of the "other mechanisms" referred to in Class II carcinogenesis by Dr. Kroes. KROES, R. replied that they could include, for example:-

1. hyper- or hypo-stimulation of the immune system
2. hormonal or anti-hormonal actions
3. co-carcinogenic action
4. microsomal enzyme induction
5. "irritating" processes such as bladder stones.

KESSLER, I. I. It is important to be aware of the dilemma faced by regulatory authorities towards weak or very weak carcinogens, and I should like to make the point that factors other than the chemical under consideration may play a role in the aetiology of carcinogenesis and I suggest that perhaps more attention should be paid to the characteristics of the host who might be susceptible.

AGTHE, C. I support strongly the view that not only findings from animal studies must be taken into consideration, but the available epidemiological evidence must also be assessed before any regulatory decision is reached.

Discussion following POULSEN, E. and general discussion

SCHLATTER, C. In outlining the position in Switzerland it should be noted that possible benefit is not taken into consideration in giving approval to a new product, and even were this so it would be difficult to assess possible benefit. Though an individual must be given as much freedom of choice and personal responsibility as possible it is not reasonable to expect the consumer to assess the chronic effects on health of ingesting various compounds and therefore authority must intervene to give guidance.

BLUMENTHAL, H. In the U.S., as in most other countries, the regulating authority is constrained by the laws of the land, and in any assessment of a product economies are not considered, but, of course, need must be shown. May I remind the audience that in the U.S. no carcinogen can be used at any level as a food additive [Delaney].

FAIRWEATHER, F. The U.K. system of assessment is carried out by the Food Additives and Contaminants Committee and this Committee is made up of representatives of industry and of academics. If a need for a particular compound is established the toxicology of the compound is assessed by a committee of the Department of Health, whose views were then considered by the Food Additive and Contaminants Committee. At present, a review of sweeteners is taking place.

ALLEN, R. J. A. I am concerned about the use of sweeteners in fluoride toothpaste. It must be realised that if toothpaste did not taste sweet it would not be acceptable to the user and the fluoride benefit would be lost. I wonder whether if saccharin and cyclamate were banned it might be necessary to sweeten toothpaste with sucrose!

GRENBY, T. I wonder whether the carcinogenicity of sweeteners other than saccharin and cyclamate had been evaluated. ROUSSOS, G. G. Up to the present there was no evidence of carcinogenicity in the sweeteners neohesperidine and dihydrochalcone. ARPE, H. J. Up to now acetsulfane-K had shown no carcinogenic effects.

FAIRWEATHER, F. Finally it is my pleasure to thank the organising committee of ERGOB and Professor Guggenheim in particular for the friendly atmosphere, kindness and courtesy shown, not forgetting the cuisine. I should also like to express the gratitude of the participants to those concern-ed with the organisation and administration of the symposium.